THE LACRIMAL SYSTEM

THE LACRIMAL SYSTEM

Benjamin Milder, M.D.
Associate Professor of Clinical Ophthalmology
Washington University School of Medicine
Saint Louis, Missouri

Bernardo A. Weil, M.D.
(Editor for Spanish edition)
Consulting Surgeon
Buenos Aires Children's Hospital
Buenos Aires, Argentina

With Eight Contributors

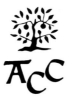

APPLETON-CENTURY-CROFTS/Norwalk, Connecticut

Notice: Our knowledge in the clinical sciences is constantly changing. As new information becomes available, changes in treatment and in the use of drugs become necessary. The author(s) and the publisher of this volume have taken care to make certain that the doses of drugs and schedules of treatment are correct and compatible with the standards generally accepted at the time of publication. The reader is advised to consult carefully the instruction and information material included in the package insert of each drug or therapeutic agent before administration. This advice is especially important when using new or infrequently used drugs.

Copyright © 1983 by Appleton-Century-Crofts
A Publishing Division of Prentice-Hall, Inc.

All rights reserved. This book, or any parts thereof, may not be used or reproduced in any manner without written permission. For information, address Appleton-Century-Crofts, 25 Van Zant Street, East Norwalk, Connecticut 06855.

83 84 85 86 87 88 / 10 9 8 7 6 5 4 3 2 1

Prentice-Hall International, Inc., London
Prentice-Hall of Australia, Pty. Ltd., Sydney
Prentice-Hall Canada, Inc.
Prentice-Hall of India Private Limited, New Delhi
Prentice-Hall of Japan, Inc., Tokyo
Prentice-Hall of Southeast Asia (Pte.) Ltd., Singapore
Whitehall Books Ltd., Wellington, New Zealand
Editora Prentice-Hall do Brasil Ltda., Rio de Janeiro

Library of Congress Cataloging in Publication Data
Main entry under title:
The Lacrimal system.
  Bibliography: p.
  Includes index.
  1. Lacrimal organs—Diseases. 2. Lacrimal organs.
I. Milder, Benjamin, 1915–   . [DNLM: 1. Lacrimal
apparatus. 2. Lacrimal apparatus diseases. WW 208
L146]
RE201.L33 1983   617.7′64   82-24507
ISBN 0-8385-5597-7

Cover and text design: Jean M. Sabato
Production: Carol Pierce

PRINTED IN THE UNITED STATES OF AMERICA

CONTENTS

PREFACE

Diversity is the common denominator for all books which embody the contributions of multiple authors. This volume is no exception. Respected colleagues from both hemispheres have lent their expertise in lacrimal disease to this effort and have spiced the chapters with their own styles.

Diversity in language, in content and pedagogic approach does not constitute a problem. Rather, the reader is afforded an opportunity to savor varying points of view and to appreciate the fact that, around the globe, physicians can reach the same goals by different paths.

Benjamin Milder, M.D., U.S.A.
Bernardo A. Weil, M.D., Argentina

.

ACKNOWLEDGMENTS

No author can hope to possess all of the skills necessary to bring to fruition a volume such as this.

It is a privilege and an honor to acknowledge our deep gratitude to those renowned experts in the field of dacryology who have given their time, effort and knowledge to the chapters of this book.

The guidance and patience of Executive Editor, Doreen Berne, of Appleton-Century-Crofts were invaluable aids to the authors. Our typist, Judy Hulla, performed feats of magic in deciphering our illegible scribbling.

Our thanks and appreciation are extended to our friends who provided technical assistance: Bernd Silver in photography and Morton Smith in pathology.

And, finally, to our respective spouses, whose patience, love and understanding provided the inspiration to push on whenever we seemed about to be overwhelmed by the project.

CONTRIBUTORS

H. Jane Blackman, M.D.
Clinical Assistant Professor of Ophthalmology
Georgetown University Medical Center
Washington, D.C. (U.S.A.)

Juan Murube-del-Castillo, M.D.
Professor and Chairman, Departmento
de Oftalmologia
Centro Especial Ramón y Cajal
Madrid (Spain)

Byron H. Demorest, M.D.
Clinical Professor of Ophthalmology
University of California at Davis
Sacramento, California (U.S.A.)

Michael A. Lemp, M.D.
Clinical Professor of Ophthalmology
Georgetown University Medical Center
Washington, D.C. (U.S.A.)

John V. Linberg, M.D.
Assistant Professor of Ophthalmology
Louisiana State University Medical Center
New Orleans, Louisiana (U.S.A.)

Bernd Silver, M.D.
Associate Professor of Clinical Ophthalmology
Washington University School of Medicine
Saint Louis, Missouri (U.S.A.)

Morton E. Smith, M.D.
Professor of Ophthalmology
Washington University School of Medicine
Saint Louis, Missouri (U.S.A.)

N. J. van Haeringen, Ph.D.
The Netherlands Ophthalmic Research
Institute
Amsterdam, The Netherlands

Abraham Werb, M.D., F.R.C.S., D.O.M.S.
Ophthalmic Surgeon
London, England

INTRODUCTION

The first question which an author of a textbook must ask himself—for, most assuredly, it is the first question which a publisher will ask—is: What is your purpose in writing this book? The reader and publisher deserve a clear, candid answer.

Dacryology, the study of the lacrimal system and its abnormalities, is inevitably viewed as one of the lesser disciplines in the broad spectrum of opthalmology. Despite the many recent contributions in the field of lacrimal physiology and the chemistry of tears, dacryology remains as a small star in the firmament of ophthalmologic knowledge, and, from time to time, becomes lost in the exponential growth of ophthalmology.

In the past twenty years, no more than a half-dozen books have been published in the field of dacryology. Some have been collections of papers read at quadrennial meetings of the International Congress of Ophthalmology. Others have been ably distilled from the wide ranging experiences of leaders in this field. From these efforts, ophthalmologists have been able to formulate principles and techniques in the management of lacrimal problems.

It is not the intention of this volume to retrace these steps and repeat the accomplishments of our colleagues. Rather, we shall endeavor to bring together in this one volume the many aspects of dacryology which have come to the fore in recent decades.

It would be unworthy and unrealistic, at the outset, to omit recognition of the contributions of such giants in this field as Lester Jones, Veirs, Pico, Radnot, Yamaguchi, Murube, Werb, and all those who have laid the foundation of our present knowledge. It is upon this solid foundation that we shall build.

This volume is not intended to be a "how I do it" text. It will endeavor to marshall the knowledge of recent decades, to incorporate new ideas and to give the clinician an overview of the field—from the history of dacryology to the present researches.

In the Old Testament's Book of Genesis, when the good citizens of Babel sought to erect their tower, little did they realize the impact which their confusion of languages would have on our exchanges of information in dacryology. For, despite the many multi-lingual abstracts and summaries available in the literature, problems in communication remain. One must guard, constantly, against the parochial point of view. A second purpose of this volume, then, is to take a step forward in redressing Babel syndrome and to recognize the accomplishments of our colleagues in other parts of the world. This volume will be published in English and Spanish editions.

No textbook can be "definitive." Clinical experiences and clinical results differ. Contributions from the research laboratories are so diverse and accumulate with such rapidity that any volume such as this can be no more than an "update," a synthesis of current knowledge in orderly form. Hopefully, it will serve as a clinically accessible resource, a fountainhead spanning a brief period until newer knowledge can by synthesized into a newer fountainhead.

THE LACRIMAL SYSTEM

PART 1

BASIC DACRYOLOGY

1

A HISTORY OF DACRYOLOGY

JUAN MURUBE-DEL-CASTILLO

What is dacryology? From early times, primitive man was aware of two dacryologic facts: the flow of reflex and psychic tears was omnipresent in his life, and dacryocystitis was so frequent as to be considered an endemic state in his community. Over the millennia, knowledge of the lacrimal system was so fragmented that it could scarcely have been considered a scientific discipline. From the time of Aristotle and throughout the dark ages, "science" consisted of a nonscientific reliance on the ancient authorities—the Aristotles, the Hippocrates, the Galens—without the independent, experimental questioning that we recognize as essential to modern scientific thought. As this was the case with every science and with every phase of study of the human body, so it was with dacryology.

Throughout those years, bits and pieces of knowledge about the lacrimal gland accumulated parallel with information about the lacrimal pathways. However, the most important part of the science of dacryology concerns what goes on between those two structures in the mare lacrimale, where tears play the metabolic, refractive, and other roles for which they were created. Up to this time, such knowledge has remained dispersed through keratology, contactology, refractology, biochemistry, and the neurophysiology of lacrimal secretion. Recent books devoted to this corpus dacryologicum, as

well as the work of physicians devoting themselves exclusively to this field, are evidence that dacryology is emerging as a new specialty.

ANATOMY

The earliest knowledge of the lacrimal apparatus was limited to the medial canthus, partly because the lacrimal puncta were grossly visible to observers and partly because of the frequent inflammatory pathology in this area, usually accompanied by tearing. Thus, this medial canthal region was, and remains, known as the "lacrimal area." The pre-Christian Greeks took note of the caruncle, a name given to that structure by the Roman, Celsus (first century AD). It was subsequently called "the lacrimal caruncle" because of its supposed important role in lacrimal function.

Galen (second century AD) believed that tears arose from two glands which emptied through the lacrimal puncta. He also reported another gland in the orbit but did not relate this to the lacrimal process. The orbital part of the main lacrimal gland has been called "Galen's gland."

Fifteen centuries later, Steno (1622) discovered the lacrimal gland ductules but thought that their function was drainage of the orbit.

The anatomy of the gland, as we know it, is attributed to Rosenmüller in 1797, and the palpebral portion of the gland is sometimes known as "Rosenmüller's gland."

The meibomian glands were first described by Casserius in 1609 and then by Meibomius in 1666. Other glands were subsequently described by Zeiss, Krause, Wolfring, Moll, Manz, and Henle over the next 200 years.

Knowledge of the innervation of the lacrimal secretory mechanism is a product of the past hundred years, being first reported by Bechterew in 1886 and Ramón y Cajal in 1899. The parasympathetic lacrimosecretory pathway, as we know it today, was described by Goldzieher in 1893.

Until the writings of Leone (1574), the lacrimal sac and duct were thought to be the secretory mechanism! However, his careful anatomic findings were not accepted for at least a century after his work. Further details of the outflow system came to light gradually during the ensuing three centuries.

The relationship of the eyelid muscles to lacrimal outflow function was first described by Duverney (1749), and further observations and studies followed over the next two centuries up to the definitive work of Lester Jones in 1955 and Nagashima in 1963. The anatomy of the mucosal folds (valves) first came to light at the end of the eighteenth century, and the investigators live on in their eponyms: Rosenmüller (1797), Taillefer (1826), Hyrtl (1847), Arlt (1855). Numerous others have been lost in the mists of lacrimal history.

The discovery of glands in the mucosa of the sac and duct was attributed first to Foltz in 1862. Cilia were found by Foltz in 1860 and other investigators since then, including Radnot who described the electron microscopy of the cilia in 1971. Amazingly, new anatomic studies continue to be reported. In 1978, Odeh-Nasrala described a sacco-orbital ligament, and Anderson in 1977 and Land and Royer in 1979 reported on the superior expansion of the tendo oculi.

EMBRYOLOGY

The hypothesis that the primordium of the lacrimal gland comes from an epithelial depression of the conjunctival fornix was first confirmed by Keibel in 1908 and more recently by Mann (1943) and Genís Gálvez (1970). Ontogenesis of the accessory lacrimal glands was studied by Falchi in 1905, and further studies were reported through this century up to Mann in 1943.

Von Baer in 1828 and Burdach in 1837 are credited with the first reported studies of the embryology of the lacrimal excretory pathways. Current concepts originated with Born (1876–1883), who found that the excretory pathways arose from a depression in the epiblast lining of the bottom of the orbitobuccalis sulcus.

Especially interesting has been the evolution of theories regarding the formation of the canaliculi. Von Kölliker (1861–1880) was the first to report on embryology of the canaliculi, and during the latter part of the nineteenth century, widely conflicting views were the order of the day. Valude (1888) felt that the canaliculi arose from two independent roots of the conjunctival epithelium, which then reached along the lid margins toward the lacrimal sac. Halben (1903) felt that the canaliculi developed from a slit on the medial lid margin, which then fused to form an enclosed tubule. Born (1876) and Cabannes (1896) were the first to recognize that the superior end of the embryonal lacrimal cord bifurcates, with each end of the bifurcation reaching its respective eyelid and later canalizing.

PHYSIOLOGY

Origins of Lacrimal Secretion

Until the seventeenth century, it was thought that the conjunctiva was intrinsically moist, and attention was paid only to hypersecretory states. The Corpus Hippocratum (fifth century BC) reported that tears came from the brain, and despite Galen's theory of two tear glands each issuing tears through a punctum, the idea that tears emanated from the brain held sway until about 300 years ago. In the ninth century, Hunain reported that tears came from the brain when a person sneezed. Al-Rhazes (tenth century AD) felt that the brain secreted tears when one felt sad, and Casserius (1609) postulated that tears flowed through the lamina cribosa.

In 1662 Steno identified the ductules of the lacrimal gland but thought that these drained the orbit. As far as we know, Janin (1792) was the first to deduce that the lacrimal gland secreted tears. Martini (1844) observed that the eye could remain moist after surgical extirpation of the gland and postulated an accessory mechanism. He was unaware of accessory lacrimal gland tissue and felt that the eye could remain moist by transepithelial diffusion.

Mechanisms of Lacrimal Secretion

Czermak (1860) and Goldzieher (1893) found that the main lacrimosecretory pathway (parasympathetic) followed the facial nerve, finally joining the trigeminal nerve. The role of the sympathetic pathway evolved in the later nineteenth century. Demtschemko (1872) established by electrical experimentation that the sympathetic innervation controls basic secretion, and the cranial nerves control reflex and psychic secretion. In 1942, Crespí Jaume found that the sympathetics controlled basal secretion by regulating blood flow to the lacrimal gland and that hypersecretion was influenced directly by the effect of the parasympathetics on the lacrimocytes of the glandular acini.

Basal, Reflex, and Psychic Lacrimation

The fact that reflex and psychic stimuli can influence tear production has been recognized since the beginnings of civilization, but scientific experimentation to clarify the multiple origins of reflex tearing has been reported only in the later nineteenth century and the present century (Badal, 1876–1885; de Wecker, 1899; Schirmer, 1903; and others). Psychic stimulation was being studied over this same period. In 1979, García de la Torre reported on two forms of psychic tearing—pathetic and esthetic.

The concept of basal tearing is, by comparison, relatively new, first suspected by Janin (1772) with important data added by Schirmer in 1903 and Lester Jones in 1966.

Darwin, Kirchstein, and Axenfeld, in the 1890s, established independently that basal secretion is initiated some months before birth. Gillette, Allansmith, et al. (1981) have suggested that since there is no histologic difference between the main and accessory lacrimal glands, the difference between basal and reflex secretion is one of quantity not quality.

Tear Quantity

The earliest scientific studies of tear volume were anything but scientific. In 1772, Janin placed a wine glass over the eye and obtained 1.25 g of tears in 30 minutes. He concluded that each eye secretes 60 g of tears per day! Studies in recent decades have identified basal secretion levels as 0.6 to 1.2 ml per minute (Frieberg, 1941; Nover and Jaeger, 1952; Mishima, 1966; González de la Rosa, 1981).

Physical Chemistry

Data establishing norms of tear pH, osmolarity, specific gravity, and temperature were all found in the twentieth century and have evoked little disagreement. However, wide variations in tear surface tension have been reported, depending on the measurement technique employed.

Tear Composition

Knowledge of the inorganic and protein components of tears is largely the product of the twentieth century, although the water content was studied by Frerichs in 1846 and Arlt in 1855. The discovery of glucose in tears by Wada (1921) has led to practical tear analysis tests for diabetes.

In the past decade, tear analysis has been used in the diagnosis of fucosidosis, mucolipidosis, Fabry's disease, Tay-Sachs disease, and metachromatic dystrophy, among others (Singer, 1973; Del Monte, 1974; Libert, 1976; Jordan, 1980; Carmody et al., 1973). A detailed list of tear components and the researchers who studied them is found in Chapter 4.

Function of Tears

As far back as 1637, Descartes took note of the optical, metabolic, and lubricant roles of tears. Of special interest, however, is the historical development of the multiple factors involved in the antimicrobial function of tears. Such a function was postulated as early as 1887 by Valude. In 1893 Bernheim demonstrated that tears were inactive against the gonococcus and *Micrococcus prodigious* but inhibited growth of *Bacillus subtilis* and *Streptococcus aureus*. He further demonstrated that this bacteriostatic effect was temperature sensitive. Bernheim's observations were confirmed in this century when lysozyme, the enzyme which is lytic for *Micrococcus lysodeikticus*, was discovered by Fleming in 1922. A second antimicrobial factor, isolated in 1941 by Thomson-Gallardo, was identified as beta-lysin by Ford et al. in 1976. Recently lactoferrin (Bröckhuyse, 1974) and alpha-arylsulphatase

(Watson et al., 1977) have been assigned bacteriostatic roles in tears. The role of immunoglobulins was reported on by Centifanto in 1970 and other investigators since that time.

The Tear Film

The fact that tears have three separate components, each with a separate origin, was known to Terson in 1892, but the three-layered structure of the precorneal tear film was not described until 1946 by Wolf.

The tear film break-up time (BUT, also known as TISC—tempus initii siccitatis corneae) was measured by Marx in 1921. He obtained normal values of 60 seconds. The recent studies of Lemp, Dohlman, and Holly, employing a slitlamp-fluorescein technique, have reduced this figure to 25 to 30 seconds.

Tear Excretion

Many chapters could be written about the history of the ongoing controversies regarding the forces that influence tear elimination. Initially, the caruncle was considered to play an important role. Galen (second century AD) wrote, "the caruncular body serves as a cover of the duct directed toward the nose; its role is partly to eliminate the eyes detritus to the nose in order that the dirt not flow from the bigger angle of the eye in a continuous shedding and in part humidify the eye in order to facilitate blinking." This concept held sway until the eighteenth century because of repeated observations that when the caruncle was destroyed by illness or cautery, epiphora resulted.

In 1734, Petit proposed gravity as a force carrying tears to the nose (the syphon theory). The influence of respiration was first noted by Hunauld (1735), capillarity by von Haller (1763), and canalicular peristalsis was put forth as an excretory mechanism by Richerand in 1802.

However, the major attention in the past two centuries has been given to the role of blinking as the predominant force that moves the lacrimal flux. In 1734, Petit proposed that, with lid closure, the tears in the conjunctival sac are hermetically compressed, forcing them into the canaliculi. This very simple explanation continues to have its strong adherents up to the present time.

It is surprising to learn that the lacrimal

pump theory described by Jones in 1961 was reported by Bérard in 1833. This theory, in which a negative pressure is created within the lacrimal sac with the act of blinking, was supported by the finding of muscular insertions into the sac at about the same time (Bourjot Saint Hilaire, 1835; Hyrtl, 1849). The opposite notion, that the sac is expressed during lid closure, was postulated by von Arlt in 1855 and by many authors since that time.

The canaliculi also have been the subject of divergent theories. The canalicular suction theory has had few supporters, but the proposition that tears are expressed by the canaliculi is gaining momentum ever since it was first espoused by Trasmondi in 1823. In this century, Nagashima (1958–1963) and Jones (1958) have ascribed such a role to the canaliculi. The recent high-speed photographic studies of Doane (1980) have confirmed this canalicular expression theory.

Most investigators in this field during the past two centuries have concluded that normal tear outflow is explained by a combination of two or more of these various theories. At the present time, there are two principal schools of thought. One, proposed by Nagashima and Jones, combines canalicular expression with simultaneous suction by the sac. Jones, in addition, commented on nasal aspiration as an additional factor. The other current theory suggests simultaneous expression by the canaliculus and sac (Valière Vialeix, 1961). This theory has received support from the studies of Doane (1980) (Chapter 6).

Tests of Lacrimal Function

As far back as the time of Aristotle (fourth century BC) it was known that a collyrium instilled in the eye can be perceived shortly afterward in the nose and mouth. That information remains the basis for tests of tear flux that are in use in the present century. Test materials have run the gamut from taste devices and color markers to radiopaque agents and radioactive isotopes. Saccharin was first used by Lundsgaard in 1922. Fluorescein was employed by Antonelli in 1902 and rose Bengal by Werb in 1966.

Contrast radiography, as a test of outflow function, was performed by Ploman in 1928. Del Duca (1929), Spackman (1938), and Milder-Demorest (1954) measured normal outflow times for contrast agents of various densities. Schmöger (1955) first employed aqueous contrast agents for this purpose. The use of radioactive isotopes dates back to Beiras García in 1961, and this modality was refined and described by Rossomondo et al. in 1972. He used ^{99}Tc as a marker.

It can be seen that although the study of lacrimal excretory function and the means of evaluating this mechanism has interested researchers for centuries, the final word has not yet been spoken on the subject. The events of today may very well amuse the scholars of tomorrow.

PATHOLOGY

Among the diseases that were common to primitive man—dermatitis, intestinal parasites, pulmonary diseases—dacryocystitis was preeminent. The Code of Hammurabi (second millennium BC) referred to dacryocystitis as the principal disease involving the lacrimal system. Many of these diseases were complicated by inflammation at the nasal canthus and rupture of the lacrimal sac with fistulization. Galen (second century AD) thought that the caruncle was the cause of lacrimal fistulization by blocking tear secretion, and this emphasis on the caruncle persisted through the middle ages.

Maître Jean, in 1701, was the first to postulate that stasis of tears and secretions in the tear sac were responsible for lacrimal abscess. He also thought that the tears were secreted by the lacrimal sac. It was not until 1891 that Peters established that dacryocystitis neonatorum was the result of congenital impatency of the ostium lacrimale.

TREATMENT

With each new treatment breakthrough (sulfamonamides, penicillin, corticosteroids), every generation of interns is condemned to repeat the same humorous cliche "treat the patient with ... for three days, and if there is no improvement, get a history and physical!" That cliche has, in actual fact, an honorable past, because the history of medicine is one of therapy preceding (sometimes for millennia) any available knowledge on which to base a logical treatment program.

The first medical treatment for lacrimal sac abscess was described in the Ebers Papyrus (approximately 1150 BC) and consisted of rubbing the eyes for four days with a mixture of honey, antimony, and wood powder. Pliny the Elder (23–29 AD) wrote that the fistula called aegylops required treatment with the herb *Aegylopia fatua,* or wild oat. Celsus (20–30 AD) recommended laying open the fistula to the bone and cauterizing the bone with a hot iron. Galen (second century AD) used grapevine ashes, aegylopia juice, vinegar, honey, carob, and others to treat the sac infection. In the fifth to seventh centuries, topical medications were favored, which included snail paste, incense, myrrh, and bittersweet. How many of our present nostra will seem equally far fetched to the physicians of 2022 AD?

Records from the tenth to twelfth centuries AD provided us with many reports of therapeutic devices employed by Moslem physicians of Spain, the Middle East, and Asia. Al-Ghafiqi of Cordoba (twelfth century AD) collected all of the medical information on the treatment of lacrimal sac infections and described a method of probing of the lacrimal fossa and perforating the lacrimal bone for relief of infection. However, it was not until 1710 that irrigation and probing through the puncta, as we know it, was introduced by Anel. Even then, it was recognized that probing did not provide definitive cures for dacryocystitis. The use of stents to maintain patency was initiated toward the end of the eighteenth century. Pallucci (1762) used linen thread, and nineteenth century ophthalmologists employed copper and platinum wires. Nylon, polyethylene, and silicone stents are a product of the past 30 to 40 years, beginning with the reports of Veirs in 1950.

In the mid-eighteenth century, surgeons began the procedure of destroying the lacrimal sac for dacryocystitis. Dacryocystorhinostomy was undoubtedly the occasional result of such efforts, especially by the Spanish physicians of the middle ages, but modern dacryocystorhinostomy was first performed by Montaigne in 1836.

The term "dacryocystorhinostomy" was given to us by Toti in 1904, and Toti's method of creating an osteotomy with hammer and chisel remained in vogue, surprisingly, for a half-century. Suturing of the mucosal flaps was an added embellishment introduced in 1921 by Dupuy-Dutemps and Bourguet, and in the same year Mosher modified the technique by enlarging the osteotomy with rongeurs. The dacryocystorhinostomies of today are not changed, in principle, since the 1920s. However, high-speed drills, improved sutures, better anesthesia, and better control of bleeding have led to consistently successful surgical results.

The past 50 years have seen the advent of many techniques for restoring lacrimal drainage when the sac is missing or when it is so damaged that conventional dacryocystorhinostomy is not possible. Grafts of buccal mucosa were introduced by Gómez Márquez in 1928. Skin grafts were described by Morax in 1925, and vein grafts were described by Weil in 1965. These and other heroic attempts have not stood the test of time. The operation of conjunctivo-dacryocystorhinostomy with retained tube, as introduced by Jones in 1961, is the method which has proved effective and which remains in use at this time.

Methods of dealing with epiphora due to canalicular obstruction are also of recent vintage. Prior to the late nineteenth century, such obstructions were treated, usually without success, with simple probing. Díaz Rocafull, in 1874, postulated for the first time that an indwelling stent was a necessary part of the repair of the torn canaliculus. He used a fishline obturator. Since that time, various materials have been used—metal, rubber, plastics. Lacrimal probes were used by Wagenmann in 1913, polyethylene by Callahan in 1950, polyvinyl in 1955 by Bunge, and silicone by Weil in 1967. The search goes on for the ideal stent material and for the definitive techniques for insuring patency.

Although our attention is focused, generally, on surgery of the lacrimal drainage system, no history of dacryology would be complete without a consideration of lacrimal gland surgery. Extirpation of gland was performed in 1843 by Carron du Villards for a neoplasm and in the same year by Bernard for chronic tearing, and results were described as successful.

During the second half of the nineteenth century, extirpation of the lacrimal gland—the orbital and/or the palpebral lobe—was performed successfully. In 1902 Wagenmann reported cases of xerophthalmia following extirpation of the gland, and in this century, the operation has declined as a treatment for epiphora, having been replaced by the more physiologic dacryocystorhinostomy.

HISTORY OF THE PHYSIOLOGY OF THE WET EYE

The concept of psychic tearing dates back to early history, but very little has appeared in the literature on this subject. Reflex tearing has been studied extensively during the past century based on our knowledge of the reflex pathways. Many syndromes characterized by neurogenic hypersecretion have been described. Most of the eponyms have disappeared from our daily clinical armamentarium. Some of those which remain are paroxysmal hypersecretion, the tabetic crisis of Pel (1898), Gradenigo syndrome (1904), Raeder's paratrigeminal syndrome (1924), and the Marín-Amat phenomenon (1918), in which on opening the mouth, the eyelids close and hypersecretion appears.

Crocodile tears were first reported in 1902 by Antonelli. In 1962, Jampol gave this phenomenon the name "paradoxical salivary-lacrimal reflex."

The embryo of what we now know as the science of dacryology was conceived at the same time as human culture. Dacryology was born, historically, with its mention in the first written document, the Code of Hammurabi in the second millennium BC. The infant dacryology was nurtured before and during the Middle Ages in the areas around the Mediterranean Sea and the Middle East. It developed a coordinated mind and form under the sunlight of inquiring minds and scientific investigation throughout the world. After two millennia of the common era, dacryology has reached its maturity as a scientific discipline.

2

DEVELOPMENT OF THE LACRIMAL APPARATUS

JUAN MURUBE-DEL-CASTILLO

This description of the development of the lacrimal apparatus is based on observations of the author at the Embrioteca in the Departments of Anatomy and Embryology at the Universities of Madrid, Granada, and Sevilla, and on a thorough examination of the literature including comtemporary as well as elder authors. We acknowledge, with thanks, the cooperation of Professors Jiménez Collado, Guirao Pérez, and Genís Gálvez. The literature contains very few papers on experimental embryology relating to the lacrimal system; most of the research reports have been based on static morphology. A bibliography detailing each of the works cited in this chapter appears in Murube J: Dacryologia Basica, Las Palmas, 1981:791–890.

DEVELOPMENTAL STAGES

By describing the development of the lacrimal apparatus ontogenetically, we can establish the blastodermic origin of the components of the lacrimal glands, lacrimal fossa, and the lacrimal excretory passages. Table 2-1 presents a condensed version of the relationships between size of the embryo and the stage of development.

By the twentieth day, at the end of the preembryonic stage, the ectoblastic cells thicken to form the neural plate. The neural plate becomes differentiated into parallel neural folds which form along a central neural groove.

These neural folds develop until they join, forming the neural tube, which becomes separate and distinct from the covering ectoblast or epiblast.

The epiblast contains the germ cells that will give rise to the lacrimal glands, lacrimal fossa, and the lacrimal excretory passages. The neural tube is the Anlage for the central nervous system.

FORMATION OF THE GENERAL STRUCTURE OF THE FACE

At the beginning of the fourth week, the neural tube begins to differentiate at the cephalic end, flexing ventrally to overlie the oropharyngeal plate and forming the frontal process. Below this, the pericardial sac develops, and the cavity between the frontal process and the pericardial sac is the stomodeum, the primitive oronasal cavity (Figs. 2-1–2-4).

During this period of initial development of the neural tube, the mesoderm is dividing into medial and lateral sheets. The branchial arches are formed from these lateral mesodermal sheets, the first two branchial arches being related to the development of the lacrimal apparatus. The first branchial arch gives rise to

TABLE 2-1. RELATIONSHIP BETWEEN SIZE OF EMBRYO AND STAGE OF DEVELOPMENT

Stage	Age (in days)	Size (in mm)
Preembryonic stage	1 day zygote 2-3 days morula (Fig. 2-1) 4-13 days blastula (Fig. 2-2) 14-18 days gastrula (Fig. 2-3) 19-20 days neurula	
Embryonic stage	22-48 days	1.5-30 mm
Previable fetal stage	49 days to 5 months	31-210 mm
Viable fetal stage	6-9 months	250-370 mm

almost all of the middle third and the entire lower third of the face. The second branchial arch forms the upper part of the neck. Cells of the superficial mesoblastic mass of this second branchial arch migrate toward the periocular region to form the orbicularis oculi muscles and Horner's muscle.

At the twenty-sixth day, the optic vesicles form at the cephalic end of the neural tube at either side of the prosencephalon. As these optic vesicles make contact with the overlying epiblast, the latter structure forms a lens plate which soon develops into primitive lens, detaching from the surface epiblast. The remaining surface covering will become the cornea as well as the adnexae, which will include the lacrimal apparatus.

The medial third of the face originates from the nasal and maxillary processes. These emerge from the first branchial arch. In the 28-day embryo, after the nasal processes have appeared, the olfactory plate develops at the forward lower border of the nasal process on either side of the midline. This olfactory plate gives rise to the nasal structures, including the site of the ostium of the nasolacrimal duct. The

frontal process grows downward at both sides of the nasal plate, which deepens and proliferates to form the primitive nasal cavity, separating the internal nasal processes from the external. Subsequently, both processes surround the nasal cavity, forming the nasal air passages. By

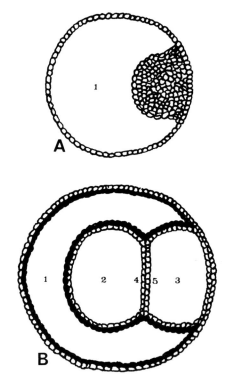

Figure 2-2. Blastula (4 to 13 days). **A.** Primary blastula. **B.** Secondary blastula. **1.** Chorionic vesicles. **2.** Endoblastic (vitelline) vesicles. **3.** Ectoblastic (amniotic) vesicles. **4.** Endoblast. **5.** Ectoblast. In black, primary mesoblast.

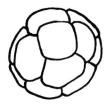

Figure 2-1. Morula (2 to 3 days). Enlarged for clarity.

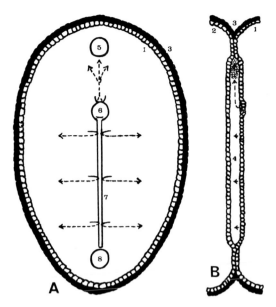

Figure 2-3. Embryonal plate of the gastrula. **A.** Dorsal view. **B.** Sagittal view. **1.** Ectoblast. **2.** Endoblast. **3.** In black, primary mesoblast. **4.** Secondary mesoblast. **5.** Buccopharyngeal membrane. **6.** Hensen's nodule. **7.** Primitive line. **8.** Anal membrane.

FORMATION OF THE LACRIMAL FOSSA REGION

In the 36-day embryo (14 mm), as the eyes begin to shift to a frontal position, the mesodermal tissue proliferates around the periocular groove, and an annular palpebral fold is formed at the depths of the circumferential palpebro-ocular sac. In the 16 mm embryo, one can already discern upper and lower eyelids, the upper eyelid from the frontal process and the lower eyelid from the maxillary. In the 35 mm embryo, the closure of the palpebral groove is completed.

In the 20 mm embryo (42 days), the epiblast which covers the frontal aspect of the optic cup starts to differentiate from that which covers the fornices and the ocular surface of the eyelids. The former evolves as the corneal epithelium, and the latter becomes the mucosal lining of the eyelids.

The lacrimal caruncle begins, at the inner angle of the eyelids, on the forty-sixth to forty-eighth day as a mesodermic extension covered by epithelium.

The plica semilunaris begins to form at the end of the second month, arising behind the internal commissure of the fused eyelids (Fig. 2-5). Three days after the plica has been formed, three or four cellular roots of epithelium develop, extend into the mesoderm, and form accessory lacrimal glands. These glands usually undergo involution but may persist in some cases. At the

the thirty-seventh day, this passage opens to communicate with the stomodeum.

The lateral wall of the nasal cavity develops three folds which become the turbinates, separated by their respective meati. This process is completed by the third month.

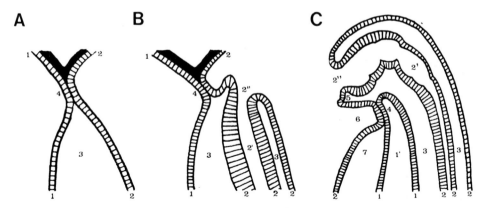

Figure 2-4. Formation of the stomodeum (8 mm embryo). **A.** Gastrula. **B.** Neurula. **C.** Flexion and invagination of the oropharyngeal membrane between the frontal processes and the pericardial sac. **1.** Endoblast. **1′** Digestive tract. **2.** Ectoblast. **2′** Neural tube. **2″** Anterior neuropore. **3.** Mesoblast. **4.** Oropharyngeal membrane. **5.** Frontal process. **6.** Stomodeum. **7.** Pericardial sac.

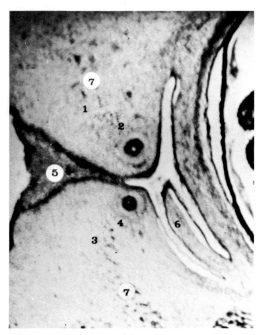

Figure 2-5. Sagittal section of the palpebro-ocular sac in 51 mm fetus. **1.** Upper eyelid. **2.** Upper canaliculus with its ectodermal and mesodermal covering. **3.** Lower eyelid. **4.** Lower canaliculus. **5.** Interpalpebral epithelium. **6.** Semilunar plica with mucous glands. **7.** Orbicular muscle of the eyelids.

nucleus and homogeneous protoplasm, deepen into the mesoderm lying in contact with the scleral surface. In the 40 to 60 mm embryo, the epithelium from this upper fornix again produces four or five ectodermal roots which invade the mesoderm less deeply than the earlier ones, forming a new glandular stratum. Thus, the primitive palpebral and orbital lobes of the main lacrimal gland are defined at this time.

In the 60 mm embryo, the glands are already clearly shaped by the ligamentous extension of the levator muscle, the upper stratum becoming the orbital portion of the gland and the lower stratum the palpebral portion (Fig. 2-6).

At the beginning of the fifth month, the acini are visible in the form of lobules (Fig. 2-7). With the maturation of the gland, the epithelium of the acini becomes nonstratified, the number of Boll's cells grows, the lobules shrink, and the vascular and nervous structures develop.

After birth, the gland continues to grow. The newborn may produce tears within the first 24 hours (basal secretion), but reflex tearing resulting from trigeminal stimulation generally does not begin for days or even weeks after birth. Tears of psychical origin begin several months later.

The origin of the accessory lacrimal glands is similar to that of the principal lacrimal gland. These accessory glands are located in the fornices and at the plica semilunaris. They begin to form at the end of the second fetal month.

The harderian glands are associated with the nictitating membrane and resemble mucilaginous crypts. In several vertebrates, they remain in extrauterine life, but in humans they disappear entirely or persist as normal muciparous glands.

The mucous glands of the conjunctiva, whose normal functioning is essential to the maintenance of the precorneal tear film, begin to differentiate from the conjunctival epithelium in the third month. Mucous crypts and/or calyciform cells appear in the conjunctival fornices, the bulbar conjunctiva, and the plica semilunaris. The calyciform cells (goblet cells) spread over the entire fetal conjunctiva. Those in the exposed bulbar conjunctiva often disappear in the adult.

The pilosebaceous glands also make their appearance at the end of the second month.

sixth or seventh month, new cells from the epithelium of the plica proliferate and invade the mesoderm to become the harderian glands.

SEPARATION OF THE EYELIDS

At the fifth month, keratinization of the ciliary border begins, and the eyelids begin to separate at the nasal end. This slow process may not be completed until the eighth or ninth month.

DEVELOPMENT OF THE SECRETORY GLANDS

In the 43-day embryo, before the eyelids are fused, epithelial cells begin to proliferate at the temporal fornix between the upper palpebral fold and the eye. Five or six compact epithelial roots of polyhedric cells, each cell with a round

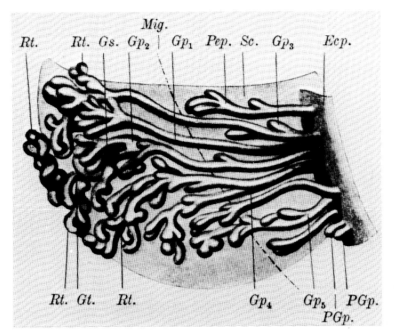

Figure 2-6. Reconstruction of the lacrimal gland of a 50 mm fetus. Six epithelial tubules penetrate an interglandular membrane formed by the lateral expansion of the levator tendon. Their ramifications form the orbital portion of the gland. The shorter tubules do not penetrate the membrane, and they give rise to the palpebral portion of the gland. **Mig**, separation between palpebral and orbital lobes of the gland; **EcP**, epithelium of superior or palpebral conjunctiva; **Sc**, sclera. (*Adapted from Speciale Cirincione, 1908.*)

The follicles of the eyelashes and the associated glands form in the lids and in the lacrimal caruncle. Each follicle develops two Zeis glands and a gland of Moll.

The meibomian (tarsal) glands begin to form in the third month. The epithelium joining the palpebral margins proliferates behind the hair follicles and produces a solid cellular root which passes between the cells of the muscle of Riolan to reach the tarsal Anlage. Subsequently, the collagen condenses around the glandular roots, forming the individual tarsal glands.

DEVELOPMENT OF THE LACRIMAL EXCRETORY PASSAGES

The lacrimal passages have an ectodermal component which forms a tubular epithelial mantle arising from the lacrimal fossa as far as the nasal cavity. This is surrounded by a mesodermal component which evolves into definitive subepithelial, fibrous, muscular, and osseous strata.

The morphologic steps in the ectodermal development are (1) the upsurge of the embryonic lacrimal plate, (2) the isolation of the embryonic lacrimal cord, (3) the progression of both ends of this cord, the lower end approaching the inferior nasal meatus and the upper one extending to become the definitive lacrimal sac and the canaliculi, (4) the segmental cavitation of the solid epithelial column, and (5) the joining of these zones of cavitation to form a continuous tubular passage (Fig. 2-8).

The mesodermal component develops in a characteristic series of steps: (1) the formation of the submucosa of the ducts, (2) the shaping of the bony fossa of the lacrimal sac and the bony canal of the lacrimonasal duct, (3) the development of the musculofibrous covering of the can-

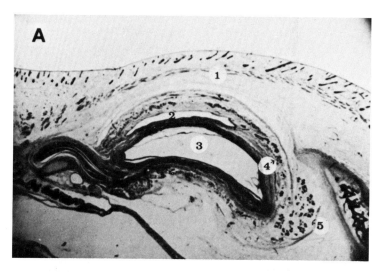

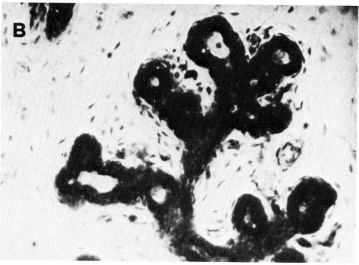

Figure 2-7. Fetus measuring 144 mm. **A.** Horizontal section of the upper part of the right orbit. **1.** Upper eyelid. **2.** Upper conjunctival fornix. **3.** Upper cap of the collapsed ocular globe. **4.** Palpebral portion of the lacrimal gland. **5.** Orbital portion of the lacrimal gland. **B.** Section of a lobule of the lacrimal gland showing acinar structure.

aliculi and of the sac, and (4) the muscular and fascial structures in the orbital parts of the excretory system.

The embryonic lacrimal plate develops at the base of the groove formed between the upper maxillary and the external nasal processes (Fig. 2-9). We believe that the cells that induce the formation of the lacrimal passages are in the maxillary lip. The proliferation which originates the embryonic lacrimal plate is seen in the 9 to 11 mm embryo. The plate does not extend the entire length of the orbitonasal groove but is limited to the most cranial part. It invaginates into the underlying mesoblast. It is two cells thick and is surrounded by a basal membrane which is continuous with the superficial epiblast. The ectomesenchymal layer that underlays the basal membrane of the epiblast

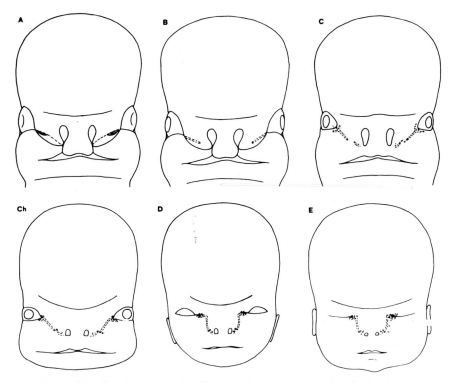

Figure 2-8. The development of the ectodermal component of the lacrimal passages. **A.** Embryonal lacrimal plate (11 to 12 mm). **B.** Embryonal lacrimal cord (13 to 14 mm). **C.** Progression of the cord, with lysis of the embryonal lacrimal pedicle (14 to 16 mm). **Ch.** Contact with nasal and conjunctival epithelium (17 to 28 mm). **D.** Epithelial fusion of nasal aspect of eyelids (28 to 35 mm). **E.** Cavitation of lacrimal passages in viable fetal stage seven to nine months.

and forms its dermis also invaginates into the mesoderm to cover the basal membrane of the embryonic lacrimal plate.

The embryonic lacrimal cord is formed, in the 35 to 36 day (25 mm) embryo, as the deepest cells of the plate remain and form a column which is subsequently separated from its pedicular attachment to the epiblast. This cellular column, the embryonic lacrimal cord, gives rise to the whole ectodermal structure of the lacrimal passages. The location of this cord deepens as the maxillary and external nasal processes fuse and continue to grow. Its sinuous path takes origin in the lower internal portion of the annular orbito-ocular groove, progresses inferiorly, forward, and deeper. It becomes depressed into the mesoderm, progressively separating itself from the surface of the face to reach the lower part of the external aspect of the primitive naris. The lacrimal cord is, from the beginning, a continuous and uninterrupted cellular column.

In the embryonic evolution of the lacrimal cord, even before the isolation of the cord is completed, all of its cells, as well as those from the surrounding mesenchyme, multiply and begin to form the definitive lacrimal passages. The most conspicuous morphologic changes occur simultaneously at the ocular and nasal ends of the cord. It appears that, at this same time, the lacrimal cord grows in the area of the future canaliculi, defining the upper end of the excretory passages.

In the 19 to 21 mm embryo, the origin of the vertical limb of each canaliculus can be identified (Fig. 2-10). The eyelid margins become elevated at the point toward which the canaliculi are directed, forming the lacrimal

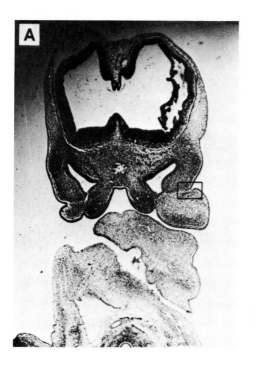

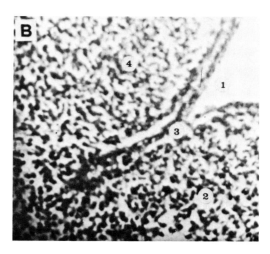

Figure 2-9. Embryo measuring 12 mm. **A.** Frontal section showing sulcus between the upper maxillary and the external nasal processes. **B.** Details of left orbitonasal sulcus. **1.** Orbitonasal sulcus. **2.** Maxillary process. **3.** Embryonal lacrimal plate. **4.** External nasal process.

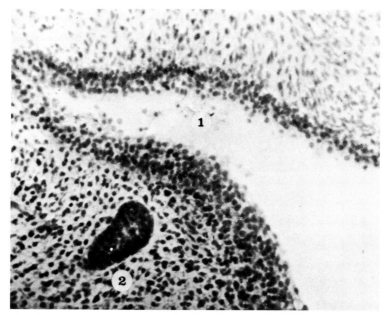

Figure 2-10. Frontal section showing beginning lid grooves in 20 mm embryo. Detail of the left medial palpebral angle showing **(2)** a section through the vertical limb of the inferior canaliculus and a **(1)** deflection of the lid margin indicating the site of the lacrimal papilla.

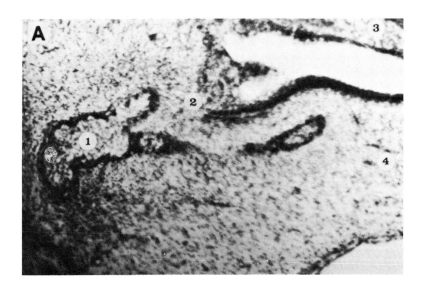

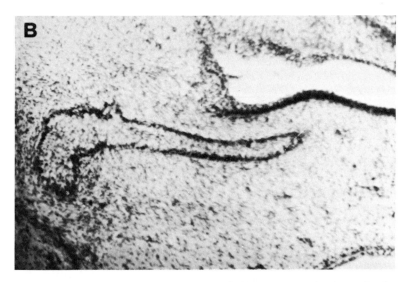

Figure 2-11. Embryo measuring 28 mm. **A.** Horizontal section immediately below the lower eyelid margin. **1.** Common canaliculus. At the lower left, the beginning of the sac-duct junction; at the right, the upper and lower canaliculi. **2.** Lacrimal caruncle. **3.** Eyeball. **4.** Lower lid. **B.** Horizontal section just below.

papillae. The palpebral furrow, which has not started to fuse yet, will take on an S shape in its medial part determined by the asymmetry of the two formative lacrimal papillae.

In the 28 to 30 mm embryo, at the end of the embryonic period, the lacrimal path con-sists of a continuous and solid structure of epithelial cells surrounded by a mesenchyme of less dense consistency. The common canaliculus, as well as its relation to the canaliculi and the lacrimal sac, can be identified (Figs. 2-11 and 2-12).

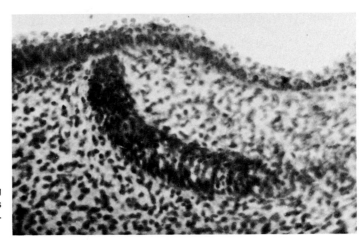

Figure 2-12. Embryo measuring 28.5 mm. Inferior canaliculus making contact with the conjunctiva at the lower lid margin.

At the beginning of the fetal period (31+ mm embryo), all of the morphologic elements that will constitute the basic structure of the lacrimal passages in the adult are already formed. These grow in length and width and undergo canalization after the end of the second month, and this cavitation process is characterized by an initial and a later identifiable period.

The transition from one phase of this development to the other is gradual and overlapping. Almost simultaneously with the cavitation of the cellular column, there begins within the nasal cavity the process of separation of both epithelial plates of the inferior meatal lamina. The space thus formed is the inferior nasal meatus. Simultaneously, in the 40 to 50 mm fetus, the basal membrane which separates the palpebral epithelium from the canalicular epithelium at the lacrimal papillae undergoes resorption. The basal membrane of the epithelium of the canaliculi is continuous with the membrane of the eyelid epithelium, and the lacrimal puncta thus formed are closed simply by a conglomerate of cells which act as a plug. Within the canaliculi, a pattern of intraluminal folds develops. During this same period, the lacrimal sac undergoes considerable growth, and the process of cavitation of the sac begins (Fig. 2-13).

The lacrimonasal duct is characterized by irregular caliber, continuous internal walls and frequent exophitic diverticuli. At about three months, the external shape of the lacrimal sacduct complex changes from its original nasal concavity to take on an S shape as it bends forward in its lower aspect to approach the epithelium of the lower meatus. The upper portion, which becomes the lacrimal sac, bends backward. At four months, the canaliculi have a fibrocollagenous envelope, which is, in turn, surrounded by longitudinal muscular fibers, and all elements of the excretory system are well defined (Fig. 2-14). The lacrimonasal duct follows a bony channel whose wall is formed by the development of the upper maxillary and lacrimal bones.

In the second half of the life of the fetus, the morphology of the lacrimal passages undergoes little change. The length of the canaliculi becomes relatively shorter, and this process continues after birth. As the process of canalization continues, the canaliculi fuse with and establish communication with the fundus of the lacrimal sac.

The development of the facial mass gradually changes the position of the lacrimonasal duct. The two chief characteristics of the later fetal development are the openings of both ends of the lacrimal passages. As the lacrimal puncta are shaped, they are directed toward the ocular surface of the eyelid margin. Initially, the

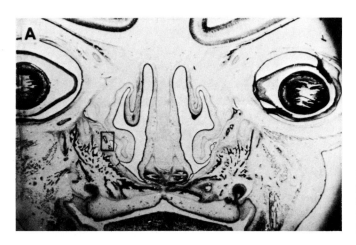

Figure 2-13. Fetus measuring 80 mm. **A.** Frontal section showing chondrification in nasal septum and turbinate and cavitation of the lacrimal pathways.

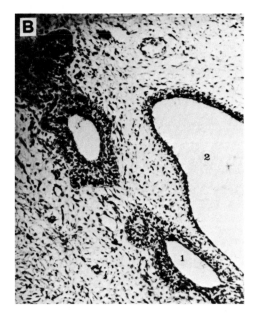

B. Details of the lowest part of the right nasolacrimal duct. Note the abundant vascularization. **1.** Nasolacrimal duct. **2.** Inferior meatus.

puncta are plugged with compressed epithelial cells, which eventually clear, forming the upper opening of the drainage system. At the lower end, between the mucosa of the terminal saccule of the lacrimonasal duct and the mucosa of the inferior nasal meatus, there is a continuous mesodermal lamina which remains until the

end of the developmental period. The ostium opens into the inferior meatus at the end of the third trimester. It seems that the perforation of the mucosa of the duct and of the nasal meatus is genetically predetermined. Depending on its location, the ostium may be rounded, oval, slit, bilobulated, or falciform.

We have studied 181 healthy full-term newborns, using a syringing technique, to determine patency of the lacrimal passages. In 131 of these, there was bilateral patency, in 46, one side was impermeable and the other open, and in four infants, both sides were blocked. Thus, 15 percent of the 362 lacrimal passages were still impermeable at birth.

DEVELOPMENT OF THE OSSEOUS STRUCTURES OF THE LACRIMAL APPARATUS

The cephalic cavities—cranial, oral, orbital, nasal, and otic—are structured progressively during the embryonic period of prenatal development. The mesoblast surrounding them separates one from the other and condenses into a desmoskeleton which will later become bone.

The bones related to the lacrimal gland and lacrimal excretory passages develop in the following way: the frontal processes will form the roof of the orbit and consequently the fossa of the lacrimal gland. The nasal processes will

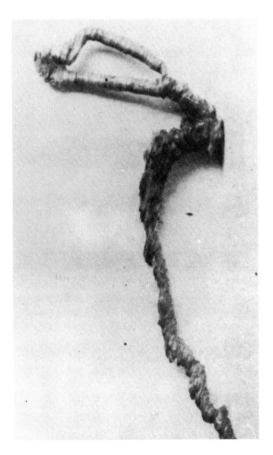

Figure 2-14. Wax reconstruction (BORN technique) of the epithelial components of the right lacrimal pathway in a five-month fetus. (Leplat, 1937.)

third will be resorbed without leaving any residual.

Ossification begins in the membranous bones. The first ossification centers related to the lacrimal apparatus appear in the sixth week of development. At two and one-half months, ossification of the maxillary begins, starting with five ossification points, two of them in the orbitonasal area and the lacrimonasal region. At four months, the different membranous bones surrounding the lacrimal apparatus are well developed.

At birth, the fossa of the lacrimal gland is deep and cone-shaped. The lacrimal sac fossa is cylindrical and is oriented forward. The bony

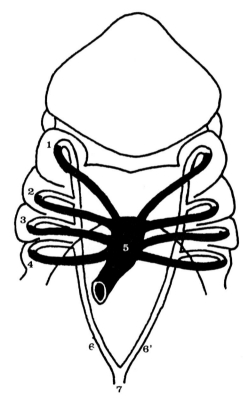

Figure 2-15. Drawing of the branchial vascular arches of the human embryo. **1.** First branchial vascular arch. **2.** Second branchial vascular arch. **3.** Third vascular arch. **4.** Fourth vascular arch. **5.** Aortic sac. **6** and **6′.** Right and left dorsal aortas. **7.** Common descending aorta.

later form the lateral mass of the ethmoid bone, the unguis, the nasal bone, and the medial portion of the upper maxillary bone, which is related to the bony lacrimal canal. Some of the bony development goes through a cartilaginous process and other parts through a membranous phase.

In the process of chondrification, the foramina serving vascular and nerve structures are formed as lacunae or bony canals. The cartilage of the nasal capsule undergoes a triple evolution: one part will remain cartilaginous, another will be substituted by bone tissue, and a lacrimonasal canal extends down and posteriorly, having a concavity directed nasally. The bones of the lacrimal canal are ossified, but their sutures are membranous. The shape and position of the bony lacrimonasal canal undergo gradual alteration as the facial bones develop.

DEVELOPMENT OF THE VASCULAR SYSTEM OF THE LACRIMAL APPARATUS

Toward the end of the third week, the aortic sac begins to form, and four vascular arches appear, one for each branchial arch (Fig. 2-15).

The evolution of the first three aortic arches is related to the formation of the head. The ventral portion of the third arch will become the carotid artery, dividing into external carotid and internal carotid. The external carotid develops two main trunks, the superficial temporal artery and the internal maxillary artery. The internal carotid divides into the middle cerebral and the ophthalmic arteries. The stapedius artery also comes from the internal carotid.

There are frequent and multiple variations of the blood supply to the lacrimal gland, and these variations are made more understandable by a knowledge of the evolution of the vascular development of the lacrimal apparatus (Fig. 2-16). One of the branches of the superficial temporal artery, the external maxillary artery, ascends to enter the orbit along the nasal capsule, where it anastomoses with the stapedial nasociliary artery, after giving rise to a naso-orbital branch. The first portion of the external maxillary artery will become the facial artery, and the anastomotic portion will become the angular artery.

The internal maxillary artery gives rise to one branch which goes to the maxillary process, where it joins the maxillomandibular branch of the internal carotid, and a second branch which ultimately supplies the lacrimal gland. The ter-

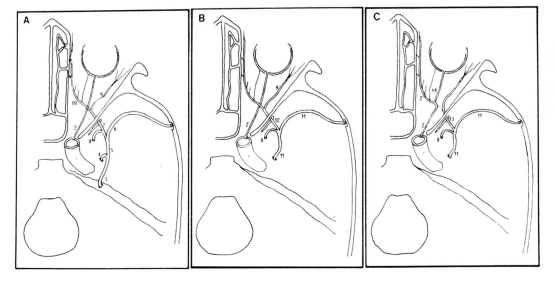

Figure 2-16. Drawing of horizontal plane through the skull and right orbit. **A.** Relationships of the stapedial and primitive ophthalmic arteries. **B.** The vascular pattern in the second half of the fetal period. **C.** The vascular pattern at the end of the fetal period. Arteries: **1.** Internal carotid. **2.** Primitive ophthalmic. **2′.** Definitive primitive ophthalmic. **3.** Stapedial. **4.** Maxillomandibular. **5.** Supraorbital. **6.** Meningeal. **7.** Orbital. **8.** Recurrent tentorial. **9. Primitive lacri**mal. **9′.** Definitive lacrimal. **10.** Primitive nasociliary. **11.** Middle meningeal. **12.** Meningo-orbital. **13.** Meningolacrimal. **14.** Central retinal artery.

minal branch of the primitive internal maxillary artery becomes the sphenopalatine artery and supplies the meati and part of the lacrimonasal duct.

The stapedial artery derives from the second aortic arch, passes through the lacuna of the auricular stapes, and enters the cranial cavity, where it branches into the maxillary-mandibular artery and the supraorbital artery. The latter gives rise to the orbital artery, which enters the sphenoidal cleft and divides into the embryonic lacrimal and nasociliary arteries. After the beginning of the third month, the stapedial trunk closes, and the maxillomandibular, supraorbital, and meningeal arteries form the middle meningeal artery.

The ophthalmic artery provides the vascularization for the retina, an extension of the cerebral ectoderm. In the embryo, the retina is supplied by branches of the stapedial artery. When the embryonic ophthalmic artery joins with the orbital branches of the stapedial trunk, the initial portion of the embryonic artery and the distal portion of the nasociliary artery will become the definitive ophthalmic artery, while the distal portion of the embryonic ophthalmic artery becomes the central artery of the retina.

DEVELOPMENT OF THE NERVE SUPPLY OF THE LACRIMAL APPARATUS

In the 22-day-old embryo, the cephalic portion of the neural tube organizes into three vesicles: prosencephalon, mesencephalon, and rhombencephalon. Ten days later, by further division, the prosencephalon subdivides into the telencephalon and diencephalon, while the rhombencephalon divides into metencephalon and myelencephalon. The lacrimal nucleus develops from the ventral aspect of the metencephalon, and its nerve becomes the efferent nerve supply to the lacrimal gland. As this nerve develops, the fibers will pass through the facial nucleus and the geniculate ganglion to terminate in the lacrimal gland.

The afferent portion of the nerve supply of the lacrimal gland is derived from the ophthalmic division of the trigeminal nerve. In the rhombencephalon, the more lateral neuroblasts form the long sensory nucleus of the trigeminal nerve, traversing the rhombencephalon to invade the mesencephalon cranially and the spinal cord caudally. This nucleus will transmit reflex stimuli to the lacrimal gland.

3

THE ANATOMY OF THE LACRIMAL SYSTEM

ABRAHAM WERB

Early anatomic descriptions of the lacrimal system make fascinating reading, but the anatomic concepts as they are known today date back only as far as Leone, who described the nasolacrimal duct (1574), and to Steensen, who described the lacrimal gland (in 1662).

In considering the gross anatomy of the lacrimal system, the two components which make up the system—the secretory system and the excretory system—will be considered separately.

THE SECRETORY SYSTEM

Different types of glands are concerned with the production of tears. The term "tear" needs qualification. The tear is a fluid sandwich which has an inner mucoid layer, an intermediate aqueous layer, and an outer oily layer. The intermediate aqueous layer is derived from two types of glands—those concerned with the constant supply of tears (basic secretion) and those responsible for the additional supply of tears on demand (reflex secretion). Maybe it is because of their different locations that there is such a discrepancy in the size of these glands in relation to their function.

The Lacrimal Gland

The lacrimal gland is the largest of the secretory group. It is located in the upper outer aspect of the orbit, in a shallow depression in the frontal bone designated as the *fossa glandulae lacrimalis.* The gland is, thus, in relation to the frontal bone superiorly. Its inferior surface rests on the eyeball and is molded by the shape of the globe (Fig. 3-1).

Because of its close relationship to the lateral border of the levator aponeurosis, the gland may have a variable form. The aponeurosis produces a deep cleft in the lacrimal gland, almost dividing the gland into two lobes—an orbital lobe above the aponeurosis and a palpebral lobe below it. Above and behind the aponeurotic cleft there is continuity of gland.

The orbital (superior) lobe, whose upper surface is molded by the frontal bone fossa in which it is located, is loosely connected to the periosteum by connective tissue fibers, sometimes referred to as "Soemmering's ligament." The inferior border is similarly connected to the sheath of the levator muscle. The anterior border is sharp, lying just behind the superior orbital margin, covered anteriorly by the orbital septum and, successively, by a thin layer of fat, orbicularis muscle fibers, and eyelid skin. The

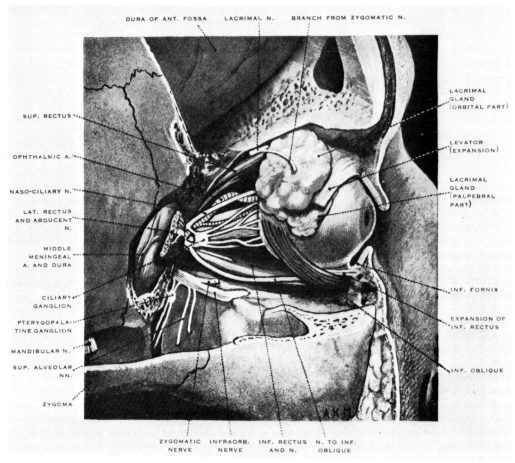

Figure 3-1. The lacrimal gland. (*From Last RJ: Wolff's Anatomy of the Eye and Orbit, 6th ed, 1968. Courtesy of H.K. Lewis & Co., Ltd.*)

posterior border of the gland is in close contact with orbital fat and has loose connective tissue attachments to contiguous orbital structures. The medial end lies on the lateral border of the levator muscle, and the lateral end is in relation to the lateral rectus muscle (Fig. 3-2).

The fluid secreted by the acini of the orbital lobe is collected into four to six ducts which traverse the palpebral lobe and which, along with the six to eight ducts of the palpebral lobe, empty into the conjunctival sac in the temporal one third of the superior conjunctival fornix. In some cases, these ductal openings may extend as far as the lateral canthus and even below (Fig. 3-3).

The palpebral (inferior) lobe of the lacri-mal gland is about half the size of the orbital lobe and is formed of several lobules. It lies below and anterior to the levator aponeurosis and, unlike the superior, extends beyond the orbital margin to lie above the superior conjunctival fornix, where its ducts open. It is this part of the gland that can be dislocated forward into the lateral palpebral aperture.

Histology of the Lacrimal Gland. The lacrimal gland is a tubuloalveolar gland with short branching tubules resembling the parotid in structure. The acini consist of two layers of cells lying on a hyaline basement membrane and surrounding a central canal. The cells in the basal layer are flat and contractile, while the

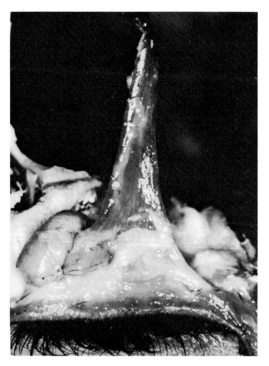

Figure 3-2. The right lacrimal gland viewed from above, showing the levator aponeurosis cleaving the lacrimal gland from below, and the superior-anterior surface molded by the lacrimal gland fossa of the frontal bone (removed). Posteriorly, the orbital and palpebral lobes are continuous.

other cells are cylindrical and contain secretory granules. The secretions of the acini pass into intermediary ducts and eventually into a definitive excretory duct. The stroma contains lymphoid elements (Fig. 3-4).

Accessory Lacrimal Glands

The glands that are responsible for the constant (basic) supply of tears are small in size but greater in number. These are the accessory lacrimal glands of Krause. More than 20 of these are found in the upper conjunctival fornix and between 6 and 8 in the lower. They are located in the substantia propria of the conjunctiva.

Another small group, described by Wolfring and bearing his name, are found near the upper border of the tarsal plate. Glandular tissue with the same structure as the lacrimal gland and those described above is also present in the plica and the caruncle (Fig. 3-5).

Goblet Cells

Two other sources contribute to the structure of the tear film. Mucin forms the deepest layer of the tear film and is secreted by goblet cells in the conjunctival surface of the upper tarsal margin as well as along the lower margin. The glands of Manz are found in the limbal conjunctiva ringing the cornea. The mucin adsorbs onto the normally hydrophobic corneal epithelium, rendering its surface hydrophilic and allowing the tear fluid to spread evenly.

Meibomian Glands

The external oily layer of the tear film is produced by the meibomian glands situated in the tarsal plates of the upper and lower lids (Fig. 3-5). Twenty-eight linear type glands are found in the upper and 18 in the lower. These glands lie side by side along the tarsus, with the long axis of each oriented at right angles to the lid margin. The glands of Zeis are found at the margin of the eyelids, and the glands of Moll are found at the roots of the eyelashes. Their function is to maintain structure of the tear film by decreasing evaporation and preventing the fluid of the lacrimal glands from overflowing the lid margins.

The significance of this anatomic arrangement becomes clear when the importance of corneal wetting is considered. The constant supply of tears is provided by those glands other than the main lacrimal gland. That gland comes into use on demand as, for example, in emotional weeping, foreign body irritation, and other reflex stimuli.

Nerve Supply of the Lacrimal Gland

The lacrimal reflex is initiated through the ophthalmic division of the trigeminal nerve by stimulation of external ocular structures, skin, or nasal mucosa (Fig. 3-6). Impulses are directed, by way of the trigeminal ganglion, to the lacrimal nucleus just above the superior salivary nucleus in the pons.

The efferent reflex pathway passes from the lacrimal nucleus through the geniculate ganglion. These centrifugal fibers join the greater superficial petrosal nerve via the nervus intermedius of the facial nerve, pass through the pterygoid canal as the vidian nerve, and synapse in the sphenopalatine ganglion. The efferent parasympathetic impulses are then

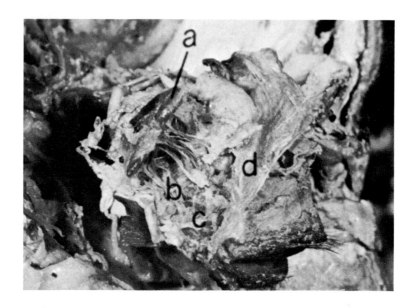

Figure 3-3. Lacrimal gland collecting ducts. In this dissection, collecting ducts (b) are seen passing from the orbital lobe (a) into the palpebral lobe (c), which lies below the lateral horn of the levator aponeurosis (d). (*From Beard C, Quickert MH: Anatomy of the Orbit, 1979. Courtesy of Aesculapius Publishing Company.*)

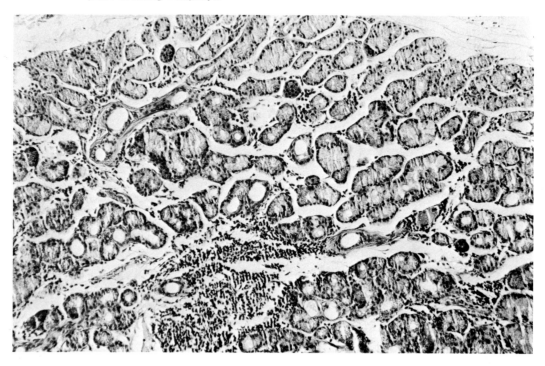

Figure 3-4. Normal lacrimal gland. (*Courtesy of ML Smith, Department of Ophthalmology, Washington University, St. Louis, Missouri.*)

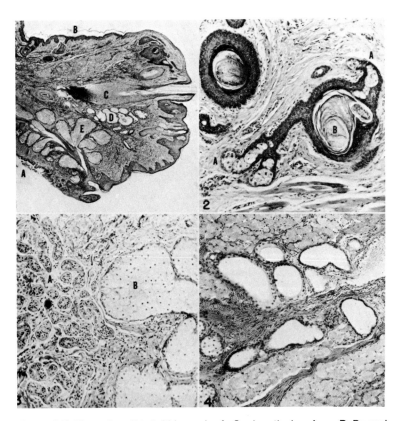

Figure 3-5. Normal eyelid. **1.** Lid margin. **A.** Conjunctival surface. **B.** Dermal surface. **C.** Hair follicle containing hair shaft. **D.** Gland of Moll. **E.** Meibomian gland. × 24. AFIP Acc. 171463. **2. A.** Glands of Zeis (sebaceous glands). **B.** Hair follicle containing hair shaft. × 125. AFIP Acc. 325133. **3. A.** Glands of Wolfring (accessory lacrimal glands). **B.** Meibomian glands (modified sebaceous glands). × 125. AFIP Acc. 482185. **4.** Gland of Moll (modified sweat glands) dilated. × 90. AFIP Neg. 103949. (*From Hogan MJ, Zimmerman LE: Ophthalmic Pathology, 2nd ed, 1962. Courtesy of W.B. Saunders Co.*)

transmitted via postganglionic fibers in the zygomatic nerve (a branch of the maxillary division of the trigeminal nerve). The zygomaticotemporal branch of this nerve gives off a recurrent branch to the lacrimal nerve, from which the efferent fibers terminate in the lacrimal gland. The sensory fibers ramify between the acini of the gland and surround the ducts.

The principal stimulus for tear secretion is mediated through this parasympathetic route. Blocking the sphenopalatine ganglion will depress tear secretion. Denervation of the efferent parasympathetic pathway will sensitize the lacrimal gland to pilocarpine and other parasympathomimetric drugs which act directly at the nerve ending.

The sympathetic fibers are derived from the postganglionic cervical sympathetic fibers, which are associated with the carotid plexus. It is uncertain whether they reach the gland along the lacrimal artery or via the pterygoid canal to the sphenopalatine ganglion and then by way of the zygomatic nerve to the lacrimal gland.

The origins for psychogenic (emotional) tearing are related to the hypothalamus, but the exact afferent pathways are not well defined. Psychogenic tearing is always bilateral.

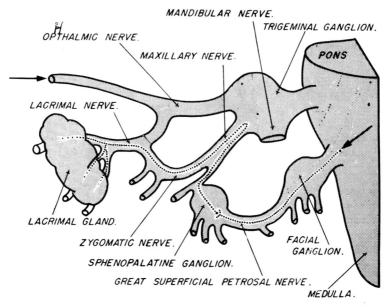

Figure 3-6. A simplified diagram of the pathway of the lacrimation reflex (*From Veirs ER: The Lacrimal System: Clinical Application, 1955. Courtesy of Grune & Stratton, Inc.*)

The nerve supply is summarized by Duke-Elder[1] as follows:

> As a general conclusion to which there are many contradictions in the literature we may surmise that the trigeminal nerve forms the afferent path of the reflex arc . . . that the efferent path is formed either by the sympathetic supply or the parasympathetic fibers associated with the facial nerve. What the precise role of these two may be must still be left to conjecture.

Vascular Supply of the Lacrimal Gland

The vascular supply of the lacrimal gland derives from the lacrimal branch of the ophthalmic artery and, sometimes, the infraorbital branch of the maxillary artery. The venous return is by way of the superior ophthalmic vein. The lymphatics of the area drain to the preauricular lymph nodes.

THE EXCRETORY SYSTEM

The elimination of tears proceeds as follows: The tears enter the punctum and pass along the canaliculus, the common canaliculus, the common opening into the lacrimal sac, and down the nasolacrimal duct into the nose. Along this course, the pathway traverses several structures, alters direction several times, and varies greatly in its accessibility to the surgeon. Direct visualization is possible only at the two ends of this drainage pathway. All that lies between, including the many variations, influences not only the pathologic processes that affect it but also the surgical approaches to relieve them.

The Punctum

The punctum is situated at the junction of the ciliary and lacrimal portions of the eyelids, on a slight elevation called the "papilla lacrimalis," in line with the sharp inner margin of the lid. Between 0.2 and 0.3 mm in diameter, the punctum is ideally a funnel-shaped structure, but other shapes exist and seem compatible with normal function. It is surrounded by a ring of connective tissue and is capable of being dilated without functional impairment. One important constant feature is its permanent patency (Fig. 3-7).

Both the upper and lower puncta are so oriented on the lid margin that they face slightly backward into the groove formed by the plica semilunaris and the globe. When the eyelids are open, there is a difference between the

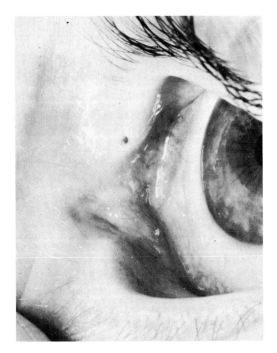

Figure 3-7. Upper punctum, showing its permanent patency (note the absence of the lower punctum).

positions of the puncta, the upper being 0.5 mm more medial than the lower. The plica is slanted to conform to this arrangement. It is placed in such a way that the upper end of the plica is slightly medial to the lower, thus accommodating both puncta in this groove. When the eyelids are closed, the upper and lower puncta are directly apposed and in contact.

During lateral movements of the eyes, the position of the puncta remains essentially stationary, but two other grooves are present to accommodate the tears. One of these grooves lies between the plica and the caruncle, the other is at the limbus. Thus, for example, in dextrorotation of the eyes, the puncta of the right eye will be in relation to the plica-caruncle groove, while the puncta of the left eye will be near the limbal groove. In primary position, both are in relation to the groove lying between the plica and the globe.

The Canaliculus
The canaliculus lies within the eyelid margin, oriented parallel with the nasal 6 to 7 mm of the margin. Each canaliculus consists of a vertical

component 2 mm in length, which may be thought of as an extension of the funnel-like punctal aperture and an 8 mm long horizontal component. At the junction of the vertical and horizontal components, the canaliculus widens to an ampulla some 1.5 to 2 mm in diameter.

The lower canaliculus has a horizontal orientation, and the upper meets it at an angle of 25°. Only when the lids are in a closed position are the two canaliculi parallel. It has been suggested that the ampulla functions as a trap for foreign bodies, more than as a part of the pumping action normally ascribed to the canaliculus. The success of the three-snip operation and, similarly, punctumplasties seems to support the notion that the ampulla and vertical components of the canaliculus are not essential to the evacuation of tears.

The canaliculus is permanently patent, although dynamically its lumen varies in cross-sectional diameter during the act of blinking. The canaliculus is lined with stratified squamous epithelium. It has variations in caliber and numerous folds that may play a role in cases of nontraumatic canalicular occlusion and during lacrimal irrigation (Fig. 3-8).

The upper and lower canaliculus join to form a common canaliculus 3 to 5 mm in length, emptying into the lacrimal sac through an opening on the lateral wall. Just before the point of entry into the lacrimal sac, the common canaliculus may have a dilated portion, called the "sinus of Maier."

The common opening enters the sac on its lateral wall at the junction of its upper third and lower two thirds and usually appears as a small dimple. Unlike the punctum and canaliculus, it is not permanently patent but appears as a slit and may have folds of tissue surrounding it. The positions of these flaps or valves are variable, and in some cases, they almost occlude the internal opening. These folds can act in trapdoor fashion, a fact which may be responsible for the inability to decompress the lacrimal sac in cases of mucocele or pyocele.

The Lacrimal Sac
The lacrimal sac is located in the bony lacrimal fossa on the anterior aspect of the medial wall of the orbit. The sac rests on a periosteal layer and is enveloped by a fascial covering which is an extension of the periosteum. The firmness of ad-

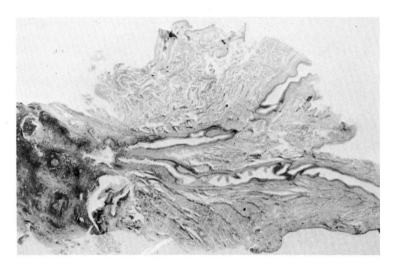

Figure 3-8. Lacrimal canaliculi. Note the numerous small mucosal valvelike folds. (*From Ann R Coll Surg Engl, 54:240, 1974.*)

hesion is greater superiorly, where the fascial covering thickens into a fibrous band, and on the deep aspect of the sac. In the fossa itself, the adhesion is much looser. The medial relations of the lacrimal sac are the structures that form the lacrimal fossa—the frontal process of the maxilla anteriorly and the lacrimal bone posteriorly (Fig. 3-9).

The lacrimal fossa is delimited by and best identified by the anterior and posterior lacrimal crests. The anterior crest may be sharp or blunt. When it is sharp, it makes the fossa appear deep and overhangs the approach to the lacrimal sac. The anterior lacrimal crest is continuous below with the inferior orbital margin. The posterior lacrimal crest becomes continuous above the superior orbital margin. Most of the lacrimal fossa is related to the middle meatus of the nose, but the upper part is contiguous to the anterior ethmoid air cells. In some instances, a large ethmoid air cell, the agar nasi, extends downward sufficiently to be interposed completely between the lacrimal fossa and the nasal cavity. The lacrimal surgeon must be alert to the position of the ethmoid air cells in his surgical approach.

The lateral aspect of the lacrimal sac is related to the lateral lacrimal fascia to which it is loosely adherent. It is in close relation to the bony origin of the inferior oblique muscle. The firm attachment of the lateral wall of the sac to the periosteum, which also receives the fibers of the inferior and superior preseptal orbicularis muscles, is of physiologic significance. According to Jones,[2] the lateral pull on this diaphragm causes negative pressure within the sac, and release results in positive pressure. This movement is said to contribute to the elimination of tears in the pump mechanism. Although there are differing concepts as to the role of the lacrimal sac and the pump mechanism, it is agreed that, at least part of the time, the lumen of the sac is collapsed and is no more than a slit.

Part or all of the fundus of the lacrimal sac is under cover of the medial canthal tendon. The tendon is inserted into a tubercle on the frontal process of the maxilla midway between the suture line joining the frontal process and nasal bone and the anterior lacrimal crest. Because the relationship of the medial canthal tendon is confined to the upper part of the lacrimal sac, abscesses or fistulas will always appear below the free margin of the canthal tendon. In fact, a swelling above the canthal tendon strongly hints at some type of tumor formation rather than inflammatory lacrimal sac disease.

Histology of the Lacrimal Drainage System

The lacrimal drainage system is lined by stratified squamous epithelium. The sac and duct

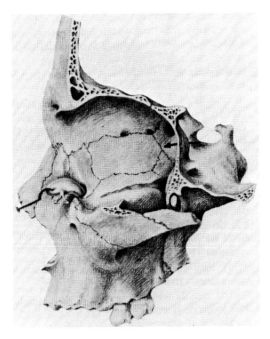

Figure 3-9. Nasal wall of the orbit. The lacrimal sac has been drawn aside to show the lacrimal fossa. (*From Murube del Castillo J: Dacriologia Basica, 1981. Courtesy of Royper.*)

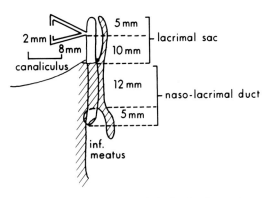

Figure 3-10. Dimensions of the lacrimal excretory system.

have two layers of epithelium, a superficial columnar layer and a deeper flat layer. The superficial layer contains goblet cells. The membranous wall of the sac consists of fibroelastic tissue.

The Nasolacrimal Duct

The nasolacrimal duct is a continuation of the sac downward to its termination at the inferior meatus of the nose (Fig. 3-10). It traverses a bony passage—the nasolacrimal canal (12 mm long)—and continues on below the nasal part as the intrameatal portion of the nasolacrimal canal (5 mm). The opening of the nasolacrimal duct is found on the anterior part of the lateral wall of the inferior meatus. The distance from the external naris to the opening of the duct is between 30 and 35 mm. The opening varies in shape as well as in size. At its lower end, it has a fold of mucous membrane, the valve of Hasner, whose probable function is to prevent reflux of air or nasal discharge into the nasolacrimal duct.

The folds in the lacrimal sac itself are prob-

ably relics of the irregularities seen in the sac of the newborn. These valves, or folds, have little effect on tear flow but probably influence the sites of obstruction.

Vascular Supply of the Lacrimal Pathways

The arterial supply to the lacrimal pathways derives from:

1. The ophthalmic artery, as the medial superior palpebral artery supplying the sac and the medial inferior palpebral artery supplying the duct
2. The angular branch of the facial artery supplying the sac
3. The internal maxillary artery

The venous plexus, under the mucous membrane of the lacrimal sac, drains to the angular and inferior orbital veins.

The angular vein is a confluence of the supraorbital and frontal veins and runs along the side of the nose lateral to the angular artery. It crosses the nasal edge of the medial canthal tendon lateral to its insertion. It communicates with the superior ophthalmic vein above and the facial vein below. The flow of blood is downward. It is a prominent structure, superficial and usually visible. Its position is of significance surgically, and it can be the source of some very troublesome bleeding. Since it is not vital, the surgeon may choose to double-ligate it and cut it, or it can be isolated and avoided at surgery. In general, the latter is the wiser step.

The lymphatic drainage from the sac is to the submaxillary lymph nodes.

Innervation of the Lacrimal Excretory Pathway

The nerve supply to the lacrimal excretory pathway is from the trigeminal nerve by way of the infratrochlear branch of the nasociliary nerve. The lower part of the duct is supplied by the anterior-superior alveolar nerve. The motor supply is through the facial nerve that supplies the orbicularis oculi. Sympathetic fibers follow the sympathetic supply to the orbit.

REFERENCES

1. Duke-Elder S: System of Ophthalmology. St. Louis, Mosby, 1952.
2. Jones LT: The Cure of Epiphora Due to Canalicular Disorders, Trauma and Surgical Failures on the Lacrimal Passages. Trans Am Acad Ophth Otolaryn 66:508, 1962.

4

CLINICAL BIOCHEMISTRY OF TEARS

N.J. VAN HAERINGEN

It is the purpose of this paper to review the literature on the composition of tears. The crucial influence of the method of sampling on the composition of this fluid is discussed; many contradictory results can be traced back to differences in specimen collection. Abnormalities caused by diseases or drug effects are emphasized, and the clinical application of tear analysis is summarized.

TEARS

Tear Film

"Tears" refers to fluid present as the precorneal film and in the conjunctival sac. The volume of tear fluid is about 5 to 10 μl.[93, 111] Most of it (95 percent or more) is produced by the lacrimal gland.[110, 112] Lesser amounts are produced by the goblet cells[41] and the accessory lacrimal glands[38] of the conjunctiva. The total mass of the latter is about one tenth of the mass of the main lacrimal gland.[5]

The normal secretion is about 1 to 2 μl/minute,[93, 121] and except for those that evap-

orate, the tears exit through the lacrimal puncta and canaliculi to the lacrimal sac, which communicates with the nasal cavity. The precorneal film is a complex layer of fluid with a thickness of 5 to 10 μm.[92] The fluid covering the conjunctiva is estimated to be somewhat thicker.[81] The film consists of a thin (0.1 to 0.2 μm) film of meibomian lipid at the air/tear interface, covering the thicker aqueous layer of tears and containing proteins,[39] metabolites,[144] electrolytes,[84, 114] and mucin.[65] An adsorption of a thin layer mucin (0.02 to 0.04 μm[65]) on the epithelial surface renders this hydrophilic, thus enabling the tears to spread over the surface of the eye immediately after a blink. Between blinks, the tear film subsequently may decrease in thickness by evaporation,[40, 92] although the lipid layer will lower the evaporation rate of water from the tear film.[68]

Production

Several drugs influence tear production and/or composition.

Decreased production of tears as a direct consequence of drug therapy has been reported after use of the β-blockers practolol[45, 148] and timolol,[96] the ganglion blockers[148] hexamethonium and chlorisondamine, phenothia-

Reprinted from Survey of Ophthalmology, 26:84-96, 1981, with permission of the author and Survey of Ophthalmology.

zines,[109–116]* the psychotropic drugs diazepam,[109] clomipramine,[109] and nialamide,[8] and the hypnotic nitrazepam.[33, 109] A combination of nitrazepam and acetylsalicylic acid even has been advocated in the treatment of epiphora.[33] There is no evidence of effect of oral contraceptives on tear production[49] or contact lens tolerance.[36]

Increased production of tears as a direct consequence of drug therapy has been reported with fluorouracil,[61] nicotinic acid and nicotinyl alcohol,[87] and bromhexine.[104] Bromhexine is claimed to be valuable in the treatment of Sjögren's syndrome.[52, 128]

Collection and Sources of Error from Sampling Methods

Collection in small glass capillary pipettes is a useful method for removing microliter quantities of tear fluid from the conjunctival sac. At normal production of about 1 μl/minute without mechanical irritation, the collection procedure for a 10 μl sample lasts 10 minutes.

Another practical method is collection of tears in absorbent material. Schirmer[113] in 1903 introduced the test named for him which measures the tear production by the moistening of a strip of blotting paper inserted 5 mm into the lower conjunctival sac for 5 minutes. All subsequent investigations described herein have been based on this method. Other absorbent materials are filter paper discs, cellulose sponges, and cotton thread, which are sometimes placed just within the conjunctival sac where they are soaked with tears.

Aside from variations caused by collection methods, the accuracy of the analytic data derived from unstimulated tears is limited by the scantiness of fluid and by variations caused by evaporation, change in the rate of secretion, and inadequate mixing.

An essential difference in composition exists between tear fluid collected in capillary pipettes or on absorbent material. In capillary pipettes only tear fluid is collected, freely floating from the tear film into the pipette by capillary suction. With filter papers or cellulose sponges placed in the conjunctival sac, not only is fluid collected but also a variable portion of the mucous layer sticking on the epithelial sur-

face and even the contents of epithelial cells, which have been disrupted by the application of the absorbent material.

Another complication of the use of filter paper material is that it has adsorbent as well as absorbent properties. This can be seen from the seldom recognized[145] poor recovery of proteins after elution in appropriate buffer solutions or saline. This incomplete elution may also occur when paper discs, soaked with tear fluid, are applied directly on agar plates in diffusion methods as used for the determination of lysozyme and immunoglobulins.

Stimulation of the production of tears is a controversial method of augmenting the quantity of a tear specimen. It has been demonstrated that the concentration of different components in the tear fluid is related to the rate of tear secretion. The concentration of proteins,[39] glycoproteins,[39] and calcium[24, 77] will decrease, but potassium[24] will increase as flow rate increases. It also has been suggested that the concentration of lysozyme is dependent on tear flow rate,[103] but this could not be confirmed by others.[9, 107] In keratoconjunctivitis sicca, abnormally high osmotic values are found using specimens of 0.1 μl tear fluid. Collection of larger volumes results in normal (lower) values.[12, 88]

The use of emotional tears[123] and tearing induced by having the patient look into the sun[113] or stimulating the gag reflex with a tongue depressor[2] are examples of noncontact methods to enhance tear production but are, for obvious reasons, of little practical value for studying basic tear film. Stimulation of the lacrimal reflex also may be induced by mechanical or chemical irritation of the mucosa of conjunctiva and nose. The Schirmer test itself is based on the mechanical reflex stimulation of tear production by insertion of the strip of paper into the conjunctival sac.[113]

Several volatile lacrimal agents can be used to induce tearing: cigarette smoke,[2] onion vapor,[2] ammonia,[30, 156] formalin,[83] and tear gas, such as benzylbromide,[120] chloracetophenon,[28, 142] bromacetone,[21] or bromtoluene.[30]

Indeed, it seems more reasonable to make use of stimulated tears if one is interested in the composition of the fluid originating from the main lacrimal glands rather than in the resting volume of ocular fluid in the conjunctival sac, which always may contain admixtures of the

---

* Koffler BH et al.: ARVO (Assocation for Research in Vision and Ophthalmology) abstracts, 1979, p. 281.

secretions of the many accessory glands and goblet cells.

Capillary sampling of stimulated tears gives samples of fluid containing primarily the secretions of the lacrimal glands with minimal contamination from other sources.[141, 142, 144]

COMPOSITION OF TEAR FLUID

The first chemical analysis of tears was recorded in 1791 by Fourcroy and Vauquelin.[48] In 1928, Ridley[103] demonstrated great concentrations of lysozyme, the bacteriolytic enzyme found by Fleming and Allison in 1922,[46] in other secretions and tissues. Since then, the number of publications on the composition of tears has increased.

The compounds present in tear fluid may be arbitrarily classified as proteins, enzymes, lipids, metabolites, electrolytes and hydrogen ions, and drugs excreted in tears.

Proteins

The total tear protein content strongly depends on the method of collection. If small amounts (10 μl) of tears are collected along the lower lid with a capillary pipette which is not allowed to touch the eye (thus avoiding any stimulation of the tear flow), levels of about 20 g/l can be found.[39] Stimulation of the tear flow results in much lower values of 3 to 7 g/l,[39] reflecting the level of the lacrimal gland fluid. Because, in practice, reflex tearing caused by pipette collection is difficult to avoid (or even is achieved deliberately), a mixture of stimulated and non-stimulated tears can be removed giving normal values in the range of 6 to 20 g/l.[14] In electrophoretic investigation under alkaline conditions, two predominant fractions in tears are found: an anodal albumin and a cathodal lysozyme fraction,[28] each of which comprises 30 to 40 percent of the total protein.[82] An intermediate fraction is subdivided into several proteins.[54, 72]

Tear Albumin.
Tear albumin is a unique protein fraction. It is electrophoretically a prealbumin, and it migrates to a position similar to serum prealbumin. However, antiserum raised to serum prealbumin does not react at all to the tear albumin.[22, 73] Hence, the names "anodal tear protein"[61] and "specific tear prealbumin"[22] have been proposed. Serum albumin is a relatively minor component of tears. Genetic polymorphism of the tear albumin has been reported.[11] In polyacrylamide gel electrophoresis, five bands are found; these are labeled 1, 2, 3, 4, and 5 in roughly decreasing order of their frequencies of occurrence. The most common type (1-1) shows a single major band 1. All of the other variant types (1-2, 1-3, 1-4, and 1-5) show, in addition to major band 1, a slower major band (2, 3, or 4) or a faster major band (5) with a staining intensity equal to that of band 1. These genetic markers in tears may prove useful for genetic investigations.

Lysozyme.
Lysozyme is a bacteriolytic protein. It is absent in tears of species other than humans and some monkeys.[43] In humans, its concentration is much higher in tears than in any other body fluid. The normal level for human tear lysozyme (HTL) is 1 to 2 g/l. This can be measured with a diffusion method similar to that of the antibiotic disc assay[21, 100] or with a spectrophotometric assay.[42, 86, 104] Both methods depend on the clearing of a suspension of *Micrococcus lysodeikticus*. This is a consequence of the selective action of lysozyme on the cell walls by enzymatically cleaving the mucopeptide N-acetyl glucosamine (β 1-4) N-acetylmuramic acid at the β (1-4)-linkage. Methods relating their values to hen's egg lysozyme (HEL), used as the standard, give normal values of 3 to 6 g/l since the specific activity of HEL is about three times less than that of HTL.[21]

HTL has been reported to be greatly decreased in tears of patients suffering from Sjögrens disease[9, 134] and ocular toxicity from long-term practolol therapy,[85, 150] thus making it a useful diagnostic aid. Other disease states, where the level of HTL is lowered more moderately are herpes simplex virus infection,[44] severe malnutrition in children,[147] and smog eye irritation.[107] It remains undecided, however, whether these lower concentrations of HTL are the result of a relatively low secretion of HTL into the reduced tear volume produced by the lacrimal gland or of an altered ratio of low lacrimal fluid volume of normal composition, mixed with relatively more of the conjunctival secre-

TABLE 4-1. SUMMARY OF ANTIMICROBIAL FACTORS IN TEARS

Compound	Evidence*	Reference
Lysozyme	+	21, 42, 86, 100, 104
Immunoglobulin A	+	89, 115
Immunoglobulin G	±	50, 89
Immunoglobulin E	+	3
Complement	+	151
Lactoferrin	+	26
Transferrin	±	26, 72, 108
Nonlysozyme antibacterial factor	?	47, 51, 127, 135
Peroxydase-thiocyanate-peroxide system	−	137
Antibiotic-producing commensal organisms	+	60

* + Present in tears; ± only present in tears after mild trauma to the conjunctiva; − not present; ? presence not proven due to shortcomings in technique[47, 51] or obsolete methods.[127]

tions. Low tear volume does not indicate low HTL concentration. Many people (particularly elderly) with small amounts of tears and sometimes suffering from "dry eye" symptoms demonstrate normal HTL levels.[9, 35, 100] Notably, a depletion of HTL and tear albumin has been demonstrated in the conjunctival secretions from patients whose lacrimal glands have been removed.[90]

The presence of nonlysozyme antibacterial factors has been reported.[47, 51, 127] These reports are based on sometimes conflicting results[135] to what is generally found by others.[21, 42, 104] For instance, an acid-heat-labile antibacterial agent was demonstrated in stimulated pooled tears, inhibiting the growth of certain strains of staphylococci.[127] HTL as measured spectrophotometrically by the clearing of a suspension of *Micrococcus lysodeikticus* was heat resistant.

In later investigations, possibly the same nonlysozymal antibacterial factor was found in normal nonstimulated tears.[51] The total antibacterial activity, measured with a gel diffusion method using lyophylized *Micrococcus lysodeikticus,* was 200 times greater than could be attributed to the amount of HTL present, as measured spectrophotometrically by the clearing reaction. The supposed antibacterial activity could be destroyed by heating, in contrast to HTL. The latter compound, however, without heating, was measured in the abnormally low value of one hundredth of the accepted norm of the population.

Beta lysin, an antibacterial substance known to be present in platelets, serum, and other body fluids, should have been demonstrated distinct from HTL in a specimen of pooled human tears.[47] The lysozyme level, however, was reported to be about 50 times less than the normal concentration. The mechanism that could account for the higher concentration of beta lysin in tears than in plasma is unknown because platelets, the major source of beta lysin, are absent in tears.

Table 4-1 summarizes the tear components which are reported to possess anti-microbial properties.

Lactoferrin. Lactoferrin, an iron-carrying protein, appears to be a major tear protein in the intermediate fraction. Its property of binding Fe(III) is 300 times stronger than the other iron-binding protein (transferrin). This is probably significant for its bacteriostatic activity in tears, making essential metal ions unavailable for microbial metabolism.[26]

Transferrin. Transferrin has been reported to be present in tears.[108] However, in some reports[26, 72] it was observed that this protein together with serum albumin and IgG could be detected only after mild trauma to the mucosal surface of the conjunctiva or in tears that were not carefully obtained.

Ceruloplasmin. Ceruloplasmin, a copper-carrying protein, can regularly be found in tears.[108] In electrophoresis the migration rate of tear ceruloplasmin varies somewhat from its serum counterpart.

Immunoglobulin A. Immunoglobulin A (IgA) is the predominant immunoglobulin in tear fluid.[89] In tears, as in other external secretions, it is attached to an additional antigenic fragment, secretory component (SC). In the human lacrimal gland, IgA appears to be synthesized by interstitial plasma cells, and after entry into the intercellular spaces, it is coupled to SC and secreted as secretory IgA (IgA-SC) through the blood-tear barrier involving intracellular transport by acinar epithelial cells into the lumen.[50]

In the conjunctiva, IgA[4] and plasma cells[5] are located in the substantia propria. Only in the acinar epithelium of the accessory lacrimal glands can SC material be found,* indicating that these are the sites of synthesis of secretory IgA of the conjunctival secretions.

Depending on the method of tear collection, IgA values are found varying from 10 to 100 mg percent. Stimulated tears containing 10 to 30 mg percent[25, 34, 83] probably reflect the concentration in the lacrimal gland fluid. Filter paper samples or unstimulated small volume samples contain greater amounts, up to 100 mg percent,[25, 67, 147] probably derived partly from the conjunctival mucosa.

Immunoglobulin G. Immunoglobulin G (IgG) is present in very low concentration in normal tears.[50, 89] However, after mild trauma to the mucosal surface of the conjunctiva or carelessly obtained tears, it can be easily detected.[72]

Immunoglobulin E. Immunoglobulin E (IgE) can be found in tear fluid collected atraumatically.[3] Values range from 26 to 144 ng/ml in tears in correlation with paired serum samples in the range of 52 to 781 ng/ml. The information on the level of immunoglobulins in tears in pathologic conditions is contradictory. In some reports, the IgA level in tears was found to be elevated in pathologic states.[20, 115] In others, the IgA level remained remarkably constant,[34, 89] but the IgG level rose. In vernal conjunctivitis, serum IgE levels were found elevated, but this was not a consistent finding in tears.[3]

---

* *Gillette TE, Allensmith MR: ARVO abstracts, 1979, p. 96.*

In practolol-induced ocular disease, only secretory IgA was found to be absent, which is perhaps indicative of damage to the lacrimal glands.[55] In the same study, however, lysozyme, determined with a semiquantitative method, was found to be normal; this is not confirmed by others.[85, 150]

Complement. Complement in tears was demonstrated in hemolytic assays up to dilutions of 1:4, whereas serum was active in this system up to 1:32.[151] In a recent study,[75a] classic complement activity could not be demonstrated, and instead a very potent anticomplementary factor was found.

Glycoproteins. Glycoproteins are contained in the tear film mucus. This may play a critical role in the lubrication of the corneal surface by rendering its hydrophobic surface more hydrophilic, permitting spreading and stabilization of the tear film. The mucus is secreted by the conjunctival goblet cells as a solution of glycoproteins (mucoids), and this sticky mixture adheres to the surface of the epithelium even though the glycoproteins are water soluble. The glycoproteins are carbohydrate-protein complexes characterized by the presence of hexosamines, hexoses, and sialic acid. In unstimulated tear fluid collected in capillary pipettes, the relative hexosamine content of the protein, which is used as indicator for glycoproteins, varies in different individuals from 0.5 to 17 percent, the hexosamine concentration from 0.05 to 3 g/l.[39] These wide ranges of hexosamine values probably reflect the variable amounts of mucus that are caught by sampling in the inhomogeneous system of mucoid-aqueous layer in the tear film. In view of the dynamic characteristics of the lacrimal system, it is unlikely that a thermodynamic equilibrium exists between the mucoid layer and the macromolecular components in the aqueous layer of the tear film.

Results achieved with pooled samples of mucoid clots, obtained in humans by collecting the mucous thread, show that three fractions of very high molecular weight glycoproteins can be separated, with a carbohydrate content of more than 50 percent.[95] Great individual variations, however, occur in the composition of carbohydrate and protein components.

Glycoproteins have been found in rabbit

TABLE 4-2. CONCENTRATION OF ANTIPROTEINASES IN PLASMA AND TEARS

Antiproteinases		Plasma	Tears	Reference
		(mg%)		
α_1-Antitrypsin	(α_1-at)	280	0.1–0.4	15
			1.5	155
			3	*
α_1-Antichymotrypsin	(α-ach)	24	1.4	155
Inter-α-trypsin inhibitor		20	0.5	155
α_2-Macroglobulin	(α_2-M)		3	15
			6	*

* Leib ML, Shuster J, Litte JM, Lorenzetti DW: ARVO abstracts, 1980, p. 102.

lacrimal gland fluid uncontaminated by fluid from other orbital glands.[78] In the acini of human lacrimal glands, mucus-secreting cells have been demonstrated, which indicates that there is another source of tear glycoproteins in addition to the conjunctival goblet cells.[39]

Using hexosamine as an indicator of mucus, it was not possible to prove a marked deficiency in mucous concentration in the so-called mucin-deficient dry eye conditions, such as ocular pemphigoid, Stevens-Johnson syndrome, and Sjögren's syndrome.[39] Perhaps the low tear volume itself or a qualitative difference in glycoprotein composition might be responsible for the instability of the tear film observed in these conditions.[66]

Glycosaminoglycans, which are complex carbohydrates also containing hexosamine (in combination with hexuronic acid), are nearly absent in tears,[17] especially in pipette samples.[39]

Antiproteinases. Antiproteinases, inhibitors of proteinases, are present in tears at levels much lower than in plasma[155] (Table 4-2), and antigenic typing indicates that the antiproteinase activity is not identical to only the α_1-at of serum.[102]

Mechanical irritation or hypersecretion of tears does not influence the normal value of α_1-at, which indicates that this protein is secreted by the lacrimal glands. The source of the other antiproteinases is unknown, and they might originate from the corneal and conjunctival surface as well.

In bacterial and viral infections of the eye and in corneal ulcerations, the levels of α_1-at and α_2-M in tear fluid are increased.[15, 154, *] Using albumin as a marker protein there is conflicting evidence suggesting that these two collagenase inhibitors are derived from plasma by a general increase in vascular permeability to proteins[15] or that they are produced locally.*

The α_1-at does not exert an inhibiting action on corneal collagenase when both compounds are present in tears of an ulcerating eye, in contrast to α_2-M which inhibits collagenases by forming tight complexes with them.[11] However, α_2-M as eyedrops possesses no ability to prevent corneal ulceration, because topical administration does not provide enough α_2-M to the corneal stroma to inhibit the collagenase present in this tissue.[13] Mouse bone collagenase is inhibited by lysozyme,[106] which suggests a possible role for tear lysozyme in the regulation of corneal collagenase.

Enzymes

Enzymes of Energy-producing Metabolisms.
Glycolytic enzymes and enzymes of the tricarboxylic acid cycle can be detected in high levels only in tear samples collected in paper strips[139] or in small (10 μl) volumes of unstimulated tears. In stimulated tears, the enzymes cannot be quantitatively measured. The lacrimal gland apparently does not secrete these enzymes, and moreover it forms a blood-tear barrier against penetration from the blood.[142] The source of these enzymes is in the conjunctiva, where they are secreted in small amounts and can be obtained during mechanical irritation.

* Leib ML, Shuster J, Litte JM, Lorenzetti DW: ARVO abstracts, 1980, p. 102.

TABLE 4-3. LYSOSOMAL DISEASES IDENTIFIED BY SPECIFIC DEFICIENCY OF CORRESPONDING LYSOSOMAL ENZYMES IN TEARS

Lysosomal Disease	Corresponding Enzyme Deficiency	Reference
Tay-Sachs ⎫ Sandhof ⎭	β-Hexosaminidase	29, 118
Fabry	α-Galactosidase	70
Fucosidosis	α-Fucosidase	81
Mannosidosis	α-Mannosidase	81
Gm-gangliosidosis	β-Galactosidase	131
Type II glycogenosis	α-Glucosidase	146
Hurler and Scheie	α-Iduronidase	146
Metachromatic leukodystrophy	Sulfatase A	146
Mucosulfatidosis	Sulfatase A	146
	Sulfatase B	146

Lactate Dehydrogenase. Lactate dehydrogenase (LDH) is the enzyme in highest concentration in tears. It can be separated electrophoretically into its five isoenzymes, showing a pattern with more of the slower migrating muscle-type isoenzymes. This is closely related to the distribution pattern of corneal tissue in contrast to serum-LDH, where the faster migrating heart-type isoenzymes prevail.[74, 138]

These findings indicate that the tear-LDH originates from the corneal epithelium.[74] Therefore, in patients suffering from various corneal diseases the distribution of the LDH isoenzymes in tears can differ from those found in healthy individuals.[75] In addition, a sixth band sometimes appears in the distribution pattern, as in tears of patients with herpes simplex or conjunctivitis. LDH-isoenzymes bound to immunoglobulins have been found in blood, and it is probable that here an analogous binding takes place in tears.

Lysosomal Enzymes. A number of lysosomal acid hydrolases are present in tears in concentrations of 2 to 10 times those in serum.[131, 143] In tear samples collected on paper strips or in small volumes of unstimulated tears, the concentrations can be higher than in stimulated tears, although the concentration in the latter case always remains at a substantial level.[142] The lacrimal gland is the main source of the lysosomal enzyme. The relatively high values are found in tear fluid collected under conditions where the epithelial cells of the conjunctiva remain intact and contain very low levels of lactate dehydrogenase or other cytoplasmic enzymes. The conjunctiva may act as a second source for lysosomal enzymes after mild trauma, such as application of a paper strip.[142]

Lysosomal enzyme activities in tears are used for diagnosis and identification of carriers of several inborn errors of metabolism. Tear enzyme analysis to demonstrate the specific deficiency of β-hexosaminidase was first proposed for the identification of Tay-Sachs disease. Subsequently, the absence or very low activity of lysosomal enzymes in a number of lysosomal storage disorders has been demonstrated (Table 4-3).

In view of the difficulties of studying other body fluids and fibroblast cultures, the idea of investigating the tear fluid is attractive because of its availability and high content of lysosomal enzymes. Moreover, easy collection by lay or paramedical personnel provides opportunities for mass screening[59] economically and practically.

However, when filter paper collection methods are used, the activity recorded depends on the state of preservation of the paper. Therefore, it is advisable to study parallel tear samples from patients and from controls stored under the same conditions. The concentration of the various lysosomal enzymes in tear fluid change in a parallel manner with each other according to the method of collection of tears. The influence of these changes can be eliminated by determining the ratio of the enzyme activity concerned to the activity of another lysosomal enzyme expected not to be defective.

The concentration of β-hexosaminidase in tears, collected on filter paper strips, also has been suggested as an index for the development and prognosis of diabetic retinopathy.[53] The tears would reflect the decreased enzyme activity of β-hexosaminidase and of other lysosomal glycosidases in the retina, showing a negative correlation with the increased plasma levels of these enzymes.

Other investigations could not support the use of β-hexosaminidase as a useful indicator for diabetic retinopathy, reporting no significant reduction in tear β-hexosaminidase levels[144] for diabetics; in fact, significantly higher levels were found in one study.[148]

Amylase. Amylase is an enzyme present in tear fluid in relatively moderate levels similar to the levels found in urine.[136] The origin is undoubtedly in the lacrimal gland. In filter paper samples[140] of tear fluid, the level is not as high as in capillary samples,[136] and the reported presence of amylase in the cornea[71] might be the consequence of contamination by tear fluid.

The isoenzyme pattern in electrophoresis is different from that of saliva and urine and similarly has a genetic basis.[136]

Peroxidase. Peroxidase (POD) is present in human tears, originating from the lacrimal gland and not from the conjunctiva.[137] Mechanical irritation with filter paper strips does not result in higher POD levels of tears collected in the paper. POD activity found in the conjunctiva[69] probably is derived from the tears. The level of tear POD varies considerably among different species; rats show very high values of 3.7×10^5 U/l, humans show 10^3 U/l, and in rabbits POD is not detectable. The existence of a POD-thiocyanate-hydrogen peroxide antibacterial system, such as has been demonstrated in milk and saliva, must be excluded in human tears because of the insufficient concentration of thiocyanate in tears.[137]

Plasminogen Activator. Plasminogen activator has been demonstrated in tear fluid, and the presence in stimulated tears[123] casts doubt on the suggestion that corneal epithelium is the source of this urokinase-like fibrinolytic activity.[98]

Collagenase. Collagenase can be found in tear fluid only in the presence of corneal ulceration from infection, chemical burns, trauma, or desiccation.[27, 63, 119] The enzyme generally is assayed by radial or linear diffusion methods, using native collagen gels or collagen dissolved in agarose.

It has been demonstrated that corneal collagenase is present as an inactive precurser, latent collagenase which can be activated by treatment with trypsin[16] and in vivo possibly by plasmin, resulting from the plasminogen activator activity in tears.[14] It is not known whether this activation takes place by conversion of proenzyme to active form or by release of an endogenous inhibitor. In the regulating mechanism of corneal collagenase in vivo, inhibitors might play a role.

Lipids

Lipids are present in small amounts in tears, as they are contained only in the very thin superficial lipid layer of the tear film. Few data of investigations of pooled samples of human tear lipids demonstrated the presence of cholesterol and cholesterol esters in the same chromatographic fractions as are found in meibomian secretion.[7] Analysis of meibomian lipids revealed the presence of all possible lipid classes, mainly hydrocarbons, wax esters, cholesterol esters, triglycerides, and in lesser amount, diglycerides, monoglycerides, free fatty acids, free cholesterol, and phospholipid.[129] However, great individual variations occur in lipid composition.

Cholesterol. Cholesterol has been reported to be present in tear fluid in concentrations of about 200 mg%, which is the same as in blood.[153] Contact lens problems, such as clouding and deposits, have been supposed by some to be correlated with abnormally high concentrations of cholesterol in tear fluid.[152] Other investigators have found quite different results, showing values of about 20 mg% cholesterol in normal tears.[66, 141] This was not correlated with high cholesterol concentrations.[141]

Cholesterol cannot be considered as a component of the tear fluid, which is secreted by the lacrimal gland. Like all lipids in biologic fluids, cholesterol has to be transported by (mainly) α- and β-lipoproteins. In normal tears the very low protein content and the absence of lipoproteins are incompatible with a cholesterol concentration of 20 mg%.

Metabolites

There are conflicting reports regarding the presence of these compounds of smaller molecular weight in tears. In general, it can be said that if the conjunctival and corneal epithelium possess a barrier function for a certain molecule, higher concentrations are found in tears collected with a method that will disrupt this barrier, such as filter paper sampling or careless manipulating of glass capillary pipettes.

Glucose. Glucose is present in minimal amounts of about 0.2 mmole/l in tear fluid collected in capillary pipettes during stimultion in normally glycemic persons. In diabetics with blood glucose levels of more than 20 mmole/l, no significant elevation in the glucose in tears is found, which demonstrates the barrier function of the corneal and conjunctival epithelium against loss of glucose from the tissues into the tear fluid.[144]

It must be the tissue fluid and not the lacrimal gland fluid that contributes to the tear glucose after mechanically irritative methods of collection. Clinical tear glucose tests[56] are in fact based on the determination of glucose from tissue fluid of the tissues surrounding the conjunctival sac. A relationship between tear glucose and blood glucose thus reflects only the equilibrium that normally exists for glucose between blood and tissue fluid.

Lactate. Lactate levels of 1 to 5 mmole/l in tears are far higher than the normal blood levels of 0.5 to 0.8 mmole/l. Pyruvate from 0.05 to 0.35 mmole/l is about the same as is normal for blood (0.1 to 0.2 mmole/l). These levels do not show significant alterations after mechanical irritation with filter paper strips.[144] The epithelium does not possess a barrier function for lactate and pyruvate. On the contrary, tears can be attributed a function in the removal of these products of metabolism. The latter was demonstrated in experiments with rabbits, where rela-

tively large amounts of lactate could be washed out from intact corneal epithelium in vivo, and after abrasion of the epithelium the amounts of lactate in the washing fluid did not increase.[76]

Urea. Urea concentrations in tear fluid and plasma have been found to be equivalent, suggesting an unrestricted passage through the blood-tear barrier in the lacrimal gland.[144] Collection on filter paper has resulted in a lowering of the urea values, an average of 0.88 of the blood values. Probably the urea concentrations in tears are lowered by increased diffusion through the damaged epithelial barrier into the tissues surrounding the anterior chamber fluid, which is known to possess a urea value of about 0.8 of the blood value.[18]

Catecholamines. Catecholamines, dopamine, epinephrine, norepinephrine, and dopa have been found in stimulated tear fluid collected with micropipettes.[156] The levels in 20 humans varied from zero values to about 1.5 μg/ml; dopamine had values as high as 280 μg/ml.

In glaucoma patients, lower values were found for these compounds, which should reflect the diminished activity of the sympathetic innervation of the eye. The determination of catecholamines in tears has been advocated as a test in glaucoma diagnosis. However, it seems not to be very useful because of the great variations observed in normal individuals.

Histamine. Histamine is present in normal tears collected with sponges in the conjunctival sac at a level of about 10 mg/ml. In vernal conjunctivitis (and not in other inflammatory eye diseases), a variable increase, sometimes to 125 mg/ml, has been observed.[1, *]

Prostaglandins. Prostaglandins are present in tears collected with paper strips from normal eyes at a level of 75 pg prostaglandin F/ml; this is a little lower than in serum.[37] In vernal conjunctivitis and in trachoma, significantly higher values were found—about 300 pg/ml of tears. As the collection method utilized paper strips, it cannot be determined if the source is in the lacrimal gland or in the conjunctiva because pros-

---

* *Yamamoto GK, et al.: ARVO abstracts, 1979, p. 277.*

TABLE 4-4. SUMMARY OF RECENT LITERATURE ON HUMAN TEAR ELECTROLYTES

	Concentration in mmole/l*						
	Na$^+$	K$^+$	Ca^{2+}	Mg^{2+}	Cl	HCO$_3$	Reference
Tears	120–170	6–26	—	—	118–138	—	126
	80–161	6–36	—	—	106–130	—	84, 91, 114
	145	24	—	—	128	26	23
	134–170	26–42	0.5–1.1	0.3–0.6	120–135	—	124
	—	—	0.4–0.8	—	—	—	133
	—	—	0.4–1.0	0.5–1.1	—	—	10
	—	—	0.4–1.1	—	—	—	78
	—	—	0.3–2.0	—	—	—	149
Serum	140	4.5	2.5	0.9	100	30	Average of normal

* The values in this table were calculated from the data of the investigations indicated by reference number.

taglandins are known to be present in ocular tissues as mediators of inflammatory processes.

Electrolytes and Hydrogen Ions

As can be seen from the data summary in Table 4-4, the positively charged electrolytes in tears are mainly sodium and potassium, and the negative ions are chloride and bicarbonate.

Sodium. Sodium in tears is about equal to that in plasma and has been found to correlate with it, suggesting a passive secretion into the tears.

Potassium. Potassium, with an average value of about 20 mmole/l, is much higher than the corresponding plasma concentration of about 5 mmole/l. This indicates an active secretion of potassium into the tears.

Calcium. Calcium is independent of the tear production and, in general, is lower than the free fraction in plasma. A correlation between tear and serum calcium concentration could not be demonstrated.[10] In cystic fibrosis patients, much higher tear calcium values, an average of 2.5 mmole/l, have been found only at slow rates, concomitant with lower tear sodium values.[24] It should be noted that in sweat secretion, calcium exerts an inhibitory effect on sodium movement by decreasing the epithelial permeability.[101] This suggests that abnormally high calcium levels in cystic fibrosis tears may exert the same pathologic effects on the sodium concentration as is seen in sweat secretion. Although, in general, calcium levels in tears are unrelated to the use of contact lenses,[149] one report draws attention to the fact that in a patient

in whom tear calcium concentration became elevated to 2 mmole/l, because of iatrogenic diminution of tearing, calcification of a soft contact lens occurred.[10]

Magnesium. Magnesium in tears is on the average a little lower than the corresponding serum value, possibly reflecting the free fraction of magnesium.[10]

Osmotic Pressure. Osmotic pressure in tears is, as in any body fluid, mainly caused by the presence of electrolytes. Measured by a dewpoint depression microtechnique requiring 5 μl samples, it is about 305 mOsm/kg, equivalent to 0.95 percent sodium chloride.[58, 125] Individual values over the waking day may range from 0.90 to 1.02 percent sodium chloride equivalents. A decrease to an average of 285 mOsm/kg, equivalent to 0.89 percent sodium chloride has been found following prolonged lid closure, which accounts for the reduced evaporation.[125]

Earlier reports in the literature indicating that in keratoconjunctivitis sicca no significant increase in osmolarity occurs[12, 88] are based on collection methods that inevitably had to induce reflex tearing in order to obtain a sufficiently large volume. However, investigations using only 0.1 μl of tear fluid[57, 58] clearly demonstrated higher osmotic values in keratoconjunctivitis sicca. This is not surprising because of the imbalance between evaporation and tear production in this disease. During contact lens adaptation, both hypertonic and hypotonic shifts of osmotic pressure may occur, but they are not of clinical significance.[132]

TABLE 4-5. SUMMARY OF DIAGNOSTIC TESTS AND DRUG ASSAYS IN TEARS

Compound	Diagnosis	Useful-ness	Reference
Lysozyme	Sjögren's disease	+	9, 134
	Practolol-induced toxicity	+	85, 150
Lysosomal enzymes	Lysosomal storage diseases	+	7, 29, 146, 131
Collagenase	Corneal ulceration	+	27, 63, 119
α1-Antitrypsin	Bacterial infections	±	15, 154†
Glucose	Diabetes mellitus	±	56
Catecholamines	Glaucoma	−	156
β-Hexosaminidase	Diabetic retinopathy	−	144, 148
Cholesterol	Hypercholesterolemia-induced contact lens problems	−	141
Tear albumin	Genetic marker	+	11

Drugs	Classification		
Phenobarbital	Anticonvulsants	+	94
Carbamazepine		+	130
Methotrexate	Chemotherapeutics	+	122
Ampicillin	Antibiotics	−	117

* Useful; ± comparatively useful; − not useful
† Leib ML, et al.: ARVO abstracts, 1980, p. 201.

Tear pH. Tear pH, measured in a closed chamber microelectrode system in small volumes of unstimulated tears, is about 7.45 in a normal population. There is a range of 7.14 to 7.82 among subjects and in a given subject at different times of the day.[31] A more acidic pH of about 7.25 is found following prolonged lid closure, possibly the result of carbon dioxide produced by the cornea and trapped in the tear pool under the eyelids.[32, 97]

The higher values reported in the literature on human tear pH[31] have to be ascribed to shortcomings in technique, mainly to substantial errors due to carbon dioxide loss during sampling.

A limited buffering capacity of tears could be demonstrated by challenging the measured pH with a standard concentration of alkali.[32] In unbuffered saline, a shift occurred of about 4.0 pH units in response to addition of 0.01N sodium hydroxide in final concentration. In tears this response shift is buffered to about 3.0 pH units.

Drugs Excreted in Tears

In the last few years there has been increasing interest in the use of saliva in therapeutic drug monitoring by predicting the free fraction of drugs in the blood from that found in saliva. Changes in the free drug levels can have important clinical consequences, since either toxic or subtherapeutic levels may exist even when the total drug concentration is within the normal range.

However, in the use of saliva, several problems hinder reliable results. These include large variations in composition and pH. Tears seem to represent a potentially more stable body fluid of low protein content and with modest variations in pH (Table 4-5). Passage of drugs from the plasma to the tears apparently takes place by diffusion of the nonprotein-bound fraction.[99] However, in regard to the presence of tight junctions between the acinar epithelial cells in the lacrimal gland, forming a blood-tear barrier, the lipid solubility may be expected to play a major role. The blood-tear barrier in this respect shows the same characteristics as that of the cell-membrane, e.g., the blood-retinal (vitreous) barrier[19] and the blood-liquor barrier.

Phenobarbital and carbamazepine are excreted in tears in about half of the corresponding plasma concentration under steady-state conditions. The correlation between tear and plasma levels for these two anticonvulsant drugs is closer than that between saliva and plasma and should offer a greater reliability of the determination of free anticonvulsant drug levels.[94, 130]

Methotrexate, an antimetabolite for chemotherapy of several malignant diseases and psoriasis, reaches tear levels of 5 percent of the corresponding plasma concentrations and appears to be in equilibrium with the unbound fraction in plasma. In contrast the saliva levels were much lower—only 5 percent of the unbound drug levels in serum.[122]

Ampicillin after oral administration is present in tears and saliva in concentrations of about 0.02 of the corresponding serum level, representing probably not only the unbound fraction but, moreover, the poor lipoid solubility of this antibiotic, which hampers its passage to the tears.[117]

REFERENCES

1. Abelson MB, Soter, NA, Simon MA, et al.: Histamine in human tears. Am J Ophthalmol 83:417, 1977
2. Allansmith MR, Drell D, Anderson RP, Newman L: Comparison of electrophoretic mobility of tear lysozyme in 50 subjects. Am J Ophthalmol 71:525, 1971
3. Allansmith MR, Hahn GS, Simon MA: Tissue, tear and serum IgE concentrations in vernal conjunctivitis. Am J Ophthalmol 81:506, 1976
4. Allansmith MR, Hutchison D: Immunoglobulins in the conjunctiva. Immunology 12:225, 1967
5. Allansmith MR, Kajiyama GA, Abelson MB, Simon MA: Plasma cell content of main and accessory lacrimal glands and conjunctiva. Am J Ophthalmol 82:819, 1976
6. Allgrove J, Clayden GS, Grant DB, Macaulay JC: Familial glucocorticoid deficiency with achalasia of the cardia and deficient tear production. Lancet 1:1284, 1978
7. Andrews JS: Human tear film lipids. I. Composition of the principal non-polar components. Exp Eye Res 10:223, 1970
8. Appelmans M, Michiels J, Verdonck M: Troubles neurovégétatifs de l'appareil visuel au cours des traitements par le psychotropes. Bull Soc Belge Ophthalmol 135:399, 1963
9. Avisar R, Menaché R, Shaked P, et al.: Lyso-zyme content of tears in patients with Sjögren's syndrome and rheumatoid arthritis. Am J Ophthalmol 87:148, 151, 1979
10. Avisar R, Savir H, Sidi Y, Pinkhas J: Tear calcium and magnesium levels of normal subjects and patients with hypocalcemia or hypercalcemia Invest Ophthalmol 16:1150, 1977
11. Azen EA: Genetic polymorphism of human anadal tear protein. Biochem Genet 14:225, 1976
12. Balik J: The lacrimal fluid in keratoconjunctivitis sicca. A quantitative and qualitative investigation. Am J Ophthalmol 35:773, 1952
13. Berman MB: The role of α-macroglobulins in corneal ulceration. In Jamieson GA, Greenwalt TJ (eds): Progress in Clinical and Biological Research. New York, Alan R Liss Inc, 1976, Vol 5, pp 225-253
14. Berman MB: Regulation of collagenase. Therapeutic considerations. Trans Ophthalmol Soc UK 98:397, 1978
15. Berman MB, Barber JC, Talamo RC, Langley CE: Corneal ulceration and the serum antiproteases. I. α_1-Antitrypsin. Invest Ophthalmol 12:759, 1973
16. Birkedal-Hansen H, Cobb CM, et al.: Trypsin activation of latent collagenase from several mammalian sources. Scand J Dent Res 83:302, 1975
17. Bleckmann H: The content of glycosaminoglycans in bovine corneal epithelium and precorneal fluid-film. Albrecht von Graefes. Arch Klin Ophthalmol 200:235, 1976
18. Bleeker GM, van Haeringen NJ, Glasius E: Urea and the vitreous barrier of the eye. Exp Eye Res 7:30, 1968
19. Bleeker GM, van Haeringen JN, Maas ER, Glasius E: Selective properties of the vitreous barrier. Exp Eye Res 7:37, 1968
20. Bluestone R, Easty DL, Goldberg LS, et al.: Lacrimal immunoglobulins and complement quantified by counterimmunoelectrophoresis. Br J Ophthalmol 59:279, 1975
21. Bonavida B, Sapse AT: Human tear lysozyme. II. Quantitative determination with standard Schirmer strips. Am J Ophthalmol 66:70, 1968
22. Bonavida B, Sapse AT, Sercarz EE: A unique lacrimal protein absent from serum and other secretions: Specific tear prealbumin. Nature 221:375, 1969
23. Bothelho SY: Tears and the lacrimal gland. Sci Am 211:78, 1964
24. Bothelho SY, Goldstein AM, Rosenlund ML: Tear sodium, potassium, chloride, and calcium at various flow rates: children with cystic fibrosis and unaffected siblings with and without corneal staining. J Pediatr 83:601, 1973

25. Bracciolini M: Le immunoglobuline delle lacrime. Ann Otal Clin Oculist 94:490, 1968

26. Broekhuyse RM: Tear lactoferrin: a bacteriostatic and complexing protein. Invest Ophthalmol 13:550, 1974

27. Brown SI: Collagenase and corneal ulcers. Invest Ophthalmol 10:203, 1971

28. Brunish R: The protein components of human tears. Arch Ophthalmol 57:554, 1957

29. Carmody PJ, Rattazzi MC, Davidson RG: Tay-Sachs disease: the use of tears for the detection of heterozygotes. Am J Hum Gen 24:30a, 1972

30. Carmody PJ, Rattazzi MC, Davidson RG: Tay-Sachs disease: the use of tears for the detection of heterozygotes. Engl J Med 289:1072, 1973

31. Carney LG, Hill RM: Human tear pH. Diurnal variations. Arch Ophthalmol 94:821, 1976

32. Carney LG, Hill RM: Human tear buffering capacity. Arch Ophthalmol 97:951, 1979

33. Carreras y Matas. M: Mogadón, Aspirina y secretión lagrimal. Rev Esp Otoneurooftalmol Neurocir 31:245, 1973

34. Chandler JW, Leder R, Kaufman HE, Caldwell JR: Quantitative determinations of complement components and immunoglobulins in tears and aqueous humor. Invest Ophthalmol 13:151, 1974

35. de Roetth AFM: Low flow of tears: the dry eye. Am J Ophthalmol 35:782, 1952

36. de Vries Reilingh A, Reiners H, van Bijsterveld OP: Contact lens tolerance and oral contraceptives. Ann Ophthalmol 10:947, 1978

37. Dhir SP, Garg SK, Sharma YR, Lath NK: Prostaglandins in human tears. Am J Ophthalmol 87:403, 1979

38. Dohlman CH: Letter: Keratoconjunctivitis sicca after lacrimal gland removal. Arch Ophthalmol 94:686, 1976

39. Dohlman CH, Friend J, Kalevar V, et al.: The glycoprotein (mucus) content of tears from normals and dry eye patients. Exp Eye Res 22:359, 1976

40. Ehlers N: The precorneal tear film. Biomicroscopical, histological and chemical investigations. Acta Ophthalmol [Suppl] 81:136 pp, 1965

41. Ehlers N, Vedel Kessing S, Norn MS: Quantitative amounts of conjunctival mucous secretion and tears. Acta Ophthalmol 50:210, 1972

42. Ensink FTE, van Haeringen NJ: Pitfalls in the assay of lysozyme in human tear fluid. Ophthal Res 9:366, 1977

43. Erickson OF, Feeney L, McEwen WK: Filter-paper electrophoresis of tears. Arch Ophthalmol 55:800, 1956

44. Eylan E, Ronen D, Romano A, Smetana O: Lysozyme tear level in patients with herpes simplex virus eye infection. Invest Ophthalmol 16:850, 1977

45. Felix RH, Ive FA, Dahl MG: Cutaneous and ocular reactions to practolol. Br Med J 4:32, 1974

46. Fleming A, Allison VD: Observations on a bacteriolytic substance ("lysozyme") found in secretions and tissues. Br J Exp Pathol 3:252, 1922

47. Ford LC, DeLange RJ, Petty RW: Identification of a nonlysozymal bactericidal factor (beta lysin) in human tears and aqueous humor. Am J Ophthalmol 81:30, 1976

48. Fourcroy AF and Vauquelin N: Examen chimique des larmes et de l'humeur des marines. Ann de Chimie 10:113 1791

49. Frankel SH, Ellis PP: Effect of oral contraceptives on tear production. Ann Ophthalmol 10:1585, 1978

50. Franklin RM, Kenyon KR, Tomasi TB: Immunohistologic studies of human lacrimal gland: localization of immunoglobulins, secretory component and lactoferrin. J Immunol 110:984, 1973

51. Friedland BR, Anderson DR, Forster RK: Non-lysozyme antibacterial factor in human tears. Am J Ophthalmol 74:52, 1972

52. Frost-Larsen K, Isager H, Manthorpe R: Sjögren's syndrome treated with bromhexine: a randomised clinical study. Br Med J 1:1579, 1978

53. Fushimi H, Tarui S: Retina, tear and serum β-N-acetylglucosaminidase activities in diabetic patients. Clin Chim Acta 71:1, 1976

54. Gachon AM, Verrelle P, Betail G, Dastugue B: Immunological and electrophoretic studies of human tear proteins. Exp Eye Res 29:539, 1979

55. Garner A, Rahi AHS: Practolol and ocular toxicity: Antibodies in serum and tears. Br J Ophthalmol 60:684, 1976

56. Gasset AR, Braverman LE, Flemming MC, et al.: Tear glucose detection of hyperglycemia. Am J Ophthalmol 65:414, 1968

57. Gilbard JP, Farris RL: Tear osmolarity and ocular surface disease in keratoconjunctivitis sicca. Arch Ophthalmol 94:1642, 1979

58. Gilbard JP, Farris RL, Santamaria J: Osmolarity of tear microvolumes in keratoconjunctivitis sicca. Arch Ophthalmol 96:677, 1978

59. Goldberg JD, Truex JH, Desnick RJ: Tay-Sachs disease: an improved, fully automated method for heterozygote identification by tear β-hexosaminidase assay. Clin Chim Acta 77:43, 1977

60. Halbert SP, Swick LS: Antibiotic-producing bacteria of the ocular flora. Am J Ophthalmol 35:73, 1952

61. Hamersley J, Luce JK, Florentz ThR, et al.: Excessive lacrimation from fluorouracil treatment. JAMA 225:747, 1973

62. Hankiewicz J, Swierczek E: Lysozyme in human body fluids. Clin Chim Acta 57:205, 1974

63. Henriquez AS, Pihlaja DJ, Dohlman CH: Surface ultrastructure in alkali-burned rabbit corneas. Am J Ophthalmol 81:324, 1976

64. Hill RM, Terry JE: Human tear cholesterol levels. Arch Ophthalmol (Paris) 36:155, 1976

65. Holly FJ: Formation and rupture of the tear film. Exp Eye Res 15:515, 1973

66. Holly FJ, Patter JT, Dohlman CH: Surface activity determination of aqueous tear components in dry eye patients and normals. Exp Eye Res 24:479, 1976

67. Horwitz BL, Christensen GR, Ritzmann SR: Diurnal profiles of tear lysozyme and gamma A globulin. Am J Ophthalmol 10:75, 1978

68. Iwata S, Lemp MA, Holly FJ, Dohlman CH: Evaporation rate of water from the precorneal tear film and cornea in the rabbit. Invest Ophthalmol 8:613, 1969

69. Iwata T, Ohkawa K, Uyama M: The fine structural localization of peroxidase activity in goblet cells of the conjunctival epithelium of rats. Invest Ophthalmol 15:40, 1976

70. Johnson DL, Del Monte MA, Cotlier E, Desnick RJ: Fabry disease: Diagnosis by α-galactosidase activities in tears. Clin Chim Acta 63:81, 1975

71. Jonadet M: Activities béta-glucuronidasique et amylasique au niveau de la cornée. Rev Pathol Comp Hyg Gen 67:453, 1964

72. Josephson AS, Lockwood DW: Immunoelectrophoretic studies of the protein components of normal tears. J Immunol 93:532, 1964

73. Josephson AS, Weiner RS: Studies of the proteins of lacrimal secretions. J Immunol 100:1080, 1968

74. Kahán IL, Ottovay E: Lactate dehydrogenase of tears and corneal epithelium. Exp Eye Res 20:129, 1975

75. Kahán IL, Ottovay E: The significance of tears' lactate dehydrogenase in health and external eye diseases. Albrecht von Graefes Arch Klin Ophthalmol 194:267, 1975

75a. Kijlstra A, Veerhuis R: The effect of an anticomplementary factor on normal human tears. Am J Ophthalmol 92:24, 1981

76. Kilp H: Über die konzentrationen einiger Metabolite in den vorderen Augenabschnitten im Modellversuch bei Kaninchen. Inaugural-Dissertation, Marburg, 1971

77. Klintworth GK, Reed JW, Hawkins HK, Incram P: Calcification of soft contact lenses in a patient with dry eye and elevated calcium concentrations in tears. Invest Ophthalmol 16:158, 1977

78. Kreuger J, Sokoloff N, Bothelho SY: Siaclic acid in rabbit lacrimal gland fluid. Invest Ophthalmol 15:479, 1976

79. Kurihashi K: Tränensekretionmessung mit der Baumwollfadenmethode. Klin Monatsbl Augenheilkd 172:876, 1978

80. Kurihashi K, Yanagihara N, Honda Y: A modified Schirmer test: The fine-thread method for measuring lacrimation. J Pediatr Ophthalmol 14:390, 1977

81. Libert J, Van Hoof F, Tondeur M: Fucosidosis: ultrastructural study of conjunctiva and skin and enzyme analysis of tears. Invest Ophthalmol 15:626, 1976

82. Liotet S: Proteins in human tears. Nouv Presse Med 8:3893, 1979

83. Liotet S, Rouchy J-P: Etude des immunoglobulines des larmes humaines. Arch: Ophthalmol (Paris) 30:799, 1970

84. Lowther GE, Miller RB, Hill RM: Tear concentrations of sodium and potassium during adaptation to contact lenses: 1. Sodium observations. Am J Ophthalmol 47:266, 1970

85. Mackie IA, Seal DV: Tear fluid lysozyme concentration: guide to practolol toxicity. Br Med J 2:732, 1975

86. Mackie IA, Seal DV: Quantitative tear lysozyme assay in units of activity per microlitre. Br J Ophthalmol 60:70, 1976

87. Marzelli FN: Ocular side effects of drugs. Food Cosmet Toxicol 6:221, 1968

88. Mastman GJ, Blades EJ, Henderson JW: The total osmotic pressure of tears in normal and various pathologic conditions. Arch Ophthalmol 65:509, 1961

89. McClellan BH, Whitney CR, Newman LP, Allansmith MR: Immunoglobulins in tears. Am J Ophthalmol 76:89, 1973

90. McEwen WK, Kimura SJ, Feeney ML: Filter-paper electrophoresis of tears. III. Human tears and their high molecular weight components. Am J Ophthalmol 45:67, 1958

91. Miller RB: Tear concentrations of sodium and potassium during adaptation to contact lenses: II. Potassium observations. Am J Ophthalmol 47:773, 1970

92. Mishima S: Some physiological aspects of the precorneal tear film. Arch Ophthalmol 73:233, 1965

93. Mishima S, Gasset A, Klyce SD Jr, Baum JL:

Determination of tear volume and tear flow. Invest Ophthalmol 5:264, 1966

94. Monaco F, Mutani R, Mastropaolo C, Tondi M: Tears as the best practical indicator of the unbound fraction of an anticonvulsant drug. Epilepsia. 20:705, 1979

95. Moore JX, Tiffany JM: Human ocular mucus. Origins and preliminary characterisation. Exp Eye Res 29:291, 1979

96. Nielsen NV, Eriksen JS: Timolol transitory manifestations of dry eyes in long-term treatment. Acta Ophthalmol 57:418, 1979

97. Norn MS: Human tear pH. Arch Ophthalmol 95:170, 1977

98. Pandolfi M, Åstedt B, Dyster-Aas K: Release of fibrinolytic enzymes from human cornea. Acta Ophthalmol 50:199, 1972

99. Pedersen KB: Excretion of some drugs in bovine tears. Acta Pharmacol Toxicol 32:455, 1973

100. Pietsch RL, Pearlman ME, Durham: Human tear lysozyme variables. Arch Ophthalmol 90:94, 1973

101. Prompt CA, Quinton PM: Functions of calcium in sweat secretion. Nature 272:171, 1978

102. Rennert OM, Kaiser D, Sollberger HK, Joller-Jemelka. S: Antiprotease activity in tears and nasal secretions. Humangenetik 23:73, 1974

103. Ridley F: An antibacterial body present in great concentration in tears and its relation to infection of the human eye. Proc Roy Soc Med 21:1495, 1928

104. Ronen D, Eylan E, Romano A, et al.: A spectrophotometric method for quantitative determination of lysozyme in human tears: description and evaluation of the method and screening of 60 healthy subjects. Invest. Ophthalmol 14:479, 1975

105. Roszman H: Behandlung verminderter Tränensekretion mit Bromhexin-Augentropfen. Dtsch med Wochenschr 99:408, 1974

106. Sakamoto S, Sakamoto M, Goldhaber P, Glimcher MJ: The inhibition of mouse bone collagenase by lysozyme. Calc Tiss Res 14:291, 1974

107. Sapse AT, Bonavida B, Stone W, Sercarz EE: Human tear lysozyme. III. Preliminary study on lysozyme levels in subjects with smog eye irritation. Am J Ophthalmol 66:76, 1968

108. Sapse AT, Bonavida B, Stone W, Sercarz EE: Proteins in human tears. I. Immunoelectrophoretic patterns. Arch Ophthalmol 81:815, 1969

109. Saraux H, Martin P, Marax S, Offret N: Hyposecrétion lacrymale et médicaments psychotropes. Ann Ocul (Paris) 209:193, 1976

110. Scherz W: Keratoconjunctivitis sicca caused by denervation of lacrimal gland. Klin Monatsbl Augenheilk 174:188, 1979

111. Scherz W, Doane MG, Dohlman CH: Tear volume in normal eyes and keratoconjunctivitis sicca. Albrecht von Graefes Arch Klin Ophthalmol 192:141, 1974

112. Scherz W, Dohlman CH: Is the lacrimal gland dispensable?: Keratoconjunctivitis sicca after lacrimal gland removal. Arch Ophthalmol 93:281, 1975

113. Schirmer O: Studien zur Psychologie und Pathologie der Tränenabsonderung und Tränenabfuhr. Albrecht von Graefes Arch Klin Ophthalmol 56:197, 1903

114. Schmidt PP, Schoessler P, Hill RM: Effects of hard contact lenses on the chloride ion of the tears. Am J Optom 51:84, 1974

115. Sen DK, Sarin GS: Immunoglobulin concentrations in human tears in ocular diseases. Br J Ophthalmol 63:297, 1979

116. Siddal JR: Ocular toxic changes associated with chlorpromazine and thioridazine. Can J Ophthalmol 1:190, 1966

117. Simon C: Antibiotikaspiegel in Serum, Speichel, Tränen- und Hautblasen-flüssigkeit. Infection [Suppl] 24:91, 1976

118. Singer JD, Cotlier E, Krimmer R: Hexosaminidase a in tears and saliva for rapid identification of Tay-Sachs disease and its carriers. Lancet 21:1116, 1973

119. Slansky HH, Dohlman CH: Collagenase and the cornea. Surv Ophthalmol 14:402, 1970

120. Smolens J, Leopold IH, Parker J: Studies of human tears. Am J Ophthalmol 32:153, 1949

121. Sørensen T, Taagehøj Jensen F: Tear flow in normal human eyes. Determination by means of radioisotope and gamma camera. Acta Ophthalmol 57:564, 1979

122. Steele WH, Stuart JFB, Whiting B, et al.: Serum, tear and salivary concentrations of methotrexate in man. Br J Clin Pharmacol 7:207, 1979

123. Storm O: Fibrinolytic activity in human tears. Scand J Clin Lab Invest 7:55, 1955

124. Tapasztó I: Pathophysiology of human tears. The preocular tear film and dry eye syndromes. Int Ophthalmol Clin 13:119, 1973

125. Terry JE, Hill RM: Human tear osmotic pressure. Diurnal variations and the closed eye. Arch Ophthalmol 96:120, 1978

126. Thaysen JH, Thorn NA: Excretion of urea, sodium, potassium and chloride in human tears. Am J Physiol 178:160, 1954

127. Thompson R, Gallardo E: The antibacterial action of tears on staphylococci. Am J Ophthalmol 24:635, 1941

128. Tiburtius H, Merker HJ: Über eine neue Be-handlungsmöglichkeit der harabgesetzten Tränenproduktion. Klin Mosatsbl Augenheilk 162:535, 1973

129. Tiffany JM: Individual variations in human meibomian lipid composition. Exp Eye Res 27:289, 1978

130. Tondi M, Mutani R, Mastropaolo C, Monaco F: Greater reliability of tear versus saliva anti-convulsant levels. Ann Neurol 4:401, 1978

131. Tsuboyama A, Miki F, Yoshida M, et al.: The use of tears for diagnosis of GM_1 gangli-osidosis. Clin Chim Acta 80:237, 1977

132. Uniacke N, Hill RM: Osmotic pressure of the tears. J Am Optom Assoc 41:932, 1970

133. Uotila MH, Soble RE, Savory J: Measure-ment of tear calcium levels. Invest Ophthal-mol 11:258, 1972

134. Van Bijsterveld OP: Diagnostic tests in the sicca syndrome. Arch Ophthalmol 82:10, 1969

135. Van Haeringen NJ: Non-lysozyme antibacte-rial factor in tears. Am J Ophthalmol 75:533, 1973

136. Van Haeringen NJ, Ensink F, Glasius E: Amy-lase in human tear fluid: Origin and charac-teristics, compared with salivary and urinary amylases. Exp Eye Res 21:395, 1975

137. Van Haeringen NJ, Ensink FTE, Glasius E: The peroxidase-thiocyanate-hydrogen perox-ide system in tear fluid and saliva of different species. Exp Eye Res 28:343, 1979

138. Van Haeringen NJ, Glasius E: Lactate dehy-drogenase in tear fluid. Exp Eye Res 18:345, 1974

139. Van Haeringen NJ, Glasius E: Enzymes of en-ergy-producing metabolism, in human tear fluid. Exp Eye Res 18:407, 1974

140. Van Haeringen NJ, Glasius E: Enzymatic studies in lacrimal secretion. Exp Eye Res 19:135, 1974

141. Van Haeringen NJ, Glasius E: Cholesterol in human tear fluid. Exp Eye Res 20:271, 1975

142. Van Haeringen NJ, Glasius E: The origin of some enzymes in tear fluid determined by comparative investigation with two collection methods. Exp Eye Res 22:267, 1976

143. Van Haeringen NJ, Glasius E: Characteristics of acid hydrolases in human tear fluid. Ophthal Res 8:367, 1976

144. Van Haeringen NJ, Glasius E: Collection method dependent concentrations of some me-tabolites in human tear fluid, with special ref-erence to glucose in hyperglycaemic condi-tions. Albrecht von Graefes Arch Klin Ophthalmol 202:1, 1977

145. Van Haeringen NJ, Vrooland JL, Glasius E: Beta-hexosaminidase activities in tears and plasma, diphosphoglycerate in blood of dia-betic patients. Clin Chim Acta 86:333, 1978

146. Van Hoof F, Libert J, Aubert-Tulkens G, Serra MV: The assay of lacrimal enzymes and the ultrastructural analysis of conjunctival biopsies: new techniques for the study of in-born lysosomal diseases. Metabolic Ophthal-mol 1:165, 1977

147. Watson RR, Reyes MA, McMurray DN: In-fluence of malnutrition on the concentration of IgA, lysozyme, amylase and aminopepti-dase in children's tears. Proc Soc Exp Biol Med 157:215, 1978

148. Whiting PH, Ross IS, Borthwick LJ: N-acetyl-β-D-glucosaminidase levels and diabetic mi-croangiopathy. Clinica Chemica Acta 97:191, 1979

149. Winder AF, Ruben M, Sheraiday GAK: Tear calcium levels and contact lens wear. Br J Ophthalmol 61:539, 1977

150. Wright P: Untoward effects associated with practolol administration: Oculomucocuta-neous syndrome. Br Med J 1:595, 1978

151. Yamamoto GK, Allansmith MR: Comple-ment in tears from normal humans. Am J Ophthalmol 88:758, 1979

152. Young WH, Hill RM: Tear cholesterol levels and contact lens adaptation. Am J Ophthal-mol 50:12, 1973

153. Young W, Hill RM: Cholesterol levels of human tears: case reports. J Am Optom Assoc 45:424, 1973

154. Zirm M, Ritzinger I: Der diagnostische und prognostische Wert einer Alpha-l-Antitrypsin-bestimmung in der Tränenflüssigkeit. Klin Monatsbl Augenheilkd 173:221, 1978

155. Zirm M, Schmut O, Hofmann H: Quantita-tive Bestimmung der Antiproteinasen in der menschlichen Tränenflüssigkeit. Albrecht von Graefes Arch Klin Ophthalmol 198:89, 1976

156. Zubareva TV, Kiseleva ZM: Catecholamine content of the lacrimal fluid of healthy people and glaucoma patients. Ophthalmologica (Basel) 175:339, 1977

5

PHYSIOLOGY OF TEARS

MICHAEL A. LEMP and H. JANE BLACKMAN

The ocular surface is covered with a watery layer called the "tear film." Tears serve a number of functions:[1]

1. They act as the anterior refracting surface of the eye, filling in irregularities in the corneal epithelium
2. They flush away noxious substances from the surface of the eye
3. They serve as a source of oxygen to the corneal and conjunctival epithelium
4. They provide a pathway for white blood cells to the central avascular cornea in the event of a corneal injury
5. They provide lubrication between the lids and the ocular surface
6. They contain antibacterial substances and antibodies
7. They serve as an exit pathway for desquamated epithelial cells and other debris

The tear film is about 7 μl in volume under normal conditions. Most of this volume is distributed over the surface in the interpalpebral area as a thin film over the cornea and conjunctiva and collected in the lacrimal rivers (tear strips) adjacent to the lid margins.

The tear film has a three-layered structure (Fig. 5-1). The innermost mucin layer is 0.02 to 0.05 μm thick and is produced primarily by the unicellular goblet cells of the conjunctiva and the goblet cell-lined crypts of Henle of the conjunctiva. It is a thin layer loosely attached to the ocular surface. It serves to provide a temporary hydrophilic covering on the hydrophobic epithelial surface, thus permitting aqueous tears to spread over the surface. Excess mucin is dissolved within the overlying aqueous tear layer and interacts with the outermost lipid layer to promote tear film stability. It is probable that lipid-contaminated mucin with altered physicochemical properties also serves to form an exit pathway for epithelial cells and debris of the tear film (see below).

By far the bulk of the tear film is taken up with the aqueous layer (7 μ). This is the product of the main and accessory lacrimal glands. Within it are dissolved all the water-soluble components of the tear film, e.g., proteins, inorganic salts, macromolecular structures, and oxygen. Under normal conditions of minimal stimulation, aqueous tear production averages about 1 μl per minute.[2,3] It has been thought that there is a distinct difference between basal tears and reflex tears, with the latter being produced by the main lacrimal gland.

The secretion of aqueous tears by the main and accessory lacrimal glands is under the control of the autonomic nervous system.[4,5] Aque-

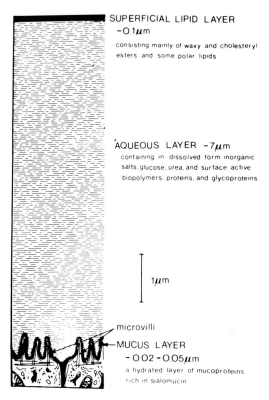

SUPERFICIAL LIPID LAYER
~0.1μm

consisting mainly of waxy and cholesteryl
esters and some polar lipids

AQUEOUS LAYER ~7μm

containing in dissolved form inorganic
salts, glucose, urea, and surface active
biopolymers, proteins, and glycoproteins

1μm

microvilli

MUCUS LAYER
~0.02-0.05μm

a hydrated layer of mucoproteins
rich in sialomucin

Figure 5-1. Proposed structure of the tear film.

ous tear production can be stimulated by the administration of cholinergic agents, such as pilocarpine, and decreased by drugs with anticholinergic effects, such as atropine, antihistamines,[6] and certain psychotropic agents.

As these glands are histologically identical,[7] it seems probable that virtually all aqueous tears are the product of some type of stimulation[8]; under normal resting conditions the stimuli are simply minimal. In response to ocular irritation or a number of other stimuli, the copious production of tears is almost immediate. The normal capacity of the conjunctival sac is about 25 to 30 μl. When its capacity is exceeded by tear production in excess of the capacity of the drainage system to drain tears, clinical tearing with overflow onto the cheeks occurs. There is a general movement of tears from the upper outer quadrant of the eye across the surface down to the medial aspect of the eye. Most of the movement of tears, however, occurs in the lacrimal river (along the eyelid margins). This general movement medially is

propelled by the blink mechanism, since, in the act of blinking, the lids close in squeegee fashion from temporal to medial.

The outermost lipid layer of the tear film is 0.1mm thick and is the product of the meibomian glands of the lids. The control mechanisms operative in the production of lipid are unknown, but there appears to be a continuous secrection of lipid material. It has been noted, however, that in infections involving the meibomian glands, there is a qualitative alteration in the lipid secretion.[9] The normally waxy long-chain cholesterol esters secreted by the meibomian glands are altered, giving rise to free fatty acids which are irritating to the surface of the eye. This breakdown of the long-chain cholesterol esters is probably effected by enzymes secreted by the microbial organisms responsible for the infection.

The three-layered structure of the tear film is part of a dynamic system involving the lids and epithelial surface.[10] The lids play an important role in the formation and maintenance of the tear film. The tear film tends to thin between blinks owing, in part, to a secondary retraction of this film into the fornices and also to evaporation. Eventually a critical thinness is reached. At this point lipid contaminates the mucin-covered epithelium, causing a retraction of the tear film from this hydrophobic area.[11] If a blink is further prevented, numerous so-called dry spots (Fig. 5-2) will develop and will enlarge and coalesce, forming larger areas of discontinuity in the tear film. Normally, a new blink resurfaces the tear film, establishing a new three-layer structure of normal thickness. The tear film, therefore, tends toward disruption between blinks and is reformed by periodic blinking. Interference with the function of the lids leads to localized areas of drying, such as is seen in exposure keratitis. In addition to periodic blinking, there must be reasonable congruity between the lids and the ocular surface in order for normal tear film to be established. The presence of elevations on the ocular surface interferes with the apposition of the lids to the ocular surface immediately adjacent, as occurs with pinguecula, pterygia, or ocular surface tumors. When localized areas of drying occur in the peripheral cornea adjacent to such an elevation, they are called "dellen."

In addition to an adequate secretion of tear film components and periodic blinking, the in-

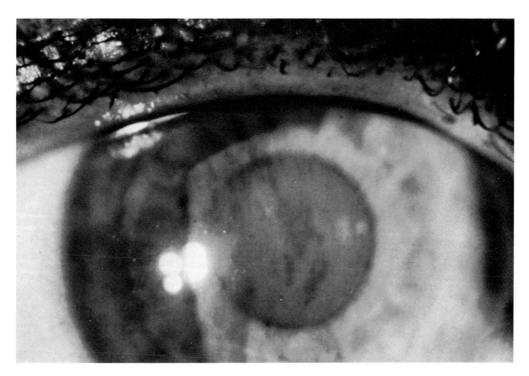

Figure 5-2. Dry spot formation.

tegrity of the epithelium of the cornea and con-junctiva is important in the establishment and maintenance of a normal tear film. The epithelial surface is thrown into a series of projections known as "microplica" or "microvilli." These increase the surface area of the eye enormously and provide a much greater area for attachment of the tear film. Abnormalities of the corneal surface that interfere with these microprojections interfere with attachment of the tear film to the epithelium and result in localized areas of drying. These are seen, for example, in anesthetic corneas in which there is a disturbance in the turnover of epithelial cells. Localized drying is also seen in areas of epithelial scarring and any type of raised epithelial irregularity.

As mucin is secreted by the conjunctival goblet cells, much of it seems to play a role in the formation of a hydrophilic mucin layer important in the formation of a tear film over the surface of the eye. It is probable, however, that mucin is eventually contaminated by the lipid of the tear film and assumes different physicochemical properties. These properties promote aggregation of macromolecules on the surface of the eye and give rise to a mucin network[12] (Fig. 5-3). This mucin network is responsible for trapping and removing desquamating epithelium, small foreign bodies, and microbial elements of the tear film. As blinking continues, this mucin network is further compressed and results in the formation of a mucin thread usually found in the inferior cul de sac. Eventually, this thread makes its way toward the medial canthus and works its way out of the eye onto the skin as a dry mucous seed.

TEAR DRAINAGE

As tears are constantly produced, some of the volume is lost in the way of evaporation from the ocular surface. The bulk of tears, however, drains out through the superior and inferior puncta into the canaliculi, thence into the lacrimal sac, and finally into the nasolacrimal duct leading to the inferior nasal meatus. Tear drainage is intimately involved with an intact blinking mechanism. As blinks occur, tears are propelled along the superior and inferior lacri-

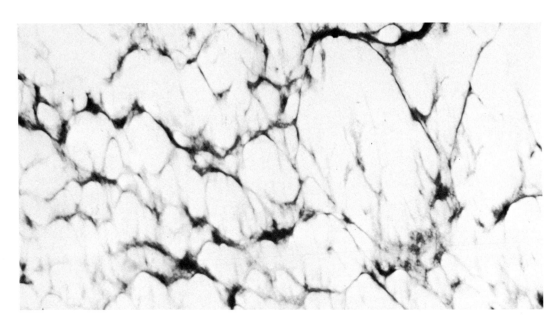

Figure 5-3. Mucin network. (*Photograph courtesy of A. Adams, M.D.*)

mal rivers toward the puncta by the action of the orbicularis muscle.[13] There is evidence to suggest that the orbicularis causes a contraction of the canaliculi and possibly the nasolacrimal sac, causing a vacuum.[14] With relaxation, tears can be seen to rush in through the puncta into the canaliculi (Fig. 5-4). There is an actual sphincterlike closure of the puncta associated with a blink.[15] Moreover, the lids can be seen to move medially about 1 mm in association with a blink. Both superior and inferior puncta are important in the drainage of tears. Should, however, one of the puncta become occluded, the remaining single punctum is sufficient for adequate tear drainage under normal conditions. (For a further discussion of the physiology of tear excretion, see Chapter 6.)

IMMUNE REACTIONS OF THE TEARS

The tears contain several mechanisms for combating inflammatory reaction of the external eye. These include specific humoral and cellular responses as well as nonspecific means of handling microbial or other noxious challenges. Biopsy of the normal, nonstimulated conjunctiva shows no inflammatory T or B lymphocytic infiltrates.[16] Most cells are fixed tissue cells present in the normal conjunctiva but which participate in certain anaphylactic responses. Immunoglobulins IgM, IgG, IgD, IgA, and IgE are present in the subepithelial tissue of the normal conjunctiva and tears, whereas the stroma of the cornea does not contain IgM.[17] The immunoglobulin IgA is the predominant one in tears. With stimulation, protective mechanisms increase beneath the epithelium, on the epithelial surface, and in the tears. In active disease processes, the conjunctival hyperemia with transudation or exudation brings in soluble substances as well as varying proportions of inflammatory cells. Transudation of fluids helps increase the levels of immunoglobulins, e.g., IgE, IgA, and IgG, which have specific functions in allergic processes or in the prevention of bacterial adherence to epithelial cell surfaces.[18] In allergic conjunctivitis, the level of IgE in the tears increases relative to the level seen in the serum.[19]

Papillary hypertrophy is an accumulation of inflammatory cells in the superficial layers of the palpebral conjunctiva. In follicular hypertrophy, the follicle is an organized collection of B lymphocytes located centrally with peripheral T lymphocytes which respond to chronic, toxic, or certain viral infections. In general, in bacterial conjunctivitis, the clinical appearance

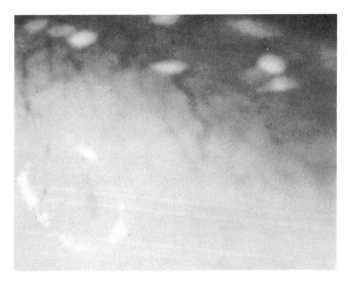

Figure 5-4. Open punctum, upper lid.

includes a purulent exudate due to masses of the predominant cell, the neutrophil. In some viral infections, such as those caused by the adenoviral group, and in hay fever conjunctivitis, the predominant infiltrate seen on scraping is the monocyte. In chlamydial disease, the early response is primarily neutrophilic, but later in untreated eyes, the inflammatory cells are mixed mononuclear leukocytes and neutrophils. Allergic ocular disease may produce large numbers of eosinophils as well as some mast cells, as seen in scrapings of patients with vernal keratoconjunctivitis. On the other hand, only scattered to absent eosinophils might be seen in the scrapings of patients with atopic conjunctivitis or hay fever conjunctivitis.[20]

Localized immunity is also provided by immunoglobins, such as secretory IgA, i.e., two molecules of IgA coupled by its secretory component. Whereas the IgA is synthesized by local plasma cells in the lacrimal gland, the secretory component is produced by the epithelial acinar cells.[21] The lacrimal gland may release a chemotactic factor for IgA-committed B lymphocytes that helps ensure that the majority of these cells are available to the secretory immune system.[22]

Other factors that may aid in the resistance of the external eye to noxious stimuli are lysozyme, lactoferrin, serum complement, and other substances released by inflammatory cells. Lysozyme is an enzyme that cleaves mucopeptides of certain bacterial cell walls, not including *Staphylococcus aureus.* Lysozyme is produced by the lacrimal glands.[23] Lactoferrin is bacteriostatic by its quality of being able to bind some metals so that they cannot be used by microorganisms.[24] Lymphokines, i.e., substances released by inflammatory cells to modulate the behavior of other inflammatory cells, may alter the response of the external eye. Lymphokines may be chemotactic for some inflammatory cells or may suppress humoral or cellular reactions or other specific functions. The definite roles of other factors, such as the Langerhans cells, i.e., dendritic cells of the macrophage family which are present in the conjunctiva and cornea,[25] the eosinophil granule major basic protein,[26] and the relatively cool environment of the external eye, are unknown at the present time.

REFERENCES

1. Holly FJ, Lemp MA: Tear physiology and dry eyes, Surv Ophthalmol 22:69, 1977
2. Mishima S, Gasset A, Klyce SD Jr, Baum JL: Determination of tear volume and tear flow. Invest Ophthalmol 5:264, 1966
3. Puffer MJ, Neault RW & Brubaker RE: Basal precorneal tear turnover in the human eye. Am J Ophthalmol 89:369, 1980
4. Erickson OF, Hatler R, Berg M: Autonomic drug studies on patients with deficient tearing. Stanford Med Bull 18:138, 1960

5. Goldstein AM, DePalou A, Botelho SY: Inhibition and facilitation of pilocarpine-induced lacrimal flow by norepinephrine. Invest Ophthalmol 6:498, 1967

6. Koffler B, Lemp MA: The effect of chlorpheniramine maleate on aqueous tear production. Ann Ophthalmol 12:217, 1980

7. Gillette TE, Allansmith MR, Greiner JV, Janusz M: Histologic and immunohistologic comparison of main and accessory lacrimal tissue. Am J Ophthalmol 89:724, 1980

8. Jordan A, Baum J: Basic tear flow, does it exit? Ophthalmol 87:920, 1980

9. van Bysterfeld OP: Lipolytic activity of *Staph. aureus* from different sources. J Med Microbiol 9:225, 1976

10. Holly FJ: Formation and rupture of the tear film. Exp Eye Res 15:515, 1973

11. Lemp MA: Breakup of the tear film. Int Ophthalmol Clin 13:97, 1973

12. Adams AD: The morphology of human conjunctival mucus. Arch Ophthalmol 97:730, 1979

13. Rorengien B: On lacrimal drainage. Ophthalmologica 164 (b):409, 1972

14. Maurice DM: The dynamics and drainage of tears. Int Ophthalmol Clin 13:103, 1973

15. Lemp MA, Weiler HH: How do tears exit? Invest Ophthalmol. In press

16. Belfort R, Jr, Mendes NF: T- and B-lymphocytes in the human conjunctiva and lacrimal gland. In Silverstein A, O'Connor GR, (eds): Immunology and Immunopathology of the Eye. New York, Masson, 1979, pp 287-291

17. Allansmith MR, Whitney C, McClellan B, et al.: Immunoglobulins in the eye: location, type and amount. Arch Ophthalmol 89:36, 1973

18. Friedlander MH: Allergy and Immunology of the Eye. Hagerstown, MD, Harper & Row, 1979, p 56

19. Allansmith MR, Hahn G, Simon MA: Tissue tear and serum IgE in vernal conjunctivitis. Am J Ophthalmol 81:506, 1976

20. Lang RM, Friedlander MH: Conjunctival scrapings in vernal and hay fever conjunctivitis. Presented at the Ocular Microbiology and Immunology Meeting, October 1980

21. Franklin RM, Kenyon KR, Tomasi TB, Jr: Immunohistologic studies of human lacrimal gland: localization of immunoglobulins, secretory component and lactoferrin. J Immunol 110:984, 1973

22. Franklin RM: A mechanism for localization of IgA-producing cells in the lacrimal gland. Suran, A., Gery, I, Nussenblatt RB, (eds): Proceedings of Immunology of the Eye Workshop. III: Sp Suppl Immunology Abstracts 1981, p 143

23. Horwitz BL, Christensen GR, Ritzmann SR: Diurnal profiles of tear lysozyme and gamma A globulin. Ann Ophthalmol 10:75, 1978

24. Broekhuyse RM: Tear lactoferrin: a bacteriostatic and complexing protein. Invest Ophthalmol 13:550, 1974

25. Rodrigues MM, Rowden G, Hackett J, Bakos I: Langerhans cells in the normal conjunctiva and peripheral cornea of selected species. Invest Ophthalmol 21:759, 1981

26. Udell Il, Gleich GJ, Allansmith MR, Ackerman SJ, Abelson MB: Eosinophil granule, major basic protein, and Charcot-Leyden crystal protein in human tears. Am J Ophthalmol, 92:824, 1981

6

PHYSIOLOGY OF LACRIMAL EXCRETION

BENJAMIN MILDER

The health of the cornea, its optical function as the most important refracting surface of the eye, and freedom from unpleasant symptoms—all these require a normal tear secretion, a normal mechanism for the elimination of tears, and a balance between the two. If the rate of tear secretion exceeds the outflow capability, the result will be an excess accumulation of tears on the cornea and along the lid margins and an annoying overflow of tears down the face. If the secretion rate is inadequate relative to the outflow capability, the result is much more serious—the dry eye syndrome, with its potential for corneal damage.

In order to maintain this balance between the secretion and excretion, several factors are involved in the elimination of tears from the conjunctival sac. These factors include:

1. The anatomy of the eyelid margins
2. Evaporation
3. Gravity
4. Capillary attraction
5. Intranasal air movement
6. The rate of tear secretion
7. The orbicularis oculi muscles (the act of blinking)
8. The competence of mucosal folds or valves

The act of blinking is generally agreed to be the most significant physiologic factor in tear outflow, and this will be considered in some detail.

ANATOMY OF LID MARGINS AND LACRIMAL PUNCTA

In normal tear drainage, the tears move along the eyelid margins in the form of a narrow concave meniscus. If the lid margins are not in correct apposition to the globe, there will be an increase in the reservoir of tears at the line between the globe and the eyelid margin. With each blink, the sweeping movement of the upper lid tends to distribute a precorneal film of uniform thickness, and the excess of tears is squeezed out onto the face. Thus, small degrees of ectropion of the lid margin may be responsible for a large amount of annoying epiphora, even in the presence of adequate orbicularis function.

The lacrimal papilla is located on the posterior aspect of the margin of the eyelid at the nasal end of the tarsus about 6 mm from the nasal canthus. At its summit is located the lacrimal punctum, 0.2 to 0.3 mm in diameter, slightly funnel-shaped, and inverted toward the eye. Anatomic integrity of the punctum is essential to normal outflow function. The punctal opening must be adequate and in correct relation to the eye. It is axiomatic that if you can see the punctum without touching the eyelid, it is out of position. Further, if the lower lid punctum is exposed to view when the patient looks upward, its position in relation to the globe in blinking will probably not be adequate for normal tear elimination.

Some patients who have malposition or occlusion of the lower lid punctum are free of epiphora. This observation has led to an improved understanding of the relative roles of the upper and lower puncta in normal tear excretion. It is now felt that, in half of the population, the upper punctum plays the major outflow role or shares it equally with the lower.[1] While this does not necessarily mean that in such cases a person will be free of symptoms if the lower punctum is nonfunctional, such instances do occur.

EVAPORATION

Under normal conditions, 10 to 25 percent of tears are lost by evaporation.[2] The remainder leave the eye by way of the excretory passages. The superficial lipid layer of the tear film, elaborated by the meibomian glands, acts as a barrier to evaporation. This layer comprises only 1 percent of the total thickness of the tear film[3] (See Fig. 5-1.) but its protective function depends less on its thickness than on its uniform distribution by the act of blinking. As the eyelids open in the relaxation phase of blink, the oily film is dragged along more slowly than the aqueous layer and covers it uniformly.[4]

Insufficiency of the oily layer, for any reason, or failure of the normal blinking mechanism will expose the aqueous layer to as much as a 10- to 20-fold increase in the rate of evaporation.[2]

The more rapid the flow of tears, the less significant is the rate of evaporation. With the eyes open, there is always some evaporation taking place, with the result that the tears become hypertonic to the corneal epithelium. Thus, there is an osmotic gradient from cornea to tear film, and evaporation plays a role in

corneal deturgescence, maintaining optical clarity.[5]

GRAVITY

The role of gravity as one of the mechanisms for the elimination of tears has attracted far more speculation than experimentation. From the speculations of Petit in the eighteenth century[6] to the present, few studies have addressed this question. Murube,[7] in 1978, attempted to evaluate the influence of gravity on lacrimal drainage by recording the flow of a radiopaque contrast agent instilled into the lacrimal sac. He used a thin, oily contrast medium having the same density as tears but greater viscosity, and found that the mixture was eliminated from the lacrimal sac and nasolacrimal duct in 6 minutes. If the same procedure was repeated with the nostrils plugged and a corneal-conjunctival anesthetic administered to eliminate blinking, the evacuation rate was much slower, demonstrating the generally accepted principle that orbicularis action plays a significant role. Since he did not perform this experiment with nasal occlusion alone, it was not possible to assess the role of air currents in the nose. The initial experiment was then repeated with the patient in a supine position using normal blinking. There was no elimination of the contrast agent. Under the conditions of this experiment, Murube had demonstrated that gravity, in fact, influences outflow function.

However, when he repeated these tests using an aqueous fluorescein instilled into the conjunctival sac, the fluorescein dye disappearance rate was normal.

Murube reasoned that the forces other than gravity that normally influence tear elimination are adequate for tears with low viscosity (i.e., normal tears), but when evacuation of the system is made more difficult by a solution of higher viscosity (as would be the case with thin mucus in the lacrimal sac and nasolacrimal duct), the usual physiologic forces may not be adequate if gravity is not added thereto.

Summing up, it is apparent that normal outflow function takes place independent of the action of gravity, even though gravity can be demonstrated to play a role in some abnormal situations. As with each of the mechanisms that influence the elimination of tears, there will be variations between individuals.

CAPILLARY ATTRACTION

Capillarity is a property of adhesiveness between a liquid and a solid. In tubes of small caliber, capillarity is a force responsible for movement of a column of liquid in the tube. Essential to capillarity is a small-caliber rigid tube. This condition is fulfilled nicely by the lacrimal punctum and the vertical limb of the canaliculus. Thus, capillarity functions as an outflow modality, drawing tears from the lacus and the marginal tear strip into the canalicular system.

It is difficult to determine the importance of capillarity in normal outflow function. On the one hand, annoying tear retention is observed not infrequently in patients whose puncta are patulous as a result of overly aggressive dilating efforts, even when the position of that dilated punctum is undisturbed.

On the other hand, in cases of punctal stenosis, a three-snip or punch punctumplasty may be curative despite the surgically enlarged punctum. It may be that, in these surgical enlargements of the punctum, the relief of the epiphora is because the opening is on the posterior surface of the lid and dips into the tear lake.

It appears that the role of capillarity may vary from patient to patient, as is the case with the other physiologic outflow mechanisms.

INTRANASAL CONVECTION CURRENTS

The movement of air within the nasal cavity has been described as playing a role in tear excretion. Proponents suggest that convection currents during respiration aid in sucking tears down the nasolacrimal duct. Whether or not such air movement has a significance in normal tear flow is open to question.[8, 9]

One could reason that if the valvular system of the nasolacrimal duct is competent, it should prevent reflux of air into the duct, and, therefore, the movement of air in the nose could not play a role in normal tear elimination. Using this same reasoning, however, changes in air pressure within the nose could play a role if the valve system were not airtight.

Kuribayashi[10] observed the ostium of the nasolacrimal duct and the plica semilunaris (valve of Hasner) and found that narrowing of the ostium and closure of the valve coincided with eyelid closure in the act of blinking, and the reverse occurred as the lids relaxed. These observations support the concept that, in the relaxation phase of blinking, tears which have been aspirated into the lacrimal sac are driven down the duct. The simultaneous opening of ostium and plica semilunaris would be compatible with such a flow. At the same time, the opening of the ostium and plica would allow for the possibility that air movement would also have an influence in drawing tears down the duct toward the nose. Conversely, closure of Hasner's valve would tend to prevent the reflux of air into the nasolacrimal duct.

An occasional patient reports feeling air issuing from the puncta when blowing his nose, and this observation is not unusual following dacryocystorhinostomy, where, even if the action of the eyelid muscles on the canaliculi is the prime factor in tear outflow, air currents may play a role.

Thus, it would appear that, under certain circumstances, air movements within a nose do impinge on the outflow passages and could be a factor in facilitating tear outflow. Such a mechanism would represent a departure from normal tear excretion physiology.

ORBICULARIS OCULI (THE ACT OF BLINKING)

The importance of the muscles of the eyelids in tear outflow has long been the subject of contemplation and experimentation. As long ago as the beginning of the nineteenth century, there was general acceptance of the act of blinking as the primary physiologic force. For many years, there was no consensus on how the eyelid muscles accomplished this task. Is the lacrimal sac compressed or dilated in the act of blinking?

Arlt, in 1855, postulated that the sac is compressed in blinking, and this notion was supported by the radiographic studies of Ploman in 1928.[11]

The opposite view, that the sac is dilated

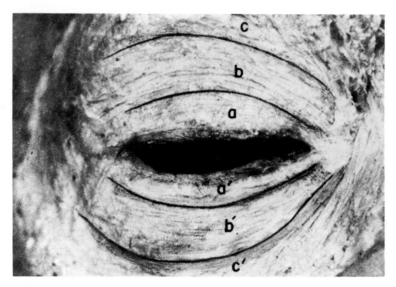

Figure 6-1. Orbicularis oculi muscle: **a-a'**. Upper and lower pretarsal fibers. **b-b'**. Upper and lower preseptal fibers. **c-c'**. Upper and lower orbital fibers (covering the orbital septum). (*From Jones LE and Wobig J: Surgery of the Eyelids and Lacrimal System, 1976. Courtesy of Aesculapius Publishing Company.*)

when the orbicularis muscles contract, also goes back to the last century, first attributed to Hyrtl in 1863 and supported by Schirmer in 1903.[12]

Are the canaliculi the principal instrument in the dynamics of tear flow? Are they dilated or compressed in the act of blinking? These questions, too, have intrigued investigators. Some 25 years ago, Lester Jones appeared to have resolved all of the conflicting theories and elucidated the relative roles of the canaliculi, the lacrimal sac, and the orbicularis muscles. His description of the mechanics of tear flow was based on his excellent anatomic studies of the orbicularis muscles. Jones identified three parts to the orbicularis: (1) that overlying the tarsus, (2) that overlying the orbital septum, and (3) that overlying the orbital margins and beyond[13] (Figs. 6-1 and 6-2).

Jones found that the preseptal portion of the orbicularis muscle of the lower eyelid is inserted into the fascia of the lacrimal sac, while the upper eyelid preseptal muscle fibers are inserted anteriorly into the medial canthal tendon and posteriorly to the lacrimal fascia.

The pretarsal muscle fibers are divided into superficial and deep heads, the former joining the upper pretarsal fibers to form the medial-canthal tendon, and the latter deep head embracing the ampulla of each canaliculus and inserting behind the posterior lacrimal crest.

From these dissections, it is apparent that the muscle contraction in the act of blinking will produce dynamic alterations in the canaliculus as well as the lacrimal sac. From his observations, Jones[14] postulated a tear outflow mechanism which has become recognized as the lacrimal pump of Jones:

1. When the eyelids are open, the marginal tear strips cover the puncta with fluid.
2. Capillary attraction pulls the fluid into the ampullae.
3. As the eyelids close, the pretarsal muscles contract, pulling the tarsi medially, which empties the ampullae and shortens the canaliculi, forcing the fluid into the tear sac.
4. The preseptal muscles contract at the same time, pulling the lateral wall of the tear sac laterally. This produces a negative pressure in the sac, creating space for the fluid and assisting in drawing it into the sac.

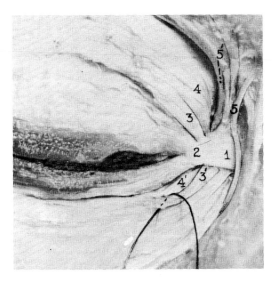

Figure 6-2. Superficial view of medial canthal orbicularis insertions: **1.** medial canthal tendon. **2.** Junction of superficial heads of pretarsal muscle to form common tendon. **3** and **3′.** Superficial fibers of preseptal muscles. **4** and **4′.** Deep fibers of preseptal muscles. **5** and **5′.** Angular vein on anterior surface of superciliaris muscle. (*From Jones LE, Wobig J: Surgery of the Eyelids and Lacrimal System, 1976. Courtesy of Aesculapius Publishing Company.*)

5. When the eyelids open again, the elasticity of the lacrimal diaphragm returns it to a position of rest, forcing the fluid from the sac down through the nasolacrimal duct into the nose.

Jones concludes that in the act of blinking, "the positive force in the ampulla and canaliculus is many times greater than the negative force in the tear sac." This explanation, which fits well with the orbicularis anatomy, assigns a major compression role to the canaliculus and a lesser negative pressure role to the lacrimal sac. The lacrimal pump of Jones has been widely accepted during the past decade as the best explanation for the normal physiology of tear outflow. However, recent studies have again focused attention on the question of just how blinking affects the canaliculus and whether the sac dilates or collapses with eyelid closure. Doane,[15] in 1980, employed high-speed photog-

raphy to study the eyelid movements, the tear film, and the puncta in relation to the elimination of tears. On the basis of the dynamics revealed by high-speed photography, Doane has postulated a mechanism for tear outflow which is, in some ways, diametrically opposite to the lacrimal pump theory of Jones.

Doane cited the studies of Rosengren in which, by retrograde catheterization of the lacrimal sac via the nasolacrimal duct and using fluid manometry, he was able to demonstrate that a valve closure mechanism at the internal punctum prevented reflux of fluid from the lacrimal sac back into the canaliculi during the act of blinking. Rosengren also found that an increase in pressure occurred within the lacrimal sac during the closure phase of each blink. Compression of the canaliculi during the closure phase drives tears through the system. Thus, Rosengren felt that the sac functioned mainly as a reservoir, emptying under compression.

Doane's photographic studies employed speeds up to 500 frames per second with exposure times of 1/1500 .seconds to record the blinking process. He found (1) that tears flow over the cornea only with blinking, confirming the observations of many earlier investigators, (2) that the punctum and marginal tear strip both move 2 to 5 mm nasally with each blink, and (3) that the lacrimal papillae project upward from the lid margins as the act of blinking begins, and the upper and lower puncta meet by the time the lid closure is only one-third to one-half completed. With the puncta thus occluded, as the lids complete their closure, the orbicularis contraction serves to squeeze the canaliculi, forcing tears into the lacrimal sac. As the tears fill the sac, regurgitation is prevented by closure of the valve at the internal punctum. Doane's studies showed also that: (4) as the lids separate in relaxation, the puncta remain in contact until the lids are almost open, then they pop apart abruptly, and (5) after the puncta separate, there is a rapid flow of fluid into the punctal openings, lasting as long as several seconds—as if a negative pressure within the canaliculi is sucking the tears into them (Fig. 6-3). (It should be remembered that without blinking there is no movement of the tear meniscus.)

Doane's pictures thus support Rosengren's contention that there is a valvular mechanism

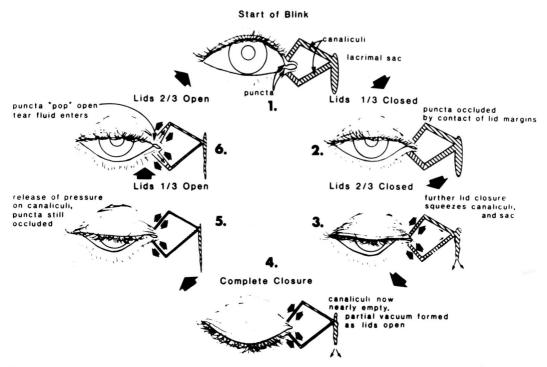

Figure 6-3. Mechanism of lacrimal drainage. (*From Doane MG: Ophthalmology 88:850, 1981.*)

in the area of the junction of canaliculi with the tear sac. This is further confirmed by Carlton and his colleagues who studied lacrimal flow using dacryoscintigraphy with technitium–99 and showed a gap between the confluence of the canaliculi and the lacrimal sac. This suggested a functional closure or valve at that point[16] (Fig. 6-4).

Doane feels that the lacrimal sac is not essential to the outflow process, since normal tear

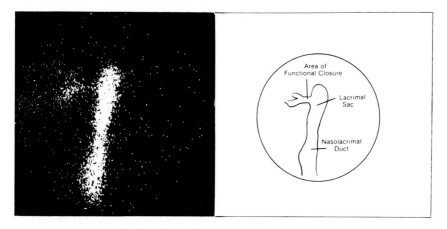

Figure 6-4. Left. Gamma camera image of nasolacrimal duct of the right eye. **Right.** Corresponding anatomic structures, showing area of functional closure. (*From Rossomondo RH, Carlton WH, Trueblood JH and Thomas RP, Arch Ophthalmol 88:524, 1972. Copyright 1972, American Medical Association.*)

outflow is restored after dacryocystorhinostomy. To support this contention, he cites the work of Maurice,[17] who measured pressures within the sac and found positive pressure values with the act of blinking, suggesting that the sac is compressed during the contraction phase. Finally, Doane has commented on the observations of numerous investigators that, after DCR, the nasal mucosa is sucked into the sac with each blink. Although other investigators have cited this as evidence for negative pressure within the sac, Doane points out that, in blinking, the compression phase of the canaliculi lasts only 0.04 second and the relaxation phase a much longer 0.18 second. He feels that what investigators are observing is that the nasal mucosal suction effect is being seen during the relaxation phase. Thus, the decrease in pressure within the sac occurs during relaxation.

From his observations, Doane has evolved his own explanation for the physiologic mechanism of lacrimal outflow:[15]

At the start of the blink, the canaliculi are already filled with tear fluid (up to approximately 1.5 microliters). If excess fluid is available in the tear strips, as with reflex tearing, the sac may also be contributory in drawing in fluid, as associated with the Krehbiel flow. As the upper lid begins its descent for the blink, the region of the lid margins containing the puncta elevate, and meet forcefully by the time the lid is halfway down. The puncta are thereby occluded, and the remaining portion of the lid closure acts to compress the canaliculi and sac, forcing the contained fluid to be expelled via the nasolacrimal duct into the nose. Thus, at the instant of maximum lid closure, the volume of fluid within the system is at its minimum. As the lids start their opening phase, the compressive force ends and the elastic walls of the canaliculi and sac attempt to return to their original shape and contained volume. Valving action at the inner end of the canaliculi, and also in the nasolacrimal duct, prevents fluid and air from being drawn back into them, and since the puncta are still occluded at this stage by the contact of the medial lid margins, a partial vacuum is formed within the system. Eventually, the parting movement of the lids becomes sufficient to force the punctal areas apart, exposing the suction force to the adjacent tear fluid in the menisci. There is then a rapid flow of fluid into the canaliculi during the 1-3 seconds immediately following the blink. If the valving action at the inner end of the canaliculi is not completely effective (and if the valving in the nasolacrimal duct is functional), the lowered pressure in the lacrimal sac will continue to draw in fluid for many seconds between blinks, provided that excess fluid is available. Thus, the system is once again primed with fluid, ready for the expulsive action of the next lid closure.

Since normal, non-reflex tear secretion amounts to something less than 1 microliter/min, and the canaliculi alone can transport more than this in one blink, the system is operating nearly empty most of the time. It appears not unreasonable that these low volumes are absorbed by the mucosal surface of the nasolacrimal duct, with little actual expulsion into the nose, as has been suggested by Maurice.

Doane's concept, while attractive and plausible, involves several assumptions not readily confirmed by his photographic studies: (1) Are the puncta sealed when they are in apposition? (2) How closed is the valve at the internal punctum? (3) How closed is the valve of Hasner during lid closure?

The anatomic observations of Jones and the photographic studies of Doane have much in common. The disposition of the deep, pretarsal orbicularis fibers explains Doane's observation of the propulsion of the lacrimal papillae in blinking. The two investigators are in agreement that the chief propulsive force lies with the compression and nasal movement of the canaliculi, and they agree that there is a valve-type effect preventing reflux from the sac. Jones has stressed the ingress of tears at the punctum as being due to capillarity, while Doane has reasonably accounted for a negative pressure as a force aspirating tears into the canaliculus from the marginal tear strip. The chief difference is the one that existed 150 years ago: Does the orbicularis contraction compress the lacrimal sac, or does it dilate the sac, producing a negative pressure? The weight of experimental evidence lies with the advocates of compression—but the next century of research will undoubtedly add more fuel to the debate.

Although the physiologic mechanisms described above are essential to normal tear drainage, these mechanisms—chiefly, the orbicularis muscles—function with varying degrees of efficiency. Whether or not an individual has symptomatic epiphora will depend on multiple factors, including orbicularis efficiency, valvular competence, rate of evaporation, and, finally, the rate of tear secretion. We have all seen the elderly patient who has grossly poor orbicularis tone or ectropion, yet has no annoying epiphora because his Schirmer test values are minimal.

In a study of the primary Jones fluorescein dye test (that is, spontaneous recovery of fluorescein solution within the nose, without irrigation), Zappia and Milder found, in a study of 200 normal individuals, that average Schirmer test values were greater than 10 mm in 61 percent of the population.[18] When the primary Jones test was positive within 1 minute, 84 percent of the patients had Schirmer test values of 10 mm or more. When the fluorescein appeared in the nose in 2 minutes, only 53 percent had Schirmer values of 10 mm or more, and at 5 minutes, only 45 percent had the same Schirmer result. Obviously, the greater the tear secretion, the more readily can the outflow system be traversed.[18]

FUNCTIONAL BLOCK

While the lacrimal outflow function is under discussion, it is appropriate to introduce the concept of functional block, a concept first introduced by Demorest and Milder in 1955 to describe the failure of lacrimal outflow despite a patent lacrimal system, distinguishing this group of problems from those that are the result of complete obstruction in the lacrimal pathway.[19]

Such interference with normal tear outflow, in a patent system, may result from a variety of pathologic processes. Failure of orbicularis muscle function, whether neurogenic in origin or simply a loss of muscle tone with age, will result in epiphora. Other impediments to normal outflow may result from partial stenosis anywhere within the outflow system, from polyps, tumors, or dacryoliths.

The diagnosis and treatment of functional block are discussed in Chapter 9.

REFERENCES

1. Jones LT, Wobig JL: Surgery of the Eyelids and Lacrimal System. Birmingham, Aesculapius, 1976, p 149

2. Mishima S: Some physiologic aspects of the pre-corneal tear film. Arch Ophthalmol 73:233, 1965

3. Holly FJ, Lemp MA: Tear physiology and dry eyes. Surv Ophthalmol 22:69, 1977

4. Brown SI, and Dervichian DG: Hydrodynamics of blinking. Arch Ophthalmol 82:541, 1969

5. Milder B: In Moses RA (ed): Adler's Physiology of the eye. St.Louis, Mosby, 1981, p 19

6. Petit JL: Sur la fistule lacrymale. Memoires de l'Academie des Sciences de Paris, 1734, p 34

7. Murube J: On gravity as one of the compelling forces in tear flow. In Yamaguchi M (ed): Recent Advances on the Lacrimal System. Tokyo, Asahi Press, 1978 p 51

8. Hounauld FJ: Some thoughts on the operation of the fistula lacrimalis. Phil Trans for 1735–1736, 39:54, 1938. Cited in Castillo J: In Yamaguchi M (ed.): Recent Advances on the Lacrimal System. Tokyo, Asahi Press, 1978, p 50

9. Hasner. Wien Med. Wochenschr. 15:388, 1865. Cited in Duke-Elder, S: Systems of Ophthalmology. St. Louis, Mosby, 1968, Vol. 4, p 431

10. Kuribayashi. Cited in Murube J: On gravity as one of the compelling forces in tear flow. In Yamaguchi M (ed.): Recent Advances on the Lacrimal System, Tokyo, Asahi Press, 1978, p 58

11. Ploman KC, Ergel A, Knutsson F: Acta Ophthalmol 6:55, 1928. Cited in Duke-Elder S: Systems of Ophthalmology. St. Louis, Mosby, 1968, Vol 4, p 430

12. Duke-Elder S: Systems of Ophthalmology. St. Louis, Mosby, 1968, Vol 4, p 430

13. Jones LT, Wobig JL: Surgery of the Eyelids and Lacrimal System. Birmingham, Aesculapius, 1976, pp 44-55

14. Jones LT: Epiphora II: Its relation to the anatomical structures and surgery of the medial canthal region. Am J Ophthalmol, 43:209, 1957.

15. Doane MG: Blinking and the mechanics of the lacrimal drainage system. Ophthalmology, 88:844, 1981

16. Carlton WH, Trueblood JH, and Rossomondo RM: Clinical evaluation of microscintigraphy of the lacrimal drainage apparatus. J Nucl Med 14:89, 1973

17. Maurice DM: The dynamics and drainage of tears. Int Ophthalmol Clin 13:103, 1973

18. Zappia R, Milder B: Lacrimal drainage function I. The Jones fluorescein test. Am J Ophthalmol 74:154, 1972

19. Demorest BH, Milder B: Dacryocystography. II. The pathologic lacrimal apparatus. Arch Ophthalmol 54:410, 1955

7

PHARMACOLOGY AND THERAPEUTICS

BYRON H. DEMOREST

BASIC PHARMACOLOGIC CONSIDERATIONS OF TOPICAL AND SYSTEMIC DRUGS USED IN THERAPY OF DISEASES OF THE LACRIMAL SYSTEM

Antimicrobial and anti-inflammatory agents available for topical use in diseases affecting the lacrimal apparatus are varied. Medications used to treat infections of the lacrimal tract are the least toxic chemotherapeutic and antibiotic substances that exert either a bacteriostatic or a bactericidal action against pathogenic organisms.[1-3] Topical drugs for ocular use in bacterial infections fall into several subgroups including the sulfonamides, the aminoglycosides, the tetracyclines, chloramphenicol, and erythromycin. For viral and mycotic infections, agents are available for topical use in the eye. Their indication for lacrimal tract infections is limited. In fact, the antiviral agents can cause cicatricial stenosis of the puncta and canaliculi with prolonged use.

Systemic antibiotics should be utilized for acute infections of the lacrimal gland and lacrimal sac. Antibiotics of choice here include penicillin, the cephalosporins, erythromycin, the tetracyclines, and gentamicin.[2,3]

In certain instances, anti-inflammatory agents, notably the adrenocorticosteroids, are advised. Most often these are used as an adjunct to antimicrobial therapy.

There are numerous artificial tears, lubricants, and other preparations offered by drug manufacturers and used with mixed results for therapy of the dry eye. These are listed along with diagnostic agents helpful in the evaluation of lacrimal problems.

Topical Antibacterial Agents

Antibacterial drugs are effective against most bacteria causing lacrimal tract disease. The most common organisms seen are staphylococci, streptococci, pneumococci, and the diphtheroids. Gram-negative bacteria, such as *Klebsiella, Haemophilus,* and *Pseudomonas,* also have been reported to cause lacrimal infections.

The Sulfonamides. This group of antibacterial agents has been available for almost 50 years. They have remained popular because of their ease of preparation, stability in solution, effectiveness against ocular pathogens, and comfort when applied topically to the eye. Allergic reactions to topical sulfas can occur.

The chemotherapeutic action of the sulfonamides is predominantly as a competitive antimetabolite. The sulfas are, therefore, bacteriostatic rather than bactericidal. Sulfonamides are effective against *Staphylococcus aureus, Diplo-*

coccus pneumoniae, Haemophilus aegyptius, Haemophilus influenzae, and *Neisseria catarrhalis.* The *Actinomyces, Brucella, Clostridium,* chlamydial infective organisms or TRIC viruses, and certain fungi are also inhibited by sulfonamides.

Sulfonamide preparations for topical ocular use include:

- *Sulfacetamide sodium* in solutions of 10, 15, and 30 percent and topical ointments of 10 percent and 30 percent.
- *Sulfadiazine* as 5 percent ointment.
- *Sulfathiazole* as 5 percent ointment.
- *Sulfisoxazole* in a 4 percent solution and 4 percent ointment

The Aminoglycosides. These antibiotics are popular for ophthalmic use. They are effective when applied topically and can readily be prepared for use in the eye. They have a broad spectrum of bactericidal antibiotic activity against both gram-positive and gram-negative organisms.

Escherichia, Enterobacter, Klebsiella, Salmonella, Shigella, and *Proteus* are those organisms listed as being predominantly sensitive to aminoglycosides; however, staphylococci and streptococci are also somewhat sensitive.

The most frequently used ocular aminoglycosides are:

- *Neomycin sulfate* is a common ingredient of many mixed ophthalmic topical solutions. Neomycin can cause ocular sensitivity in certain individuals, and cross-sensitivity to the remaining aminoglycosides may occur should sensitivity to this agent develop. The usual combination medications using neomycin are mixtures of polymyxin B 5000 U/g + bacitracin 400 U/g + neomycin 5 mg/g in ointments and solutions.
- *Gentamicin sulfate* is available in solutions and ointments with 3 mg/ml (0.3 percent solution).
- *Tobramycin* is available as a 0.3 percent solution.

The Tetracyclines. These are broad-spectrum antibacterial agents produced by several species of *Streptomyces.* Their action is largely bacteriostatic. For ophthalmic use, two antibiotics from this group are available. They are tetracycline

hydrochloride (Achromycin) and chlortetracycline (Aureomycin).

Tetracyclines are indicated for treatment of infections caused by the TRIC (trachoma and inclusion conjunctivitis) agents. They are also agents of choice for infections by rickettsiae and *Haemophilus ducreyi.* Prolonged systemic use may cause overgrowth of mycotic organisms or development of resistant strains of Staphylococcus.

Topical ocular preparations of tetracyclines are:

- *Tetracycline hydrochloride* in 1 percent ophthalmic ointment.
- *Chlortetracycline* in 1 percent ophthalmic ointment.

Chloramphenicol. Chloramphenicol has a broad spectrum of activity and is particularly useful topically as an eye preparation because its popularity as a systemic agent has lessened. Systemic utilization has been documented to cause severe aplastic anemia and death. Topically, it has an action resembling that of the tetracyclines but rarely causes cross-sensitization to tetracycline.

Topical preparations include:

- *Chloromycetin* in 1 percent ophthalmic ointment and 0.5 percent solution in a 5-ml container

Erythromycin. Erythromycin is one of the safest bactericidal antibiotics for systemic or topical use. It appears to impede the protein synthesis of bacteria. Erythromycin is effective against most gram-positive bacteria but is not useful against gram-negative organisms. In the eye, it is most often used to treat staphylococcal, streptococcal, and pneumococcal infections. It is also effective against chlamydiae and is a drug of choice for ophthalmia neonatorum. It is available as a 0.5 percent ophthalmic ointment.

Topical Antifungal Agents

Fungi cause infections, notably *Actinomyces* canaliculitis, of the lacrimal drainage system. Occasionally, it is possible to culture or see fungi in dacryoliths of the sac or casts of the nasolacrimal duct. Unfortunately, topical use of antifungal preparations is only weakly effective in the therapy of mycotic disease of the lacrimal tract.

Topical angifungal agents include:

- *Amphotericin B*—2.5 to 10 mg/ml solution in distilled water or 5 percent dextrose in water. This agent has the broadest spectrum of all antifungal agents, with action against *Blastomyces, Candida, Coccidioides, Cryptococcus,* and *Histoplasma.*
- *Nystatin* as an ointment with 100,000 U/g is active against *Aspergillus* and *Candida.*
- *Flucytosine* in 1 percent solution. The highest activity of this agent is against *Candida* and *Cryptococcus:*

Two other agents are used for mycotic infections.

- *Pimaricin* in 5 percent solution is active predominantly against *Fusarium.*
- *Miconazole* in 1 percent solution is active against *Candida* and *Aspergillus.*

Topical Antiviral Agents

Secondary involvement of the lacrimal drainage system can occur with viral infections of the conjunctiva and cornea.

Agents active against herpes simplex virus include:

- *5-Iodo-2-deoxyuridine* in 0.1 percent solution and 0.5 percent ointment
- *Adenine arabinoside* as 3 percent ointment
- *Trifluorothymidine* in 1 percent solution

Systemic Antibiotics

Systemic antimicrobial drugs for use in lacrimal tract infections are chosen on the basis of several criteria. Drug toxicity is an important factor, and the physician must choose the least toxic alternative for agents that will be effective. Fortunately, penetration of antibiotic drugs is not a problem in lacrimal tract disease, since good penetration occurs with all agents in this area. Identification of the infecting organisms should be done when possible, but therapy based on clinical findings should start immediately. Keep in mind that the most common infecting organisms causing dacryocystitis are the gram-positive bacteria, pneumococci, streptococci, and staphylococci. Often

a gram-stained smear of exudate from an infected gland or lacrimal drainage system will provide preliminary information about the organism. Cultures are then advised for absolute diagnosis. Sensitivity testing helps to determine the first choice of drug for the infection.

Without consulting a table or list of recommended antibiotics, it is difficult for the ophthalmologist to select the optimum antibiotic for systemic use against infections. The following outline (Table 7-1) should be helpful in this regard.

Anti-inflammatory Agents

Oral adrenocorticosteroid anti-inflammatory drugs may be indicated occasionally to reduce swelling of nonspecific inflammatory disease of the lacrimal gland. Because of ocular side effects, such as the development of cataracts and glaucoma and overgrowth of conjunctival and lacrimal tract fungi, prolonged use is discouraged. Topical use is contraindicated, since little is gained in therapy of disease of the lacrimal drainage system by the use of local steroid preparations. However, at the end of a dacryocystorhinostomy operation, some surgeons instill a corticosteroid ointment into the lacrimal sac area to minimize the postoperative inflammatory reaction.

For systemic use, prednisone is the most used and least expensive corticosteroid. Because it is a short-acting agent with low mineral corticoid activity, side effects, including sodium and water retention, are less than those seen with the use of cortisone or hydrocortisone. When employing corticosteroid therapy, it is recommended that the smallest dose possible be used. Short-term exposure to steroids is relatively safe, and when given for less than two weeks, most adverse reactions are avoided. When long-term use is indicated, every-other-day dosage has been suggested to reduce systemic side effects. Adverse reactions include peptic ulcer, hypokalemia, superinfections, suppression of growth, central nervous system effects, osteoporosis, cataracts, glaucoma, atrophy of the skin, myopathy, and systemic edema.

The usual dose of prednisone when used for anti-inflammatory activity in chronic granulomatous inflammation of the lacrimal gland is 10 to 20 mg per day in divided doses.

TABLE 7-1. ANTIBIOTICS OF CHOICE

Organism	First Choice	Alternatives
Gram-positive cocci		
Staphylococcus aureus		
Nonpenicillinase-producing	Penicillin G or V	A cephalosporin, clindamycin, vancomycin
Penicillinase-producing	Oxacillin, methicillin, nafcillin	A cephalosprorin, clindamycin, vancomycin
Streptococcus pyogenes	Penicillin G or V	Erythromycin, a cephalosporin
Streptococcus anaerobic	Penicillin G	Clindamycin, a tetracycline, erythromycin
Streptococcus pneumoniae	Penicillin G or V	A cephalosporin; erythromycin
Gram-negative cocci		
Neisseria gonorrhoeae	Penicillin G, a tetracycline	Ampicillin, cefoxitin, erythromycin
Gram-positive bacilli		
Bacillus anthracis	Penicillin G	Erythromycin, a tetracycline
Clostridium perfringens (*welchii*)	Penicillin G	Erythromycin, a tetracycline
Cornyebacterium diphtheriae	Erythromycin	Penicillin G
Enteric gram-negative bacilli		
Bacteroides		
Oropharyngeal strains	Penicillin G	Clindamycin, chloramphenicol, ampicillin, a tetracycline
Gastrointestinal strains	Clindamycin	Chloramphenicol, ampicillin, a tetracycline
Enterobacter	Gentamicin	Tobramycin, chloramphenicol, a tetracycline, carbenicillin
Escherichia coli	Gentamicin or tobramycin	Ampicillin; carbenicillin
Klebsiella pneumoniae	Gentamicin or tobramycin	A cephalosporin, a tetracycline, chloramphenicol
Proteus mirabilis	Ampicillin	Amoxicillin, a cephalosporin, gentamicin or tobramycin
Other gram-negative bacilli		
Acinetobacter (*Mima-Herellea*)	Gentamicin or tobramycin	Kanamycin, doxycycline, chloramphenicol
Haemophilus influenzae	Chloramphenicol plus ampicillin	Trimethoprim-sulfamethoxazole
Pseudomonas aeruginosa	Carbenicillin or ticarcillin with tobramycin or gentamicin	
Actinomycetes		
Actinomyces israelii (*actinomycosis*)	Penicillin G	A tetracycline
Nocardia	Trisulfapyrimidines	Trimethoprim-sulfamethoxazole

Adapted from The Medical Letter on Drugs and Therapeutics, 24:24, March 5, 1982.

Artificial Tear Solutions

Commercially available artificial tears contain surfactants and viscous agents that fall into three groups:

1. Cellulose ethers, such as methylcellulose 0.25 percent, hydroxyethylcellulose 0.2 percent and hydroxypropylmethylcellulose 0.5 percent

2. Polyvinyl alcohol 0.5 and 3 percent

3. Mucomimetic polymers—polyoxyethylene

These solutions are packaged in drop bottles with one of several different preservatives—benzalkonium chloride 0.01 percent, thimerosal 0.002 percent, or chlorobutanol 0.5 percent.[4, 5]

The addition of viscosity-producing chemicals to normal saline produces a prolonged retention time for these artificial tears, but all such drops exit from the eye after a few minutes. Tear substances may dry on the lid margin, producing crusts or a sticky residue, and some artificial tears cause distortion or blurred vision after instillation.

None of these substances is entirely successful, since the retention time is so short, and to be effective the solution must be added to the eyes constantly at intervals too frequent to be practical. However, in some few cases, instillation of such agents eight to twelve times a day may be the only means of providing symptomatic relief. A recent device for the prolongation of the effectiveness of moistening agents is the hydroxypropyl-cellulose rod. It is inserted into the cunjunctival fornix (see Chap. 13.)

Diagnostic Agents

Fluorescein. Testing lacrimal excretion with the Jones dye test or Milder's fluorescein dye disappearance test is best done with fluorescein solution. Fluorescein is available as a 2 percent solution, either in its pure form or in combination with topical anesthetics. It also is packaged as sterile filter paper slips with the ends impregnated with fluorescein. Since such solutions have been known to become easily contaminated with *Pseudomonas,* the safest method of application is the one-use 1 ml sterile container of 2 percent fluorescein solution.

Rose Bengal. Used as a 1 percent solution or in the form of impregnated filter paper strips, rose bengal is useful for staining the devitalized cells of the conjunctiva in patients who have dry eye syndrome. Although rose bengal is available as a solution, the rose bengal strips are more convenient and are recommended.

Schirmer Test Papers. Cut strips of filter paper measuring 5 by 30 mm are packaged for use in testing tear production. A marked 5-mm end of the strip is folded and inserted into the lateral one third of the conjunctival sac along the lower lid and removed after 5 minutes to demonstrate a normal range of 10 to 25 mm of wetting of the strip.

Topical Anesthetic Agents

Most surgery of the lacrimal tract can be accomplished using regional anesthesia, and topical anesthesia alone is frequently used for diagnostic and minor surgical procedures, such as irrigation, probing, and intubation. Popular agents available for such use are cocaine 5 percent, benoxinate 0.4 percent, proparacaine 0.5 percent, and tetracaine 0.5 percent. Detailed information about these agents can be found in the AMA drug evaluations.

Cocaine in a 5 percent solution is excellent for use as an intranasal surface anesthetic. It provides a profound loss of sensation and also is a strong vasoconstrictor. Because of this latter trait, it is unnecessary and even dangerous to use it in combination with epinephrine. Cocaine packs placed above and below the inferior turbinate provide anesthesia to the middle and lower portions of the nasolacrimal duct and also aid in visualization of this area. There is a rapid loss of sensation (1 minute), and anesthesia lasts for up to 2 hours.

Cocaine is not recommended for topical use in the eye as it can cause mydriasis, lid retraction, and punctate keratopathy with sloughing of the corneal epithelium. In fact, it has been used to aid in the debridement of the cornea in herpetic dendritic ulceration.

The three most frequently used topical anesthetic agents are benoxinate, proparacaine, and tetracaine. The potency and length of anesthesia with these agents may be enhanced by using a drop of 1:1000 epinephrine prior to instillation of the anesthetic. For lacrimal use, soaking a cotton applicator with the agent and placing it between the upper and lower puncta while the patient closes the eye increases the anesthetic effect.

Benoxinate hydrochloride 0.4 percent has an average anesthesia onset of about 1 minute, and its effect lasts approximately 20 to 30 minutes. Because of the latency in onset of the anesthesia, benoxinate causes stinging on instillation, but there is less punctate keratopathy than is seen with other topical agents, such as tetracaine.

Proparacaine hydrochloride in a 0.5 percent solution produces less burning on instillation than any topical ophthalmic anesthetic because it has a rapid onset of 20 seconds. The effect lasts for 15 minutes. As with all topical anesthetic agents, allergic reactions have been reported with the use of this drug.

Tetracaine hydrochloride 0.5 percent is a

potent surface anesthetic. Its onset develops slowly, and its action lasts for about 15 minutes. Allergies and corneal damage occur with prolonged use, and sulfonamides, mercury, and silver salts should not be used concomitantly.

TOXICOLOGIC REVIEW OF SYSTEMIC AND LOCAL DRUGS AFFECTING THE LACRIMAL SYSTEM

Several classes of topical ophthalmic medications produce toxic changes in the lacrimal tract. The most frequent offenders are the miotics (notably the anticholinesterases) plus antiviral and other drugs, such as topical antimicrobials, that may cause allergic or cicatricial changes in mucous membranes. Certain systemic drugs also have lacrimal implications. Steroids are known to decrease lysozyme production and thus allow increased growth of pathogens in the conjunctival sac. Anesthetic agents decrease tear production.[6, 7] For this reason, the eyes of individuals given general anesthesia must be closed tightly, protected with moist patches, or have ointment placed in them during prolonged surgical procedures.

The long-term use of miotics may induce epiphora in glaucoma patients. In 1951, Shaffer and Ridgway described a permanent obstruction of the nasolacrimal passages in 71 percent of patients where furmethide was used to treat glaucoma.[8] They compared this figure with the 2.5 percent of patients treated with other miotics who had increased tearing. Following their report, furmethide was withdrawn from use.

In 1980, Wobig reported to the American Academy of Ophthalmology that 15 percent of his patients needing a dacrycystorhinostomy had a history of long-term use of glaucoma medications.[9] He noted that 8 percent used pilocarpine and phospholine iodide. He found that all such patients required either a conjunctivocystorhinostomy with a Jones tube or insertion of silicone tubing through the puncta and canaliculi to open the cicatricial changes of the upper drainage system. He also noted that these patients had all teared for a considerable length of time because their ophthalmologists felt that the epiphora was due to stimula-

tion of the lacrimal gland by the miotic.

A review of reports from the National Registry of Drug-induced Ocular Side Effects reveals that "lacrimal disease, punctal stenosis, and cicatrization" have been mentioned as side effects from a large number of miotic preparations. These include furmethide, pilocarpine, echothiophate, and demecarium.[8, 10-14] In addition, some sympathomimetic agents have been incriminated, with neostigmine and epinephrine both reported as medications causing lacrimal side effects.[14, 15] Punctal occlusion may occur with these drugs, but more commonly the black casts that form in the lacrimal drainage system from oxidized epinephrine products are seen.

Antiviral agents and antimetabolites also can cause cicatricial changes in the puncta and canaliculi. The antiviral agents, idoxuridine, vidarabine, and trifluridine, have all been incriminated.[16-22] Among the antimetabolites, thiotepa is the most commonly mentioned drug causing punctal and canalicular occlusion, since it was once widely used to reduce neovascularity following pterygium surgery.[23]

If chronic epiphora occurs in patients who have a persistent need for the antiviral agents, it might be wise to consider a recommendation of Wobig, who stated that at the first hint of epiphora in herpes simplex patients who have a negative Jones I dye test, silicone tubing should be inserted into the nasolacrimal drainage system to prevent the need for a subsequent conjunctivocystorhinostomy.[9]

Dry eye syndrome similar to keratitis sicca and even Stevens-Johnson changes in the mucosa have been reported as toxic reactions to certain drugs, including such antibiotics as penicillin and neosporin and the sulfa drugs. Systemic propranolol, cromolyn, nadolol, and heparin are among other medications mentioned.[24-30] Topical timolol may also cause dry eye findings in rare instances.

There is a possibility that any medication used topically or systemically may cause toxicity, with changes in the mucous membrane of the conjunctiva and the lacrimal passages. Ophthalmologists should be aware of this threat, and dacryologists should treat patients early who develop tearing secondary to cicatricial side effects of topical drugs.

REFERENCES

1. The Medical Letter on Drugs and Therapeutics. New Rochelle, NY, Medical Letter, Inc., 1982, Vol 1, pp 21–27
2. Physicians' Desk Reference for Ophthalmology. Oradell, NJ, Medical Economics Company, 1981-82
3. AMA Drug Evaluations, 3rd ed. Littleton, MA, Publishing Sciences Group, 1977
4. Lemp MA: Artificial tear solutions. Int Ophthalmol Clin 13:221, 1973
5. Waring GO, Harris, RR: Double mask evaluation of a poloxamer artificial tear in keratoconjunctivitis sicca. Symp Ocular Ther 2:127, 1979.
6. Krupin T, Becker B: General anesthesia and the eye. Symp Ocular Ther 2:120, 1979
7. Krupin T, Cross D, Becker B: Decreased basal tear production associated with general anesthesia. Arch Ophthalmol 95:107, 1977
8. Shaffer RN, Ridgway WL: Furmethide iodide in the production of dacryostenosis. Am J Ophthalmol 34:718, 1951
9. Wobig JL: Personal communication, 1981
10. Zimmerman TJ IV: Pilocarpine. Ophthalmology 88:85, 1981
11. Ostler HB, et al.: Drug-induced cicatrization of the conjunctiva. In O'Connor GR (ed.): Immunological Diseases of the Mucous Membrane. New York, Masson, 1980, pp 149-158
12. Hiscox, PDA, McCulloch C: The effect of echothiophate iodide on systemic cholinesterase. Can J Ophthalmol 1:274, 1966
13. Andersen KE, Maibach HI: Allergic reaction of drugs used topically. Clin Toxicol 16:415, 1980
14. Tripathi RC, Tripathi BJ: Ocular toxicity in pathology of drug-induced and toxic diseases. To be published
15. Moses RA: Adler's Physiology of the Eye, 6th ed. St. Louis, Mosby, 1975, pp 21-22
16. Patterson A, Jones BR: The management of ocular herpes. Trans Ophthalmol Soc UK 87:59, 1967
17. Sugar J, et al.: Trifluorothymidine treatment of herpes simplex epithelial keratitis in comparison with idoxuridine. Ann Ophthalmol 12:611, 1980
18. Bron AJ: Mechanisms of ocular toxicity. In Garrod JW (ed.): Drug Toxicity. London, Taylor & Francis, 1979, pp 229-253
19. Laibson PR, et al.: Ara-A and IDU therapy of human superficial herpetic keratitis. Invest Ophthalmol 14:762, 1975
20. McGill JI, et al.: Adenine arabinoside in the management of herpetic keratitis. Trans Ophthalmol Soc UK 95:246, 1975
21. PDR Supplement A-1980. Oradell, NJ, Medical Economics Company, 1980, pp 56-57.
22. Trifluridine (Viroptic) for herpetic keratitis. Med Lett Drugs Ther 46:48, 1980
23. Gonzalves JOR, Magalhaes MM: O uso tio tepa no pos operatorio do pterigio e outras neoplasias conjuntivais. Rev Bras Oftal 33:829, 1974
24. Davies GE: Adverse reactions to practolol. In Turk JL, Parkers D (eds.): Drug and Immune Responsiveness. Baltimore, University Park Press, 1979, pp 199-210.
25. Idanpaan-Heikkila JE, Hastbacka J, Jarvinen, H.J.: Eye and skin reactions precede practolol peritonitis. Lancet 2:1354, 1977
26. Adverse reactions to cromolyn sodium. Drug Bulletin 9(2), US Food and Drug Administration, 1978, p. 24.
27. Krieglstein G: Nadolol: A new beta-blocking agent; dose dependent, duration of action, and comparative efficacy. Ophthalmol Reporter 5:4, 1980
28. PDR Supplement A-1980. Oradell, NJ, Medical Economics Company, 1980, pp 64–66
29. Soll, DB: Evaluation of timolol in chronic open-angle glaucoma once a day vs twice a day. Arch Ophthalmol 98:2178, 1980
30. Willcockson J, Willcockson T: Timolol: double-blind comparison with pilocarpine and open-angle glaucoma. Curr Ther Res 27: 538, 1980

8

DIAGNOSTIC TESTS OF LACRIMAL FUNCTION

BENJAMIN MILDER

It is axiomatic that accurate diagnosis is dependent upon accurate diagnostic tests, tests that can be performed with precision, that can be repeated with reliability, and that are susceptible to unambiguous interpretation. For a diagnostic test to be useful, it must be accessible to every practitioner. The materials must be readily available, the instrumentation and technique must be simple, and the procedure must not be unduly time consuming. In short, it must be a clinical tool. The difficulty with most clinical tests is that they are too "clinical," lacking the precision, reliability, and quantitative capability of more sophisticated laboratory procedures.

It is unnecessary to make apologies for the spectrum of clinical diagnostic tests used in the study of lacrimal disease. They are simple and readily available, and they have demonstrated their usefulness over the years. However, it is important to recognize their limitations and to maximize their usefulness by standardizing, insofar as possible, both the techniques and the interpretation. It has been suggested, and we would agree, that accurate clinical diagnosis

depends on the use of more than one test. In some instances, modification of a standardized test serves as additional confirmatory diagnostic evidence.

TESTS OF LACRIMAL SECRETION

Schirmer Test

Since Schirmer described his blotting paper test for lacrimal secretion in 1903,[1] it has been the most maligned of all lacrimal function tests. It is interesting that, despite the endless calumnies heaped upon Dr. Schirmer's test, it is still the most universally employed means of evaluating lacrimal secretion.

The routine Schirmer test, sometimes named the "Schirmer I" test, is performed without topical anesthesia. White filter paper, usually 41 Whatman, is cut into strips 5.0 mm wide and 50.0 mm long. The strip of filter paper is folded 5.0 mm from one end, and the short, folded end is inserted into the inferior conjunctival fornix at the junction of the middle and temporal thirds of the eyelids. The patient is instructed to close the eyes lightly. After 5 minutes, the strips are removed, and the extent of wetting is measured from the fold. Precut filter paper strips are available commercially.

Figures 8-1 through 8-4 appear on Color Plate I, between pages 78 and 79.

As with all clinical procedures, there are many individual differences in the technique of performing this Schirmer test. Some physicians prefer to have the patient keep the eyes open and rotated upward during the test. Some use litmus paper as the absorbent medium, since the extent of wetting is more readily visible because of the change in color.

In a series comparing filter paper and blue litmus paper, the author found little difference between the two. The average Schirmer I result for filter paper was 12 mm (range 1 to 27 mm) and for blue litmus paper 10 mm (range 0 to 27 mm) (Fig. 8-1, Color Plate I).

The rate of tear secretion is not uniform during the 5-minute test period. Most of the wetting of the absorbent paper takes place during the first minutes of the tests, and it has been suggested that, if the test is performed for 1 minute and the result is multiplied by 3, the final result will be closely comparable to the standard 5-minute technique.

It can be said for the method described here, as well as for all the variations in the test, that the chief essential is that the test should always be performed in the same manner for every patient, every time. The only absolute requirement for any modification of the Schirmer technique is that it be performed for both eyes simultaneously in every case.

Basic Secretion Test

It is generally held that there is *basic* and *reflex* tear secretion. Although this is still debated,[2] such a distinction is useful in rationalizing quantitative variations in tear flow. The basic secretion amounts to 0.50 to 1.25 ml per day[3] and represents that part of our lacrimal secretion which performs the essential physiologic tear functions (Chapter 5). The reflex secretion is a response to any of a wide variety of physiologic, neurologic, or psychologic stimuli. Basic secretion is reported to be elaborated by the accessory lacrimal glands of Krause and Wolfring, while the reflex tearing is said to come from the orbital and palpebral lobes of the lacrimal gland.[4] Without entering into a discussion of the site of origin of basic and reflex tears or whether they differ only in rate of secretion, it is evident that the Schirmer test as normally performed (without topical anesthesia) does not distinguish between basic and reflex secretion. When the Schirmer test results indicate excessive tear secretion, the examiner does not know what fraction of that Schirmer test result is due to basic secretion and what fraction is due to reflex secretion, since the latter could be stimulated by the paper strips themselves.

If there is excessive secretion, the Schirmer test can be modified by instilling a *topical anesthetic* into the conjunctival sac, thereby eliminating any reflex stimulus from conjunctival irritation. By subtracting this "basic secretion value" from the original Schirmer result the reflex component can be determined. For example, if the Schirmer I test result is 35.0 mm in 5 minutes, and the basic secretion test (with topical anesthesia) is 10.0 mm, the difference of 25.0 mm would represent reflex secretion. In this way, one can rule out any exaggeration of the test results arising from irritation by the paper strips.

Schirmer II Test

When the initial Schirmer test yields subnormal values, it is often desirable to assess the reflex capability of the system. To determine this, the Schirmer II test is performed by using a topical anesthestic in the conjunctival sac to eliminate the effect of local irritation. The Schirmer test is then repeated while stimulating the trigeminal nerve by lightly touching the nasal mucosa with a cotton applicator or by using, as a reflex stimulus, ammonium chloride on a cotton pledget held at the external nares. The amount by which the Schirmer test is increased in this manner represents reflex secretion.

With the modifications described, the Schirmer test serves a useful purpose in the clinical evaluation of tear secretion—notwithstanding such comments as that by Duke-Elder: ". . . the test is, of course, rough and ready, without any pretence to accurate assessment . . ."[5]

The usual range of Schirmer test results is 10 to 30 mm, decreasing progressively with age. Average values, using litmus paper, are shown in Table 8-1.

Schirmer test values in the first three decades of life are higher in females. With succeeding decades, the rate falls more rapidly in females than in males.[6]

TABLE 8-1. SCHIRMER I TEST

Age	Normal Range*
To 30 years	25+ mm
30–60 years	10–25 mm
Over 60 years	5–10 mm

* Schirmer I values of 4 mm or less may represent true hyposecretion, and values of 2 mm or less are usually associated with signs and symptoms of dry eye syndrome.

Tear Film Break-up Time

The tear film consists of a superficial oily surface, a principal aqueous layer, and a deep, thin mucin layer. The multilayered nature of the tear film has long been recognized. It remained for Lemp and his associates, in their important researches, to point out the dynamics of the interactions between these layers[7] (Chapter 5). Until their work, little attention was paid to the fact that the Schirmer test was essentially a measure of the aqueous component of the tear film. If the mucin layer is not present to render the corneal epithelium hydrophilic, signs and symptoms of the dry eye syndrome may be present even if there is adequate aqueous component.

The integrity of the mucin layer can be assessed by another clinical test, the tear film break-up time (BUT). This test is performed with the patient seated at the slit lamp microscope. One drop of fluorescein is instilled into the conjunctival sac. The patient is instructed to blink once to spread the fluorescein over the cornea, and then he is instructed to refrain from blinking. With a cobalt blue filter, the observer scans the cornea for the first appearance of dry spots, identified by fluorescein-free areas. In the cobalt-filtered blue light, these fluorescein-free areas appear black. Normal tear film break-up time is 15 to 30 seconds or longer, and a BUT of less than 10 seconds suggests mucin deficiency. If the BUT is subnormal and the patient has dry eye symptoms, mucomimetic agents would be the treatment of choice as replacement therapy.

Rose Bengal Test

Rose bengal stains devitalized epithelial cells. If tear secretion is deficient, the application of a 1 percent solution of rose bengal to the eye will result in staining of the abnormal epithelium of the conjunctiva, particularly in the interpalpebral space. The intensity and extent of staining can be graded on a scale of 0 to 4+. The heavier staining areas (3+ to 4+) are found in clinically significant lacrimal hyposecretion. Thus, the rose bengal test is, indirectly, a measure of tear secretion (Fig. 8-2, Color Plate I).

Tear Lysozyme Determination

Lysozyme is a long-chain, high molecular weight, proteolytic enzyme which has bacteriostatic activity. It is found in most tissues and secretions. In human tears, it makes up 21 to 23 percent of the total protein of tears.[8] In excessive tear formation, lysozyme levels are decreased by dilution. However, in reduced or absent tear secretion, as in Sjögren's syndrome, lysozyme levels are characteristically much reduced.

The tear lysozyme level can be measured by a bacterial growth inhibition test, using the bacterium *Micrococcus lysodeikticus*.[9] This method of determination of lysozyme employs a 6.0 mm filter paper disc, placed in the conjunctival sac to absorb tear fluid. The inhibition of bacterial growth around the disc is then measured as an expression of lysozyme activity. Results are recorded in units of activity per microliter of tears. Fifty or more units per microliter is normal.

TESTS OF LACRIMAL EXCRETION

Abnormalities in the tear drainage process are more than a nuisance. The accumulation of excess tears in the conjunctival sac and on the cornea can be responsible for infections, blepharitis, and disturbances in vision. We have seen surgeons and dentists completely disabled by epiphora.

The normal elimination of tears involves several physiologic mechanisms to carry away that portion of the tears not lost by evaporation. On the average, about 25 percent of tears are lost by evaporation. The physiologic mechanisms of tear excretion include the squeegee effect of lid closure during blinking, the capillary action of the puncta, the shortening of the canaliculi with blinking, and the influence of blinking on the sac during the orbicularis contraction. According to Jones,[10] this pumping action is responsible for the aspiration of tears into the sac and the evacuation of tears into the nasolacrimal duct. In addition, there are lesser physiologic influences, such as gravity and convection currents of air in the nasal passages. Murube has performed experiments that have suggested to him that gravity plays a greater role in normal tear outflow than has previously been considered.[11]

Up to the present time, no one single clinical test is able to separate these several elements of the tear drainage mechanism and to localize the site of impairment of outflow function. Therefore, we must use several lacrimal excretion tests in order to obtain adequate diagnostic information.

It is convenient to think of the outflow system as having an *upper* and *lower* part. The upper part is made up of the lid margins, puncta, canaliculi, and common canaliculus, while the lower part consists of the lacrimal sac, nasolacrimal duct, and plica semilunaris. Such a separation is arbitrary but convenient for diagnostic purposes.

We shall discuss several tests of tear excretion that combine the virtues necessary for a useful clinical evaluation. These tests require no complicated instrumentation, they are simple to perform and easy to interpret. Finally, we shall combine these tests so that they provide an orderly diagnostic plan.

Jones Fluorescein Tests

Jones Primary Dye Test. In the Jones primary dye test, fluorescein is instilled into the conjunctival sac, and, if the excretory system is normal, the dye can be recovered from the nose within a period of 5 minutes. As with all clinical procedures, there are individual variations in technique and materials.

In our method, the patient is seated in an ophthalmic chair, and the inferior meatus and turbinate are sprayed with 4 percent cocaine hydrochloride or with 4 percent lidocaine hydrochloride. One drop of 2 percent fluorescein solution, from a sterile container, is instilled into the conjunctival sac of each eye. The nose is examined at 2 minutes and again at 5 minutes for evidence of spontaneous flow of the flu-

orescein from the conjunctival sac into the nose. This is accomplished by introducing a cotton-tipped, wire nasal applicator into the inferior meatus of the nose under direct visualization, employing a nasal speculum. A binocular, indirect ophthalmoscope provides excellent paraaxial illumination for this procedure. The applicator is moved up into the vault of the inferior meatus and then swept posteriorly and across the floor of the nose before it is removed. If any fluorescein staining appears on the cotton swab, at either 2 or 5 minutes, the test is considered a *positive* primary Jones test and is indicative of normal tear excretion. If fluorescein is not recovered on the cotton applicator, further attempts to verify the presence of fluorescein in the nose can be made by having the patient blow into a tissue or by using a cobalt blue light to examine the region of the inferior meatus and turbinate. It is even possible to irrigate a small amount of clear saline into the inferior meatus to determine if fluorescein can be recovered in this manner.

False positive results are very rare with the Jones primary dye test. Therefore, a positive result is a clear indication of normal tear outflow. However, false negative test results are less rare, and because of technical problems, the examiner may be unable to verify the presence of fluorescein in the nose even if the outflow system is normal. Therefore, although a positive test means normal outflow, a negative test does not completely rule out the possibility that the system is normal.

Jones Secondary Dye Test. If, after 5 minutes, no dye is recovered in the primary test, the remaining fluorescein is flushed from the conjunctival sac with clear irrigating solution. The puncta are then anesthetized with a topical anesthetic in the usual manner as for lacrimal irrigation. Following this anesthesia, clear saline or other irrigating solution is flushed through the nasolacrimal system. The lacrimal cannula is introduced into the lower canaliculus, the patient's head is tilted forward over a basin, and a solution is flushed through the lacrimal system (Fig. 8-3, Color Plate I).

If this irrigant emerges from the nose stained with fluorescein, the secondary dye test is considered to be positive. If the irrigant comes through clear, the secondary dye test is negative. A positive secondary dye test verifies that the fluorescein originally instilled into the conjunctival sac had migrated into the lacrimal sac or, at least, into the horizontal limb of the canaliculus. Such a positive secondary dye test proves that the upper system is functioning and that the lower system is patent. A negative secondary dye test indicates that no fluorescein had entered the excretory system, and, therefore, the upper system is malfunctioning.

The secondary dye test is a measure of patency of the lower system but does not evaluate its function, since the irrigant is instilled under pressure. If one obtains a positive primary Jones test, the excretory system may be considered to be normal. However, since a positive primary test cannot always be elicited in some apparently normal individuals, the combination of a negative primary dye test and a positive secondary dye test may indicate partial outflow obstruction but may also be compatible with normal outflow function in some cases.

The validity of the primary Jones test as an index of normal lacrimal excretory function has been verified in several ways. One interesting observation has been the difference in primary dye test results in bilaterally normal outflow systems as compared with unilateral normals. The tendency for lacrimal disease to occur bilaterally is well recognized. Therefore, in those patients who have clinical evidence of outflow impairment on one side, it would be expected that the opposite, apparently normal, side might harbor evidences of latent malfunction. In one study of 200 patients having normal lacrimal outflow systems, it was found that, for bilateral normals, more than 80 percent had positive primary dye tests. However, in those who had unilateral lacrimal disease, the normal side of these patients yielded only 58 percent positive primary dye tests. Even more striking, if the primary dye test was limited to a 2-minute duration, positive primary dye tests were found in 70 percent of bilateral normals but only 29 percent of unilateral normals.[12] This observation supports the validity of the primary Jones test as an index of normal outflow.

It would seem reasonable that the rate of tear secretion could influence tests of lacrimal excretion. A high rate of lacrimal secretion would aid in the flushing action of the fluorescein solution in the primary dye test. In order to study this question, a series of normal patients underwent Jones dye tests after having had a preliminary Schirmer test. The distribution of Schirmer values corresponds closely with known normal values. When the primary Jones dye test results were correlated with the Schirmer tests for each patient, a direct relationship was found between the Schirmer test result and the rapidity with which the primary dye test was found to be positive. The higher Schirmer test values were associated with the most rapidly positive dye tests. Conversely, the slower the primary dye test, the greater was the number of hyposecretors.[12]

Fluorescein Dye Disappearance Test

Fluorescein, or other colored solutions, will disappear from the eye when the lacrimal excretory system is normal but will remain in the conjunctival sac for an abnormal length of time when outflow is impaired or when the outflow system is completely obstructed. This simple test or observation has a higher degree of reliability than any other lacrimal outflow test. However, it does not distinguish between impairment in the upper and lower portions of the outflow system. For example, an everted punctum would yield the same fluorescein retention in the eye as would a complete nasolacrimal duct obstruction. However, this test can be employed in conjunction with the primary and secondary dye tests of Jones to increase the clinician's diagnostic yield.

For the fluorescein disappearance test, it is essential to introduce into the conjunctival sac a standard volume of a standard concentration of fluorescein. Since we employed a single drop of 2 percent fluorescein solution in the primary dye test of Jones, this same drop serves for the fluorescein dye disappearance evaluation. It is necessary only to examine the bulbar conjunctiva and the tear strip along the lower lid margin to evaluate the amount of retained fluorescein. This can be graded from 0 to 4+ retention (Fig. 8-4, Color Plate I). Where the retained fluorescein after 5 minutes is 0 or 1+, the outflow system is normal. Where the retained fluorescein is 3+ or 4+, the outflow is impaired. A 2+ retention is borderline, usually indicative of some impairment. The fluorescein which escapes from the conjunctival sac onto the skin of the eyelid does not influence the test in any sig-

TABLE 8-2. FLUORESCEIN DYE DISAPPEARANCE IN NORMAL SUBJECTS

	FDD Positive (0/1+ Retention)	FDD Negative (2+/4+ Retention)	Totals
If Jones I is:			
Positive at 1 minute	111 (97%)	3 (3%)	114
Positive at 5 minutes	19 (91%)	2 (9%)	21
Total	130 (96%)	5 (4%)	135
If Jones II is:			
Positive	33 (79%)	9 (21%)	42
If Jones I and II are:			
Negative	0	0	0
Totals	163	14	177

nificant fashion. In known bilateral normal systems, the fluorescein dye disappearance was positive (that is, no fluorescein remained in the conjunctival sac after 5 minutes) in more than 90 percent of patients. A false positive dye disappearance test in the presence of impaired outflow is extremely uncommon. When the primary dye test of Jones was positive, the dye disappearance test was also positive in 96 percent of normals, essentially a 1:1 correlation. In patients with known abnormal lacrimal outflow, 45 percent of secondary dye tests were positive, but only 14 percent of fluorescein dye disappearance tests were positive. These data confirm the fact that a positive secondary dye test of Jones is not an indicator of whether the system functions normally in lacrimal excretion, but it does define normal function for the upper system and patency for the lower system.[12]

In the Yamaguchi[13] modification of the fluorescein dye disappearance test, a 5.0 mm disc of fluorescein filter paper is placed on the upper temporal quadrant of the bulbar conjunctiva. After normal blinking for 2 or 3 minutes, the paper is removed from the conjunctival sac. In this manner, fluorescein dissolves into the tear fluid without gross staining of the eyelids. The fluorescein concentration is then read from the fluorescein color in the marginal tear strip. Using this method, the time required for disappearance of the fluorescein from the marginal tear strips is normally 15 to 20 minutes, somewhat shorter in the very young patient. In the patients with obstruction of the puncta or canaliculi, the fluorescein concentra-

tion remains unchanged, and after several minutes, the epiphora causes the fluorescein to stain the eyelids. In obstructive dacryocystitis, the fluorescein disappears quite slowly from the marginal tear strip, and some fluorescein retention can be detected for as long as 150 minutes after instillation of the fluorescein.

The Yamaguchi technique would seem to be somewhat more meticulous and orderly than that described by the authors. However, when the dye disappearance time is determined from staining of the bulbar conjunctiva, the tests can be accomplished clinically within 5 minutes. When the fluorescein concentration is determined from the intensity of fluorescein in the lid margin tear strip, 15 to 25 minutes or longer is required to perform the test.[14] A survey of normal patients revealed that the fluorescein dye disappearance test, as performed by the authors, has a reliability factor of 96 percent (Table 8-2). Thus, it is a useful, rapid, clinical test which can be performed as a part of the Jones dye test procedure or as a rapid, simple screening test. Combining the information from the Jones and the fluorescein dye disappearance tests produces a high yield of diagnostic information.

The flow sheet (Fig. 8-5) shows that a positive primary dye test of Jones is satisfactory to establish the fact of normal lacrimal excretion. A positive secondary dye test, when combined with the disappearance of fluorescein from the eye, is strongly indicative of normal outflow function. However, a positive secondary dye test when combined with retention of fluores-

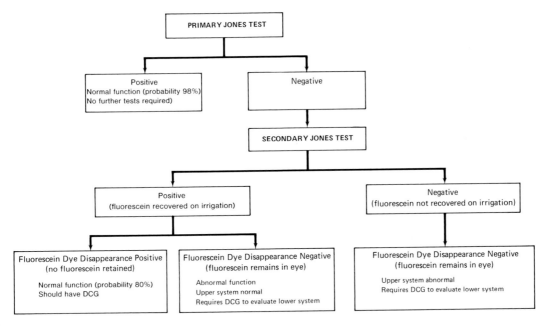

NOTE:
Where the excretory system cannot be irrigated successfully, the Primary Jones, Secondary Jones, and the Fluorescein Dye Disappearance tests will all be negative, and definitive study will rest with probing and DCG.

Figure 8-5. Flow sheet: Clinical interpretation of tests of lacrimal excretory function in a patent system.

cein in the eye is indicative of a functional block. As the chart indicates, in such cases, further attempts at localization must be undertaken by dacryocystography.

Taste Tests of Lacrimal Excretion

Sweetening agents, such as glucose solution, have been instilled into the conjunctival sac as a test of lacrimal excretion. If the patient reports that he can taste the agent instilled into the conjunctival sac, this is presumptive evidence of normal tear outflow. The time interval may be as long as 30 minutes. One of the difficulties with this test is that it cannot be performed on both eyes simultaneously; a second problem is the length of time required to derive the necessary information. However, the greatest drawback is that the test is completely subjective.

Dacryocystography

Roentgenography of the lacrimal excretory passages after instilling a radiopaque contrast agent is one of the most useful lacrimal function tests. Microscintigraphy is a method of sequential imaging of the lacrimal excretory system

after instilling into the conjunctival sac a single drop of a radioactive tracer, such as technitium–99. Although microscintigraphy requires more sophisticated instrumentation than is available for most clinicians, it is a useful method of evaluating lacrimal excretory function with a minimum of hazards. Dacryocystography and microscintigraphy are considered in Chapter 9.

RECENT DEVELOPMENTS

Several interesting developments which have been reported in the past few years are testimony to the evanescent nature of textbooks. While these tests have not yet fulfilled our definition of a useful clinical tool, they could, with further refinements, find their way into the diagnostic armamentarium.

Dacryoscopy. Although attempts at direct visualization of the lacrimal excretory system are not new, the diagnostic possibilities of this technique have been advanced by the recent development of a miniature endoscope[15] having approximately the same caliber as a II Bowman probe. It provides a 61° field of view with 30× magnification of the image. Internal illumination is provided by a 0.5 mm fiberoptic probe, which is inserted into the lacrimal sac through the free canaliculus. Further refinements are underway.

Thermography. Temperature differences at the surface of the skin can be detected by employing an instrument which combines a high-speed infrared scanner, a display unit, and a color monitor.[16] The device is sensitive to temperature differences of 0.5C. Cold water is instilled into the system through a catheter in one canaliculus. Differences can be demonstrated between a low-grade dacryocystitis on one side and a normal lacrimal sac on the other.

Chemiluminescence. Visualization of the lacrimal drainage system by the instillation of a chemiluminescent material may, in time, provide an alternative to dacryocystography.[17] The method employed in this study consisted of an activator (diphenylphthalate) in a glass ampule suspended within a plastic wand which contained dimethylphthalate and tertiary butyl alcohol. When these chemicals mix, an intense green luminescence is produced. Using cadaver models, this technique compared favorably with dacryocystography in locating the site of experimentally produced obstruction in the drainage system. Such a device could prove to be a useful adjunct during surgery.

REFERENCES

1. Schirmer O: Studien zur Physiologie und Pathologie der Tränenabsorderung und Tränenabfuhr. Albrecht von Graefes Arch Klin Ophthalmol 56:197, 1903
2. Jordan A, Baum J: Basic tear flow, does it exist? Ophthalmology 87:920, 1980
3. Adler FH: In Moses RA (ed): Physiology of the Eye, 7th ed. St. Louis, Mosby, 1981
4. Jones LT: The lacrimal secretory system and its treatment. Am J Ophthalmol 62:47, 1966
5. Duke-Elder S: System of Ophthalmology. St. Louis, Mosby, 1952, Vol 5, p S202
6. Henderson JW, Prough WA: Influence of dye and sex on flow of tears. Arch Ophthalmol 43:224, 1950
7. Lemp MA, et al: The pre-corneal tear film: factors in spreading and maintaining a continuous tear film over the corneal surface. Arch Ophthalmol 83:89, 1970
8. Adler FH: In Moses RA (ed): Physiology of the Eye, 7th ed St. Louis, Mosby, 1981, p. 21
9. Mackie IA, Seal DV: Beta-blockers eye complaints and tear secretion (letter). Lancet, 2:1027, 1977
10. Jones LT: The cure of epiphora due to canalicular disorders, trauma and surgical failures on the lacrimal passages. Trans Am Acad Ophthalmol Otolaryngol 66:506, 1962
11. Murube J: On gravity as one of the impelling forces of lacrimal flow. In: Yamaguchi M. (ed): Recent Advances on the Lacrimal System. Tokyo, Asaki Press, 1978, pp 51-61
12. Zappia R, Milder B: Lacrimal drainage function. I. The Jones fluorescein test. Am J Ophthalmol 74:154, 1972
13. Yamaguchi M (ed): Recent Advances on the Lacrimal System. Tokyo, Asaki Press, 1978, p 216
14. Yamaguchi M (ed): Recent Advances on the Lacrimal System. Tokyo, Asaki Press, 1978, p 220
15. Cohen SW, et al: Dacryoscopy. Ophthalmic Surg 10:57, 1979
16. Raflo GT, Chart P, Hurwitz JJ: Thermographic evaluation of the human lacrimal drainage system, Ophthalmic Surg 13:119, 1982
17. Raflo GT, Hurwitz JJ: Assessment of the efficacy of chemiluminescent evaluation of the human lacrimal drainage system. Ophthalmic Surg 13:36, 1982

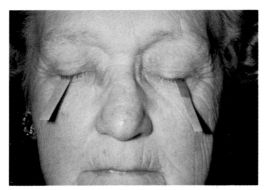

Figure 8-1. Schirmer test using blue litmus paper.

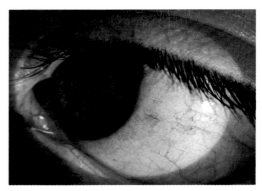

Figure 8-2. Rose bengal staining.

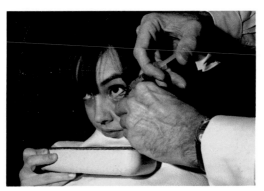

Figure 8-3. Jones secondary dye test—instilling clear irrigant into the excretory system.

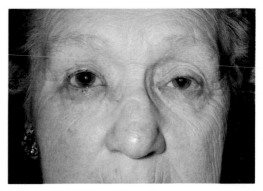

Figure 8-4. Fluorescein dye disappearance test. OD has 4 + retention (nasolacrimal duct obstruction). OS has trace retention (normal).

9

DACRYOCYSTOGRAPHY

BENJAMIN MILDER

The legendary surgeons of the early years of this century, the men with the golden hands—where have they gone? What is responsible for the decline of the virtuoso surgeon, he of the delicate sense of touch and unfailing surgical intuition? The fact is that he has not left but that there are now so many of him that highly skilled surgery is the rule rather than the exception in the operating theaters of the world.

The cloak of mystery has fallen away from the problems of the lacrimal system. The tentative attitude of our earlier colleagues toward lacrimal surgery was not so much a matter of the paucity of patients as it was of the paucity of knowledge of the lacrimal system. Lacrimal surgery has become accessible because in ophthalmology, as in all fields of medicine and surgery, therapeutic advances have followed the development of improved diagnostic tools. Particularly, the ability to visualize organs and organ systems has been an essential ingredient in finding surgical answers to medical problems. Such visualization, whether it be done by endoscopy, photography, or radiographic means, has been the major factor in the decline of the mystique of those virtuoso surgeons who were beyond the province of the larger body of practitioners. Now, direct visualization of the lacrimal system by dacryocystography is avail-

able to complement other diagnostic tests, and the entire field of lacrimal surgery has been brought within the competence of all trained ophthalmologists.

Although radiography of the lacrimal system was attempted as far back as 1909 by Ewing,[1] the term "dacryocystography" first appeared in medical literature in 1954.[2] The availability of this diagnostic tool was made possible by careful delineation of the normal roentgenographic appearance of the lacrimal system and by simplifying the technique. The awareness of this useful diagnostic device gathered momentum slowly and in the past 20 years has blossomed, as evidenced by the increasing numbers of books and papers from medical centers throughout the world and by the plethora of changes, refinements, and alternative methods that have been described. Those techniques that have found their way into the clinical diagnostic armamentarium and are discussed in this chapter include:

- Dacryocystography with oily contrast medium
- Dacryocystography with aqueous contrast medium
- Macrodacryocystography
- Distention dacryocystography

- Subtraction dacryocystography
- Lacrimal microscintigraphy (nuclear scanning)

CONTRAST DACRYOCYSTOGRAPHY

Dacryocystography with Oil-based Contrast Medium

The first attempt at dacryocystography, by Ewing, involved retrograde filling of the nasolacrimal duct with bismuth paste. Subsequently, the system was filled from above with iodized oils. It was felt, initially, that high viscosity media were necessary to obtain adequate contrast visualization of the system. However, because of difficulties of instilling such contrast agents, this diagnostic device lay dormant for the first half of our century until the advent of low viscosity oily media triggered renewed interest in dacryocystography.

Early studies by this author demonstrated that dacryocystography could supply information regarding the *excretory function* of the system as well as the pathologic anatomy and would provide a permanent visual record of both of these parameters.[3] The full benefits of this clinical tool will be achieved only if both of these areas are explored.

Technique. Two of the authors[2a] studied a wide variety of oily and aqueous radioopaque contrast media, and it was concluded that a low-viscosity, iodized oil would be most suitable to obtain the information required. Ethyl iodophenylundecylate (Pantopaque*) is such a contrast agent. It is easily manipulated, readily drawn into a syringe, and instilled without undue pressure into the lacrimal system through an ordinary lacrimal cannula. In a series of more than 2,500 dacryocystograms, no single case of toxicity or hypersensitivity to this agent has been encountered. Inadvertent extravasation of the contrast agent into the subcutaneous tissues has occurred in less than 0.5 percent of cases, and in each instance, the contrast medium has been absorbed uneventfully without residual scarring.

Dacryocystography is performed with the patient seated upright at a roentgen head unit.

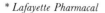

* *Lafayette Pharmacal*

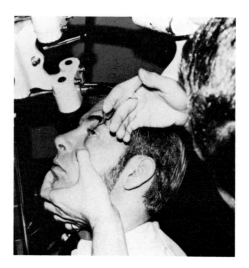

Figure 9-1. Instillation of oil-based contrast medium.

Anesthesia is effected by instilling one drop of a topical anesthetic into each eye and then inserting cotton pledgets soaked in the anesthetic between the puncta. The patient is instructed to keep the eyes closed for a period of 2 minutes, during which time the puncta and proximal canaliculi are well anesthetized. The lacrimal sac is then irrigated gently with saline in order to remove any accumulated secretions, and if the sac is found to be distended, it is decompressed digitally before instilling the contrast agent. Dacryocystography should not be performed in the presence of acute or subacute dacryocystitis.

The patient's head is positioned for the first x-ray picture, then is tilted back, and 1 ml of Pantopaque is instilled into the excretory system of the suspected abnormal side, using a straight lacrimal cannula (Fig. 9-1). On completion of instillation of the contrast medium, the cannula is withdrawn, and the head is positioned immediately for the first exposure, a posteroanterior (Caldwell) view, which is made by placing the forehead and nose against the upright cassette holder and angling the roentgen tube 15° downward. A lateral exposure is made immediately therafter (Fig. 9-2). The entire sequence, including instillation of the contrast medium, can be accomplished within 15 seconds. As the cannula is withdrawn and the patient blinks, tiny droplets of contrast medium

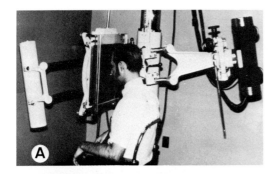

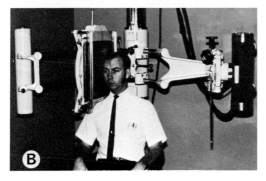

Figure 9-2. Dacryocystography. **A.** Patient positioned for posteroanterior (Caldwell) exposure. **B.** Lateral exposure.

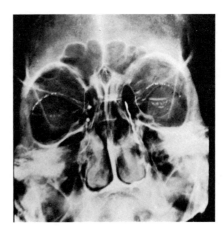

Figure 9-3. Palpebral fissure outlined by contrast agent on cilia.

will adhere to the cilia. If the patient is instructed to keep the eyes open, the palpebral fissures will be outlined by the droplets of contrast agent (Fig. 9-3).

The side having the suspected pathology is examined first, but the opposite side is *always* studied for comparison. When the same procedure is repeated for the opposite side, the face is rotated 15° for the lateral view so as to avoid superimposing the two contrast shadows. Finally, and most importantly, a single posteroanterior view is taken after 30 minutes in order to assess the amount of residual contrast medium remaining in the lacrimal sac and nasolacrimal duct.

The length of time required for 1 ml of contrast agent to pass through the excretory system will depend upon the viscosity of the agent. Using Pantopaque, studies in normal individuals showed that the lacrimal sac will be emptied within 15 minutes, and the nasolacrimal duct will show little residual after 30 minutes. Having established the rate at which this

particular contrast medium empties from a normal system, the 30-minutes follow-up film thus provides key information as to the excretory function of the system. Any substantial residual of contrast agent in the lacrimal sac or in the lacrimal duct signifies impaired outflow, even if there is radiographic evidence of patency. On the other hand, if most of the contrast agent has passed through unimpeded and appears in the nasal cavity, failure to visualize all parts of the outflow system in the initial films is compatible with normal function.

The Normal Dacryocystogram. In the normal dacryocystogram employing Pantopaque, it is unusual to obtain good visualization of the canaliculi or the common canaliculus. If both canaliculi are well visualized, it is likely that there is increased back pressure within the system, indicating some impediment to normal outflow. The same is true for significant filling of the lacrimal sac above the common canaliculus. In the erect patient, there is normally insufficient back pressure to obtain retrograde filling of the cupola of the lacrimal sac. Thus, good visualization of the upper sac is also indicative of some interference with outflow.

In order to assess the extent of filling of the cupola of the sac, it is important to locate the point of entrance of the common canaliculus into the sac. Since the common canaliculus is located immediately posterior to the medial canthal tendon and since it empties into the lat-

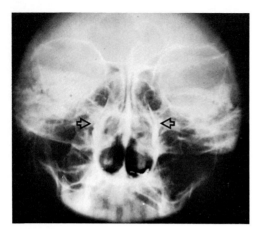

Figure 9-4. Normal sac and duct (posteroanterior view). Note the slender sac shadow, its contour conforming to the bony lacrimal fossa. Sac-duct junction is shown by arrows.

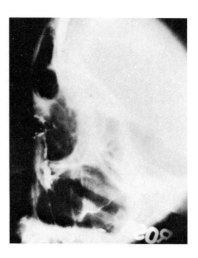

Figure 9-5. Normal sac and duct (lateral view). Sac-duct junction is at the level of the inferior orbital margin.

eral aspect of the lacrimal sac at the junction of its middle and upper third, the practice of outlining the palpebral fissure with droplets of oil on the cilia enables one to locate the position of the medial canthus and, thus, of the common canaliculus.

The normal lacrimal sac is seen, in the posteroanterior view, as a straight or gently curving contrast shadow with its concavity directed laterally, since the lacrimal sac lies within a slightly concave bony lacrimal fossa (Fig. 9-4). Since the vast majority of obstructions in the outflow system occur at the junction of the lacrimal sac and nasolacrimal duct, the location of the sac-duct junction becomes important. The sac shadow tends to be wider at its lowest portion. At the junction of the lacrimal sac and nasolacrimal duct, this widening may take the form of an angulation at the temporal side, identified anatomically as the sinus of Arlt. More often than not, the lacrimal sac and duct are represented by a continuous contrast shadow. When the sinus of Arlt cannot be identified on the roentgenogram, the sac-duct junction can be located by noting the point at which the inferior bony orbital margin intersects the vertical column of contrast medium.

The nasolacrimal duct, in the posteroanterior view, presents in its upper third as a much wider contrast shadow than the lacrimal sac, and the irregularity of its outline suggests

mucosal folds. The midportion of the duct is visualized poorly or not at all, apparently as a result of interruption of the flow of the oily agent by a larger mucosal fold, the spiral valve of Hyrtl (or a fold sometimes identified as the valve of Taillefer). In some instances the spiral configuration of the contrast shadow can be made out clearly. In the lower third of the nasolacrimal duct, the shadow again broadens out at the ostium of the membranous duct.

In the lateral view, the sac and duct have an irregular ribbonlike configuration (Fig. 9-5). In the lateral view, as in the posteroanterior view, the intersection between the floor of the orbit and the contrast medium identifies the sac-duct junction, and an accumulation of contrast medium will be found in the nasopharynx in each patent system. As has been noted previously, nonvisualization of the lacrimal system can occur in a normal patient if all of the contrast medium has moved quickly through the system into the nasopharynx.

The only complication encountered when using this method of dacryocystography has been the rare infiltration of the subcutaneous tissues with the oily contrast medium (Fig. 9-6). As noted these have cleared uneventfully.

Complete Obstruction. If there is complete obstruction of the outflow system at the common

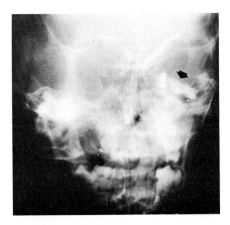

Figure 9-6. Complication of dacryocystography —inadvertent subcutaneous extravasation of contrast agent, left side.

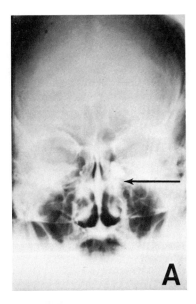

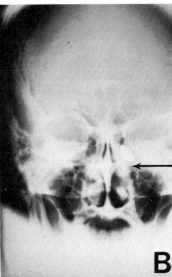

Figure 9-8. Complete obstruction of nasolacrimal system, left side. **A.** At 0 minutes. **B.** At 30 minutes (no change).

canaliculus or internal punctum, the two canaliculi will be well outlined, but no contrast medium will be found in the sac or duct (Fig. 9-7). However, if the complete obstruction lies at the sac-duct junction or in the nasolacrimal duct, the lacrimal sac will frequently be distended, with no contrast medium found in the nose, and the level of obstruction will be clearly delineated. The 30-minute follow-up film will usually show little or no change in the picture. However, when the sac is markedly atonic, there may appear to be some decrease in contrast medium as the result of pooling of the oily

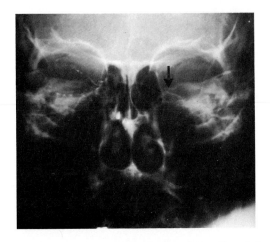

Figure 9-7. Common canaliculus obstruction, left side.

agent in the lacrimal sac or duct (Fig. 9-8). In some instances, postinflammatory scarring will reduce the sac lumen, and valuable information is thus obtained for surgical planning.

In 85 percent of cases of dacryocystitis, the obstruction will occur at the sac-duct junction. Some, however, occur in the mid- or lower duct,

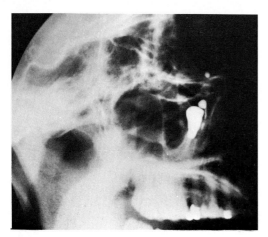

Figure 9-9. Obstruction in lower nasolacrimal duct, lateral view.

and these cases are not infrequently the result of facial fractures involving the bony nasolacrimal canal (Fig. 9-9). It is necessary to identify these low nasolacrimal obstructions, since the usual dacryocystorhinostomy technique would leave the patient with an undesirable cul de sac, capable of sustaining infection.

In a complete obstruction, it is important to note whether the sac is simply distended or whether it is, in addition, displaced from its normal position. A lateral displacement of the sac could indicate a fracture or other disturbance in the area of the lacrimal fossa or could suggest an extrinsic mass displacing the sac. Such differentiations cannot be made by palpation or by irrigating the lacrimal sac. Dacryocystography is essential here.

In the presence of obstructions, partial or complete, the outline of the sac may reveal a diverticulum or a lacrimal sac fistula, both of which would require modification of the surgical approach. Acquired diverticula, resulting from repeated bouts of dacryocystitis, will tend to dissect laterally along the inferior orbital margin. If there has been previous incision and drainage of the sac, or if there was a spontaneous rupture, the sac may herniate forward, and this anterior herniation or diverticulum can be identified in the lateral film. In the absence of roentgenographic confirmation, these diverticula and fistulae could escape detection during the surgery and be responsible for the failure of a dacryocystorhinostomy (Figs. 9-10 and 9-11).

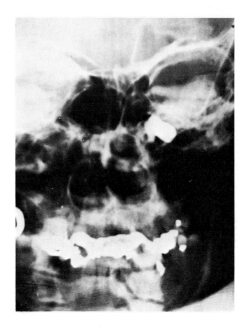

Figure 9-10. Lateral diverticulum (posteroanterior view).

Functional Block. The most troublesome diagnostic lacrimal problems for the physician are those in which the patient has a complaint of tearing in the presence of a patent excretory system. It is obvious that the mere ability to irrigate the lacrimal system successfully provides

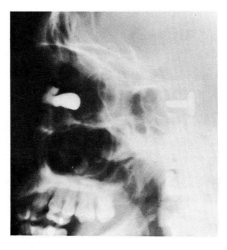

Figure 9-11. Anterior herniation of sac (lateral view).

no indication of its functional state. The classic example of this distinction between patency and normal function is found in peripheral facial paralysis (Bell's palsy), where the lacrimal system is anatomically intact but does not function to eliminate tears because of failure of the orbicularis-controlled lacrimal pump. Most frequently, such functional block cases are the result of one or more episodes of dacryocystitis and represent a partial obstruction with dilatation and atonicity of the lacrimal sac. The patient will have epiphora and some spontaneous reflux of mucus into the conjunctival sac, and often mucus or mucopus can be expressed by digital pressure over the sac. In some cases of functional block, however, the patient may have no findings on examination other than the presence of laking of tears.

The most valuable use of the dacryocystogram is in identifying the site of pathology in a patient who complains of tearing in the presence of a patent excretory system. The most common roentgenographic findings are those of a *dilated lacrimal sac or upper duct*, with some contrast medium present in the nose on the initial films. The follow-up film in 30 minutes will show little change in the residual contrast agent in the lacrimal sac, although the duct may be empty. A significant quantity of residual contrast medium at 30 minutes is strong evidence of functional failure of the system. Some 30 percent of patients who have persisting epiphora in the presence of a patent excretory system will have a functional block, confirmed by dacryocystography (Fig. 9-12).

Dacryocystography thus provides a clear-cut method of distinguishing between a normal system and a nonfunctioning patent system. In the absence of infection, most clinicians tend to be overly cautious in recommending surgery for a patient with epiphora. However, if roentgenograms show evidence of abnormal retention within the system, one can anticipate relief of the symptoms by surgical means.

In one of every six cases of functional block, dacryocystography will reveal the presence of a *dacryolith*. Lacrimal sac stones are non-calcific accumulations of cellular debris, inspissated mucus and fungi. Such stones are radiolucent and these as well as other benign masses within the sac, such as polyps, can readily be outlined by dacryocystography. Characteristically, a

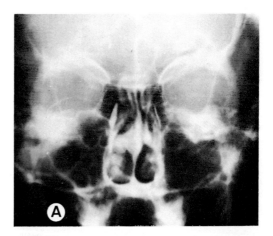

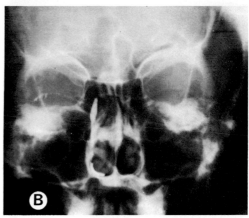

Figure 9-12. Functional block, right side. Note contrast agent in the nose. **A.** At 0 minutes. **B.** At 30 minutes. System is patent but sac does not empty.

stone within the lacrimal sac will appear on the x-ray film as a duplication of the lacrimal sac shadow embracing a central area of relucency. The most characteristic picture is seen in the lateral view where the sac is lightly outlined and there is a large clear central area of radiolucency. The sac shadow will usually show little change after 30 minutes since effective pumping action is compromised by the mass within the sac (Fig. 9-13).

Malignant *tumors* of the sac are uncommon but have a characteristic clinical picture which includes recurrent episodes of dacryocystitis, an irreducible mass with or without bleeding from the lacrimal puncta, persisting epiphora and an

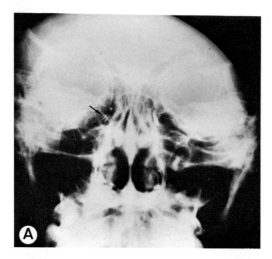

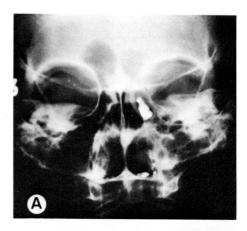

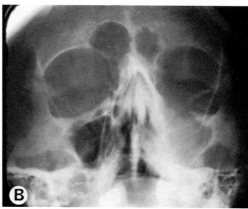

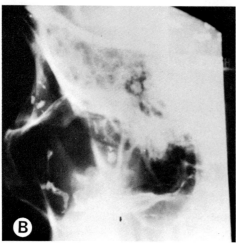

Figure 9-14. Epidermoid carcinoma, left. **A.** Posteroanterior view showing a dilated sac due to extrinsic impingement in the region of the sac-duct junction; the system is patent.
B. Waters view, taken 2 weeks after dacryocystorhinostomy, showing cloudy antrum and destruction of inferior orbital margin.

Figure 9-13. Dacryolith, right side. **A.** Posteroanterior view. Note reduplication of lacrimal sac shadow, with central radiolucent area (arrow). **B.** Lateral view. Note rounded outline of sac, with central radiolucent area.

abnormal configuration of the sac when visualized on the dacryocystogram.

When the tumor mass is extrinsic to the sac, as in the case of an ethmoid mucocele eroding through the lacrimal fossa, the sac will not only be displaced laterally but its normal concave outline will be reversed by the impinging mass.

Malignant tumors may erode through the sac and produce staining of the surrounding tissues. The sac shadow itself may be mottled and

irregular, reflecting the irregularities of the mass within the sac (Fig. 9-14). Radiographic visualization of such tumors is essential in surgical planning.

In *older persons,* a not uncommon clinical picture is the presence of epiphora, not explained by any evidence of external disease, with a freely patent excretory system. In such instances, the dacryocystograms may spare the patient the annoyance of repeated probings and other manipulations, to say nothing of possible fruitless surgery. If the dacryocystogram is normal, other causes must be sought for the tearing. Most frequently, the functional evaluation with the dacryocystogram will prove that the problem is merely one of a diminishing lacrimal pump action.

Dacryocystography is also useful in evaluating the postdacryocystorhinostomy patient who continues to have symptoms. The surgical anastomosis may remain patent, but at times a large atonic sac or diverticulum may interfere with normal emptying. When a dacryocystorhinostomy has failed, dacryocystography is essential in planning repeat surgery. In some instances, the puncta or canaliculi are responsible for persistent tearing after dacryocystorhinostomy. In these instances, the normal outflow demonstrated by the dacryocystogram will enable the surgeon to direct his further care appropriately. In other cases, the surgical failure may be the result of a large remaining atonic lacrimal sac. If this is identified by dacryocystography, reoperation is indicated, with mobilization and resection of the redundant lacrimal sac. Figure 9-15 illustrates a patient in whom preoperative dacryocystograms were not done. The diverticulum, undetected, was responsible for failure of the dacryocystorhinostomy.

In children who have epiphora associated with dacryocystitis due to congenital lacrimal obstruction, irrigation and probing is the procedure of choice. The majority of these children can be treated successfully by one or two probings. If they do not respond by a second probing, a dacryocystogram will provide information regarding the site of obstruction and the anatomy of the excretory passages. In children, dacryocystography is performed under general anesthesia in the radiology department of the hospital. The contrast medium is instilled with the child lying on the x-ray table, and the child is then turned prone for a posteroanterior film and a lateral exposure. Confirmation of complete obstruction of the lacrimal system in a child would substantiate the indication for dacryocystorhinostomy.

In summary, dacryocystography is a valuable clinical diagnostic technique that is easily performed, that subjects the patient to minimum discomfort and negligible risk, and that yields information unobtainable by any other diagnostic method. It is useful in localizing partial or complete obstructions within the naso-

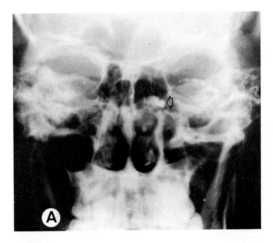

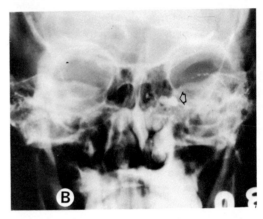

Figure 9-15. Dacrocystorhinostomy failure, left side, postoperative dacryocystograms. **A.** At 0 minutes, showing sac and lateral diverticulum (arrow). **B.** At 30 minutes, the sac has emptied, but lateral diverticulum persists (arrow). In this patient, preoperative dacryocystograms had not been obtained.

lacrimal excretory system and in identifying the etiologic factors involved. It is invaluable in patients who have functional block in a patent system. The technique will identify lacrimal stones, tumors, diverticula, fistulae, and the sequelae of trauma.

The lacrimal excretory system is a delicate and anatomically intricate membranous system. It is logical that dacryocystography will yield more and better diagnostic information than the blind manipulation of rigid instruments in a nonrigid system, and it would seem to be unreasonable to undertake surgical modification of this system without such preoperative visual evaluation. With the current availability of a battery of diagnostic tests and of a simple method for dacryocystography, every ophthalmic surgeon can have the golden hands.

DACRYOCYSTOGRAPHY WITH AQUEOUS CONTRAST MEDIUM

When aqueous contrast media are used for dacryocystography, the technique can be similar to that described previously for ethyl iodoundecylate (Pantopaque*). That is, it can be instilled into the lacrimal system by syringe through a lacrimal cannula. It has been pointed out that Pantopaque drains from the lacrimal sac within 15 minutes and from the nasolacrimal duct in 30 minutes. Since aqueous contrast media, such as iodipamide meglumine,† are miscible with tears and since emptying time for aqueous solutions within the excretory system has been determined to be 60 seconds,[4] it is essential that aqueous dacryocystography be performed using zero time exposures. Therefore, the use of syringe-cannula methods of instilling aqueous agents is unsatisfactory, since all or most of the material may be in the nasopharynx before the necessary posteroanterior and lateral views can be taken.

The inferior canaliculus is intubated with polyethylene tubing which is taped to the forehead, and the tube is affixed to a syringe so that the x-ray exposures can be made *while* the system is being filled with the contrast material. It is often necessary when using aqueous contrast agents to occlude the punctum of the upper lid in order to fill the system adequately. Such precautions are unnecessary when using iodized oils.

In our view, a properly performed dacryocystogram requires that both sides be studied simultaneously. This can be accomplished with the polyethylene intubation technique but not when the aqueous agent is delivered from a syringe-cannula combination.

The most frequently cited objection to the use of iodized oils for dacryocystography has been that the test does not properly simulate

---

* Lafayette Pharmacal.
† Sinografin, E.R. Squibb & Sons.

normal tear outflow since the material is being introduced under pressure. However, the same reservation holds true for aqueous agents even though they require a lesser degree of artificial pressure. This artifact in technique can be avoided only in visualization of the lacrimal system by a nuclear scanning technique (lacrimal microscintigraphy), where one drop of radionuclide material is placed in the conjunctival sac, and its progress into the system is followed with a gamma camera.

Despite the fact that aqueous contrast agents pass quite rapidly through the excretory system, the several advantages cited for this method undoubtedly will raise a question in the minds of the readers: "Why do the authors continue to prefer a low-viscosity iodized oil for dacryocystography?" This is a reasonable question, and there are two reasonable answers. As we have noted, dacryocystography should attempt to elicit two types of information: the pathologic anatomy of the excretory system and the functional state of that system. In order to evaluate the functional state, one must have accurate baseline data with appropriate supporting evidence. Since this evidence is not clearly spelled out in regard to the aqueous contrast media, the physician who performs an occasional dacryocystogram does not have a sound basis for interpreting function. It is true that the studies of Jones and Linn[4] have demonstrated that aqueous solutions pass through the system in 1 minute, but this has not been translated into aqueous dacryocystography. We have performed aqueous dacryocystograms using zero minute and 2-minute readings for function, but an insufficient number of these tests has been performed to draw firm conclusions. If one does not attempt to evaluate the functional state when performing dacryocystography, the examination does not yield all possible information.

The second reason for preferring a low-viscosity iodized oil as contrast agent is that since it is not miscible with tears, the bolus of oily contrast material moves through the excretory system without dilution. Therefore, changes in the density of the radiopaque shadow on the film can be read accurately, as can changes in the amount of retained contrast material. On the other hand, aqueous solutions are diluted by the tear flow, and, therefore, interpretation of the dacryocystogram will vary with varia-

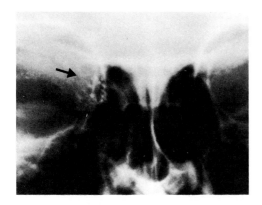 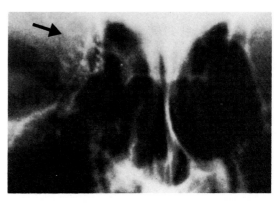

Figure 9-16. Left. Malignant melanoma, right lacrimal sac, with extension into upper orbit. Oval outline, with mottling of the contrast agent and poorly defined limits of the tumor. **Right.** Same dacryocystogram, enlarged 2x.

tions in tear secretion. For this reason, since normal emptying time for low-viscosity agents is known and since the instillation can be accomplished more simply using the syringe-canula technique, we continue to prefer the low-viscosity oil.

MACRODACRYOCYSTOGRAPHY

In 1964, Campbell[5] described a technique for obtaining a magnified view of the lacrimal outflow system employing radiopaque contrast agents. This technique, macrodacryocystography, consisted of having the patient lie prone on a Perspex table with the x-ray tube placed above the patient's head and the x-ray cassette placed on the floor under the table. This method was not only unwieldy but failed to provide opportunities for simultaneous bilateral study and for evaluation of outflow function. It required a high-viscosity contrast agent.

A simplified technique for macrodacryocystography was described in 1977,[6] in which the unexposed plate was placed on a chair beneath the patient's head at a distance of 30 inches. The patient's head was supported by a head extender, and the x-ray tube was placed 30 inches above the patient. While this method had the advantage of requiring no special table, it retained all of the problems of the original technique.

Macrodacryocystography raises several in-teresting questions. If the examiner desired an enlarged view of the lacrimal excretory system, why would he not employ the more widely used low-viscosity iodized oil or the aqueous techniques and view the films with a hand magnifying lens? Why would one forego the opportunity to study lacrimal outflow function in order to achieve a magnified view of the pathologic anatomy?

Figure 9-16 (left) illustrates a malignant melanoma with extravasation of the contrast agent through the lacrimal sac superiorly. On the right, the same picture has been magnified two times, providing the same information that would be available through macrodacryocystography.

SUBTRACTION MACRODACRYOCYSTOGRAPHY

In 1974, Lloyd and Wilham[7] described an interesting and useful modification of dacryocystography. By employing subtraction radiograph techniques to provide bone-free visualization of the excretory system, they were able to produce excellent visualization of the canaliculi and common canaliculus. They employed simultaneous catheterization of both excretory systems. By using a hand-operated serial changer set beneath the skull table, they could take a sequence of four films during injection of the low-viscosity iodized oil contrast medium, thus producing sequential studies of the system. A control film was taken prior to injection for subtraction studies. With this method, visualization of the canaliculi was improved through elimination of the bony ethmoid structures. Films were taken during injection for maximum distention of the lacrimal passages. With this method, no attempt was made to study lacrimal function, and the chief purpose was to provide optimum visualization of the pathologic anatomy of the canaliculi and common canaliculus.

DISTENTION DACRYOCYSTOGRAPHY

Iba and Hanafee[8] used a tapered Teflon catheter for instilling a low-viscosity iodized oil. The contrast agent was introduced under pressure with the patient in a sitting position, and roentgen exposures were made as the contrast agent was being injected. A series of posteroanterior, Waters, Riese, and lateral projections were used. In this manner, the system is seen consistently in a distended state, and the authors feel that a maximum amount of information regarding pathologic anatomy can be obtained in this fashion. A similar distention method was used subsequently to evaluate the variations in the normal lacrimal excretory system.[9]

CINEDACRYOCYSTOGRAPHY

Studies of the outflow function, using cinematography, have been reported in the literature from time to time. In one such study,[10] an aqueous iodine agent, Urografin, was instilled into the conjunctival sac, and a motion picture record was made of its movement through the system while, at the same time, the examiner conducted a fluoroscopic examination. This free-flow method (as opposed to the injection method described previously) utilized an image-intensifier apparatus with a 5-inch screen. This small screen provides excellent definition, and the author felt that this was the optimal method for studying the physiology of lacrimal outflow. There are obvious barriers to its use as a routine clinical diagnostic tool, chiefly, the sophisticated apparatus required.

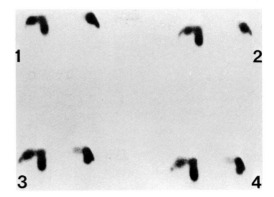

Figure 9-17. Microscintigraphy at (1) 60 seconds, (2) 2 minutes, (3) 5 minutes, (4) 10 minutes. Sequential films show progressive emptying of the sac and filling of the nasolacrimal duct.

MICROSCINTIGRAPHY

Radioactive tracer materials have provided the only new diagnostic tool for imaging the lacrimal excretory system. In 1972, Rossomondo et al.[11] utilized technitium[99], instilling a single drop containing approximately 100 Ci of Tc^{99} into the conjunctival sac. The patient was seated before a gamma camera. A special tapered microcollimator with an aperture of 0.043 inch allowed for close positioning of the patient's eye to the pinhole. Serial photographs were made at 2-second intervals for the first 20 seconds, and every 40 seconds thereafter (Fig. 9-17). The field of view of each photograph extended from the middle of the cornea to the nasal midline.

Studying a series of normal subjects, it was found that one quantitative parameter was the time required for the radioactive material to enter the lacrimal sac, and a second quantitative index was the time required for the material to reach the bottom of the nasolacrimal duct. In studies of normal subjects, the median transit time for the material to reach the lacrimal sac was 6 seconds (range 4 to 43 seconds), and the median time to reach the bottom of the nasolacrimal duct was 43 seconds (4 to 323 seconds). Despite the rather broad range of normal times, this method is useful in evaluating lacrimal outflow function if it is performed simultaneously on both sides so that a suspected abnormal can be compared with the clinically normal side. One of its chief advantages is that the radiation dose is about 2 percent of that received in an anteroposterior x-ray. On the other hand, it does not delineate either normal or abnormal anatomy clearly and so does not substitute for other radiographic methods. One interesting and useful finding from the study of outflow physiology by microscintigraphy was the consistent gap between the confluence of the canaliculi and the point of entry into the lacrimal sac. This finding suggested that the region of the common canaliculus must be functionally closed most of the time, since the tracer material readily traverses this apparently closed section. The authors suggested that, in blinking, the lacrimal pump apparatus might open that part of the common canaliculus briefly, allowing tears to be pumped into the lacrimal sac.

SUMMARY

It would be an abuse of an overworked cliche to say that dacryocystography is "an idea whose time has come." In truth, its time came many decades ago, and it required the intervening years for the clinician to take possession of it. One final word of advice and caution: the person who reads and interprets the dacryocystogram should be the ophthalmologist who has examined the patient and who has performed the diagnostic tests.

REFERENCES

1. Ewing AE: Roentgen ray demonstration of the lacrimal abscess cavity. Am Ophthalmol 24:1, 1909
2. Milder B, Demorest BH: Dacryocystography. I. The normal lacrimal apparatus. Arch Ophthalmol 51:180, 1954
2a. ———. Dacryocystography. I. The normal lacrimal apparatus. Ach Ophthalmol 51:181, 1954
3. Demorest BH, Milder B: Dacryocystography II. The pathologic lacrimal apparatus. Arch Ophthalmol 54:410, 1955
4. Jones LT, Linn M: Rate of lacrimal excretion. Am Ophthalmol 65:76, 1978
5. Campbell W: The radiology of the lacrimal system. Br Radiol 37:1, 1964
6. Arnold DG, et al: A simplified method for microdacryocystography. Ann Ophthalmol 9:305, 1977
7. Lloyd GA, et al.: Subtraction macrodacryocystography. Br Radiol 47:379, 1974
8. Iba GB, Hanafee WN: Distention dacryocystography. Radiology 90:1020, 1968
9. Rodriguez HP, Kittleson AC: Distension dacryocystography. Radiology, 109:317, 1973
10. Epstein E: Cinedacryocystography. Trans Ophthalmol Soc UK, 81:284, 1961
11. Rossomondo RM, Carlton WH, Trueblood JH, Thomas RP: A new method of evaluating lacrimal drainage. Arch Ophthalmol 88:523, 1972

PART 2

CLINICAL DACRYOLOGY

10

CONGENITAL DISORDERS OF THE LACRIMAL SYSTEM

BERNARDO A. WEIL

SECRETORY SYSTEM

Ophthalmologists recognize that not all hereditary diseases are present at birth. Conversely, not all congenital diseases are products of mendelian inheritance. In fact, congenital diseases are, by our usual understanding of the term, acquired diseases, albeit acquired in utero.

Ever since Gregory Mendel propounded the essentials of inheritance and subsequent generations developed knowledge of genetic mutations and chromosomal deficiencies, clinicians have laboriously gone about the business of assembling groups of signs and symptoms into clinical entities that are recognizably transmitted in accordance with the mendelian laws. At the same time, variations in fetal maturation have given rise to lacrimal disorders which are termed "congenital" but might properly be called "neonatal."

In this chapter, we consider a variety of entities affecting the newborn child—congenital, neonatal, and hereditary.

Absence of Lacrimal Gland

Congenital absence of the lacrimal gland is extremely rare. It is often associated with other

Figures 10-1, 10-2, 10-5, 10-8, 10-9, and 10-10 appear on Color Plate II, page 96.

congenital ocular anomalies, such as anophthalmos and cryptophthalmos.

Alacrima

Congenital absence of tear secretion can occur in the presence of the lacrimal gland. Such cases are usually bilateral and manifest all of the usual findings of the dry eye: keratitis, corneal ulceration, and keratinization of the conjunctiva, often with secondary infection.

Congenital Lacrimal Hyposecretion

Lacrimal hyposecretion is not as unusual as complete absence of tear secretion. Here, too, the symptoms and signs are those of the dry eye syndrome (Fig. 10-1, Color Plate II). Hyposecretion may coexist with other congenital anomalies. Reports of alacrima with histologically normal lacrimal gland[1] suggest that, at least in some cases, the problem may be a congenital innervational defect.

Innervational dysgenesis abnormality, or absence of innervation to the lacrimal gland, may result in tear secretion deficiency.

Familial dysautonomia (Riley-Day syndrome) is characterized by failure of secretion of tears. Other prominent symptoms are extreme muscular hypotonia, arterial hypertension, diminished reflexes, emotional instability, and insensitivity to pain. Corneal anesthesia may be

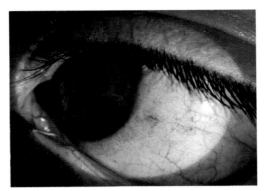

Figure 10-1. Congenital lacrimal hyposecretion. Rose bengal staining of bulbar conjunctiva.

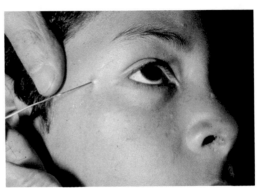

Figure 10-2. Congenital lacrimal gland fistula. *(Courtesy of J. Brzezinski, M.D.)*

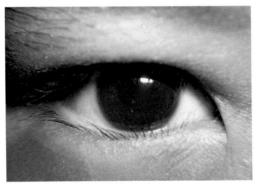

Figure 10-5. Distichiasis, congenital, nasal half of eyelid. Reflex tearing due to corneal irritation.

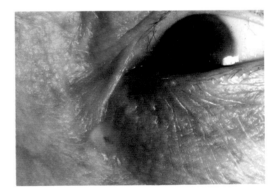

Figure 10-8. Congenital lacrimal fistula.

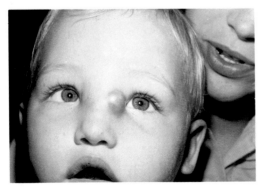

Figure 10-9. Chronic dacryocystitis, secondary to untreated congenital dacryostenosis.

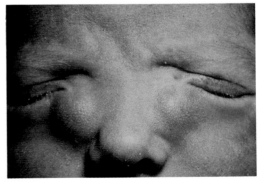

Figure 10-10. Mucoceles of lacrimal sacs in an infant.

accompanied by indolent corneal ulcers, with little or no associated inflammatory reaction.

Other Congenital Anomalies

Aberrant lacrimal tissue may be found anywhere under palpebral or bulbar conjunctival tissue. It may be present at the corneal limbus, in the plica, or in any of the external ocular structures.

Congenital fistula of the lacrimal gland may present at the lateral canthus or just above. Tears exuding through the small opening onto the skin may be responsible for localized irritation. Those stimuli which normally enhance tear secretion will also increase flow through the fistula. The treatment is surgical removal of the fistula (Fig. 10-2, Color Plate II).

EXCRETORY SYSTEM

The *lacrimal excretory passages* are often divided into *upper* and *lower* excretory passages. The upper passages include the lid margins, the lacrimal puncta and canaliculi, the common canaliculus, and the internal punctum (valve of Rosenmüller). The lower system is comprised of the lacrimal sac, nasolacrimal duct, and the plica semilunaris (valve of Hasner).

This arbitrary separation into upper and lower systems serves several useful purposes, diagnostic as well as therapeutic (Chapter 8).

Upper Lacrimal Passages

Congenital Absence of Puncta and Canaliculi. Complete absence of these structures is uncommon, but imperforate puncta are less rare. In these latter cases, the lacrimal papilla can be identified and the site of the punctum located by a shallow depression in the papilla or by a thin gray membrane occluding the punctal orifice. There may be supernumerary puncta opening into the canaliculus or more extensive anomalous canalicular defects (Fig. 10-3).

Other anomalies include supernumerary puncta and canaliculi. Most of these are symptom free because the outflow of tears is unaffected (Fig. 10-4). Abnormal length of the canaliculi is a congenital anomaly found in one of the von der Hoeve syndromes.

Congenital Eyelid Abnormalities. These may cause epiphora. Congenital entropion with distichiasis (Fig. 10-5, Color Plate II) initiates re-

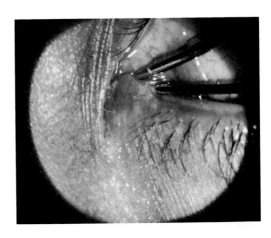

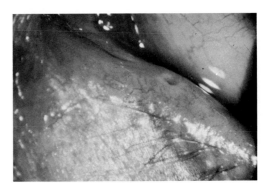

Figure 10-3. Top and **Bottom.** Canalicular anomaly—failure of closure along the eyelid margin.

flex hypersecretion of tears. Ectropion of the temporal half of the lower eyelid (Fig. 10-6) and colobomas of the nasal angle are responsible for epiphora in infants. Blepharophimosis may be associated with maldevelopment of the excretory pathways (Fig. 10-7).

Lower Lacrimal Passages

Functional Block. In Down's disease, failure of tear excretion in the presence of a patent system (functional block) is a common finding. It is probably due to the general muscular weakness.

Anatomic Block. The most common congenital lacrimal abnormality is low obstruction in the nasolacrimal duct (at Hasner's valve area) due to failure of complete canalization of the membranous nasolacrimal duct at birth. This may open spontaneously or may yield to a probing of the nasolacrimal duct.

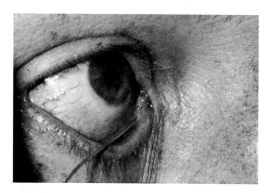

Figure 10-4. Anomalous opening into canaliculus on conjunctival aspect of the eyelid.

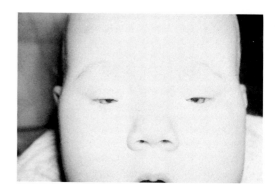

Figure 10-7. Blepharophimosis.

Congenital obstructions may also be due to a more extensive atresia of the duct or to failure of canalization of the bony nasolacrimal canal.

Diagnosis of congenital obstruction in the lower lacrimal system is not difficult. Epiphora is the first and most constant symptom. The affected eye appears wet and brilliant, and the caruncular area and lacus lacrimalis are filled with tears or mucopurulent secretion. It has been recognized that tears are secreted in the first few days of life, and we have observed puddling of tears in the affected eye, particularly when inflammation is present, within days or even hours after birth. However, it happens quite frequently that the epiphora is not noted during those first days and may not be detected until the second or third week. The epiphora increases when the infant is exposed to cold, wind, or dusty environment.

The only clinical symptom may be a persisting mild conjunctivitis which does not respond to local medications. The persistence of a chronic conjunctivitis despite treatment, particularly if only one eye is affected, should cause one to think of a possible congenital lacrimal obstruction. Pressure should be exerted over the lacrimal sac to determine if the sac contains mucus or pus, and lacrimal irrigation and probing may be necessary to confirm the diagnosis.

Although dye test diagnostic procedures for lacrimal obstruction are an accepted and widely used diagnostic device, they are particularly important in the investigation of congenital excretory problems. It is often possible to avoid any traumatic manipulation of the lacrimal system, especially in suspected unilateral congenital obstruction, by the simple instillation of one drop of fluorescein or rose bengal into the conjunctival sac of each eye. The rapid disappearance of the dye from the normal conjunctival sac as compared with the suspected abnormal sac will confirm the diagnosis of lacrimal obstruction.*

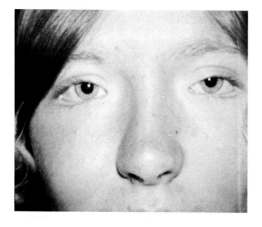

Figure 10-6. Telecanthus and ectropion of eyelids, with epiphora.

Personal preference or bias has always been a characteristic of the clinical practice of medicine. The authors, who have agreed to collaborate, have also agreed that it is unnecessary to agree on all points. In this case, one of us (B.M.) prefers to use fluorescein 2 percent, while the other (B.W.) prefers rose bengal 0.5 percent. The latter feels that the contrast is greater with rose bengal and that it could possibly avoid an additional examination under general anesthesia.

Where the diagnosis remains in doubt, we do not hesitate to perform lacrimal irrigation for diagnostic purposes. Dacryocystography is reserved for those infants in whom the diagnosis is not made or treatment has been unsuccessful after a series of diagnostic-therapeutic lacrimal probings.

Congenital Lacrimal Sac Fistula. The embryonic lacrimal plate, the anlage of the excretory passages, begins to form near the upper end of the groove between the maxillary process and the external nasal process. These processes fuse together, isolating and deepening the ectodermal lacrimal cord. If this fusion process is imperfect and cells from the upper end of the lacrimal cord are not completely isolated from surface ectoderm, they may undergo anomalous cavitation, forming a fistulous track to the skin. Such congenital lacrimal fistulas are histologically identical with the canaliculi and are sometimes referred to as a "third canaliculus."

These congenital fistulas may not canalize completely or may close spontaneously or dimple at the skin surface, 2 to 10 mm inferior to the nasal canthus. If the fistula is patent, it may produce symptoms either as a result of infection or from annoying excretion of tears and maceration of the skin (Fig. 10-8, Color Plate II).

TREATMENT OF LACRIMAL EXCRETORY PROBLEMS IN INFANTS

Over 5,000 congenital lacrimal obstructions were treated by one of the authors (B.W.) and his colleagues over a period of 20 years at the Children's Hospital of Buenos Aires, Department of Ophthalmology. The therapeutic measures described below are those which were employed in that extensive series.[2]

Acute Dacryocystitis

Acute purulent dacryocystitis, seen at birth, is extremely rare. Acute infections of the lacrimal sac usually are superimposed upon congenital mucoceles which become manifest a few hours or a few days after birth. Factors in the pathogenesis of such an acute infection include congenital obstruction in the excretory passages, partial or complete, and mucosal edema which produces obstruction at the internal punctum and prevents reflux of secretions or amniotic fluid via the canaliculi.

Pericystitis, Lacrimal Sac

When an acute dacryocystitis is not treated early or does not respond to treatment efforts, the inflammatory process may involve the perisaccular structures, with accompanying systemic symptoms. Conjunctival cultures can provide a clue for appropriate intensive antibiotic therapy. Spontaneous rupture of the sac with external fistulization may complicate the picture.

Chronic Dacryocystitis

Chronic infection involving the lacrimal sac, as a complication of congenital lacrimal obstruction, is far more common than the acute form. It may be present with little or no apparent discomfort, variable enlargement of the tear sac, and little or no mucoid secretion. In some instances, pressure over the lacrimal sac will produce almost no secretion reflux through the puncta (Fig. 10-9, Color Plate II). In other instances, the chronic dacryocystitis may take a suppurative form, presenting with a large ectatic sac which drains readily when the sac is decompressed by digital manipulation. The secretion is purulent and thick in these cases. In either event, whether the chronic dacryocystitis is accompanied by gross purulent secretion or not, an appropriate first effort should be to irrigate the sac and then perform therapeutic probing.

Mucocele

The congenital lacrimal sac mucocele is characterized by a large, smooth tumefaction without associated inflammatory signs (Fig. 10-10, Color Plate II). The mucoid nature of the sac content can be identified by transillumination of the sac. Sometimes, it is difficult or even impossible to evacuate the contents of the sac by digital pressure. Occasionally, if one inserts a probe through the upper punctum and canaliculus into the sac, the sac can be decompressed while the probe is in place, with the secretions emerging through the lower punctum.

Most important, it is mandatory to differentiate a suspected mucocele of the lacrimal sac from a congenital meningocele. Although a meningocele presenting at this site is uncommon compared to a congenital lacrimal sac mucocele, the differential diagnosis may not be simple. Neither may be reducible by pressure. Light palpation may reveal pulsation if it is a meningocele or a meningoencephalocele. Dacryocystography is an invaluable aid in making this differential diagnosis.

Dacryocystitis with Fistulization

Resolution of the acute dacryocystitis, in congenital lacrimal obstruction, may be hastened by spontaneous fistulization. Such fistulization may occur externally or internally. If the sac perforates through the skin, the local inflammatory process improves rapidly, but, of course, it does not alter the original etiologic factor of congenital nasolacrimal obstruction. There are cases, however, in which the acute dacryocystitis is resolved suddenly, without fistulization or apparent drainage, and in such cases even the previously existing epiphora may disappear. We have interpreted this type of spontaneous cure as being the result of internal fistulization of the sac into the lower portion of the nasolacrimal duct.

GENERAL PRINCIPLES
OF TREATMENT
OF CONGENITAL EPIPHORA

If the infant has epiphora with no suppuration or distention of the sac, it is unnecessary to attempt probing earlier than 3 months of age. Before that, some of the obstructions will resolve spontaneously.

Korchmaros et al.[3] reported on the rate of spontaneous opening of the nasolacrimal duct in stillborns and in 5,588 newborn infants. Using an air-syringing technique, they found that half of all of their newborns had impatent lacrimal pathways at birth and that two fifths of these were still blocked after 3 months. Although they reported no precise data on the rate of spontaneous opening of blocked ducts beyond the fourth month, their conclusion was[3]:

> It seems probable that the rate of the blocked nasolacrimal ducts decreases gradually with age. At the same time, the rate of blocked lacrimal pathways with discharge, i.e., the rate of

infantile dacryocystitis cases, increases. To prevent the complication of the infantile dacryocystitis, we have been syringing the lacrimal pathways of infants in cases of conjunctival discharge or tear flow. If syringing fails, we do not hesitate to continue the procedure with the same syringe as a cannula-probing.

After the first 6 months, the rate of success by probing diminishes gradually, and at the second year of age probing success is very low. However, the child with congenital epiphora should have a therapeutic trial with probing, no matter what the age.

On the other hand, a child who has epiphora which is evidently not congenital, that is, which does not appear until after the first 6 to 9 months, should have diagnostic dacryocystography, performed under general anesthesia. Probing should be performed during the same anesthesia. If the dacryocystogram identifies the site of obstruction and reveals no contraindications to probing in infantile or juvenile-acquired dacryocystitis, the decision as to which method of treatment is to be used will depend upon the site of the obstruction. If it is low in the duct, in the region of the plica semilunaris, the procedure of choice is probing. If the obstruction is located in the middle third or above, the chances of curing the patient with probing are relatively remote. In such cases, probing should be attempted, but dacryocystorhinostomy will usually be the ultimate treatment, just as in adult-acquired dacryocystitis.

TECHNIQUE OF PROBING

Lacrimal probing in the infant appears to the neophyte to be one of the simplest of surgical manipulations. However, it is deceptively complex for several reasons. These include the risk of making false passages and producing permanent cicatricial closure in the excretory system, damage to the lacrimal puncta resulting either in stenosis or a patulous opening that compromises the capillary attraction capability of the punctum, and inability to determine whether the probing has actually opened the excretory passage.

Although probing is a technique that must be mastered through experience, several basic principles are essential to its success:

1. Complete immobilization of the infant's head. This may be accomplished in the first 3 months of life, by immobilizing the child and having an assistant hold the head steady (Fig. 10-11). Much preferred, however, is general anesthesia with the procedure performed in the operating room.

2. The lower punctum should be dilated slowly and only moderately. The lower canaliculus is then checked for patency using a fine Bowman's probe. If there is obstruction in the canaliculus, no attempt should be made at this point to open it by sheer force.

3. The upper punctum should be dilated moderately and the lacrimal system irrigated through the upper canaliculus. A diagnostic irrigation should precede any attempt at probing, since the system may be found to be patent by irrigation, and the trauma of probing would thus be avoided. If the anesthesia is superficial, any saline that passes through the lacrimal excretory system into the nasopharynx will elicit gagging or a swallowing reflex. This can be detected easily by palpating the child's throat. In addition, the patency of the system by syringing can be confirmed by staining the irrigating solution with fluorescein and inserting a clear silicone suction tube into the nasal airway on the side under examination. The colored solution can readily be identified as it is aspirated into the clear suction tube.

If the system is not patent by syringing,

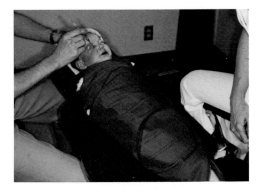

Figure 10-11. Papoose board employed to immobilize infant for lacrimal irrigation.

probing should be undertaken through the upper canaliculus. The probe should pass without great resistance through the nasolacrimal duct. There is usually mild resistance at the lower portion of the duct and this can be penetrated by light pressure on the probe. Following the probing, irrigation should be repeated to confirm that the system is, in fact, patent.

A convenient way to perform the irrigation and probing with a minimum of manipulation involves the use of the Weil infant lacrimal probing cannula. This cannulated probe has a blunt tip with a lateral fenestration. With this instrument, it is possible to pass the probe through the canaliculus, sac, and upper duct, and then irrigate lightly. If the system is not patent, simple light further pressure on the probe will achieve the desired penetration without the insertion of a second instrument. The subsequent irrigation to confirm patency is then performed with the probe still in place.

4. It is essential to confirm that the system is patent. If a question remains after the probing and subsequent irrigation, the nose should be inspected carefully for appearance of the probe. Sometimes it is necessary to introduce a slender metal instrument, such as a periosteal elevator, into the inferior meatus to feel direct contact of metal on metal. If the probe cannot be identified, the inferior turbinate can easily be deflected toward the midline by means of the periosteal elevator so as to improve the visualization of the inferior meatus.

The procedure described has the following advantages:

1. It protects the lower canaliculus from damage, since introducing the probe-cannula into the nasolacrimal duct through the lower canaliculus would require bending the canaliculus at right angles to its normal position and risking a tear.

2. It prevents false passages in the lower canaliculus and avoids excessive dilatation of the lower punctum.

3. The probing through the upper punctum and canaliculus can be performed with greater facility.

Respect for the lower punctum and canaliculus is admirably summed up by Werb: "We have been blessed with two canaliculi, the lower for the excretion of tears and the upper for the ophthalmologist."[4]

It is general practice among most ophthalmologists to suggest to the parents that the tear sac be massaged, in the hope that this will facilitate the spontaneous opening of the system. Such manipulation is rarely successful and serves little purpose beyond enabling the parents to feel that they are participating in the treatment program. When such massage is successful, it usually occurs as a result of penetration of a lightly imperforate membrane at the lower end of the duct by the increased hydrostatic pressure of the column of fluid contained within the sac and duct. If this is the mechanism by which massage or pressure over the sac can be successful in opening an imperforate membrane, the procedure is best performed by the ophthalmologist rather than the parents. In the presence of a chronic dacryocystitis, such massage could favor the development of a pericystitis.

When the probing procedure has been unsuccessful, it should be repeated. In a small percentage of cases, a second probing will succeed when the first one has failed. Usually, however, if the first attempt is unsuccessful, the second will suffer the same fate, since the location of the obstruction can vary greatly (Fig. 10-12).

At this second probing or at most a third probing, dacryocystography should be performed in order to identify the site and the nature of the obstruction. If the obstruction is at the region of the plica semilunaris and if there is no excessive ectasia of the lacrimal sac, an attempt to open this obstruction can be pursued with the cooperation of a rhinologist. Under general anesthesia, the probe is passed through the upper canaliculus, sac, and duct and pressed toward the inferior meatus. Under direct visualization, the rhinologist can see the tenting of the mucosa by the probe and remove a large part of the mucosa at that time. In some instances, a portion of the inferior turbinate is removed at the same time, or the turbinate is outfractured to provide better visualization and a greater opportunity for maintaining patency. It may be useful to introduce a silicone canalicular tube for 3 to 6 weeks in order to maintain the patency of the newly formed opening.

In the series of infants studied at the Children's Hospital of Buenos Aires, a first probing was successful in 87.8 percent of cases. If such complications as a concurrent dacryocystitis were present, the success rate dropped to 71.1 percent. Under conditions where there was no previous manipulation or trauma, no associated purulent dacryocystitis, and no associated congenital malformation, success rates in probing were 92.7 percent.

TREATMENT

Acute Dacryocystitis

In the presence of acute dacryocystitis, with or without pericystitis, probing and manipulation of the outflow system must be avoided until the acute process is brought under control. Treatment should begin with systemic antibiotics. An initial sac culture may be helpful in identifying one or more organisms so that appropriate antibiotic sensitivity tests can be employed (Chapter 7). Warm compresses, such as are employed in the treatment of acute dacryocystitis in the adult, are of little value here because of difficulties in cooperation and because of the risks of thermal burns of the skin. Similarly, the use of

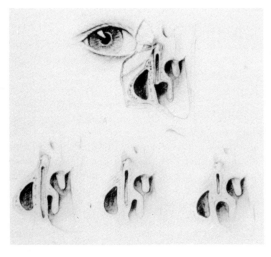

Figure 10-12. **Top.** Normal opening of the nasolacrimal duct into the vault of the inferior meatus. **Bottom.** Varieties of congenital closure of the duct.

cold compresses is of little value. However, analgesics may be employed to provide relief from discomfort associated with the tense, distended lacrimal sac. The more rapid the resolution of the acute process, the less likely will be an external fistulization of the sac. Incision and drainage of the sac during the most acute phase are not recommended. However, as the acute phase begins to resolve, if the sac is distended and fluctuant, it may be profitable to evacuate the sac by inserting a thin-walled 19-gauge needle into the sac cavity at the lower pole of the distended sac. Decompression of the distended sac in this manner is less likely to cause fistulization. If a fistula should result, the small opening has been placed in the line of incision of later dacryocystorhinostomy so that the fistula can be excised during that surgical procedure.

If the epiphora persists after the acute phase of dacryocystitis has resolved, probing should be undertaken. Infrequently, if the acute dacryocystitis persists despite medical treatment, some surgeons will elect to attempt probing during this acute phase. The procedure is fraught with dangers of disseminating the infection through false passages, with resulting orbital cellulitis. Such manipulations should be avoided.

If the acute dacryocystitis is accompanied by perisaccular inflammatory reaction, and if this does not diminish with vigorous medical treatment, it is advisable to use perisaccular injections of an antibiotic-corticosteroid combination.

Chronic Dacryocystitis

The treatment of chronic dacryocystitis, whether it is accompanied by purulent secretion or whether it exists in the form of a mucocele, is probing of the obstructed system. When suppuration is present, probing should not be delayed. In these instances, the sac should be lavaged before probing is attempted. After the probing, antibiotics should be irrigated into the lacrimal sac. Similarly, in the presence of a mucocele, probing should not be delayed, since spontaneous resolution is unlikely.

When dacryocystitis is accompanied by fistulization through the lacrimal sac, probing should be performed without delay. If the probing is successful, the fistula may close spontaneously without further treatment. However,

if the fistula persists, it should be excised at the time that dacryocystorhinostomy is performed.

DACRYOCYSTORHINOSTOMY

If one or two probings are not successful, it is inevitable that a more aggressive surgical effort will be required. Dacryocystorhinostomy has been the procedure of choice for both authors. One of us (B.W.) has performed dacryocystorhinostomy on infants from the age of 3 months onward. The other (B.M.) has performed bilateral dacryocystorhinostomies on infants as young as 7 months. There has been no subsequent residual facial asymmetry or other deformity as a result of early lacrimal surgery. It is our usual practice, if the dacryocystitis is not producing any secondary problem other than epiphora, to wait until the child is about 2 years of age before performing dacryocystorhinostomy. Indications for earlier surgery would be excessive ectasia of the sac, recurrent bouts of acute dacryocystitis, or the need to eliminate this source of infection before addressing another concurrent congenital defect.

Dacryocystorhinostomy performed on a child is not more difficult technically than it is on an adult. The nasal mucosa is usually adequately thick, the bone is thin, osteotomy is readily performed, and there are no annoying ethmoid sinus cells to interfere with the surgical procedure. Hemorrhage has not been a significant complication in more than 200 dacryocystorhinostomies performed on children under the age of 10 years.

When dacryocystitis occurs in association with other craniofacial anomalies, such as cleft palate, meningocele, or midfacial dysplasia, dacryocystorhinostomy should be performed if needed as part of a major surgical approach in this area. If there is no evidence of gross purulent secretion, it is often desirable to perform as many reconstructive procedures as possible at each surgical session.

In the past few years, some surgeons have used silicone intubation in infants as a form of treatment for congenital dacryostenosis, with or without associated infection. Such a silicone stent, left in the nasolacrimal duct for 3 to 6 weeks, may cure the obstructive problem in some cases. If there is dacryocystitis associated with pronounced distention of the lacrimal sac, such measures are unlikely to effect a cure.

CONCLUSION

It is important to close this chapter by repeating a warning: always think of the possibility of a meningocele if the tumor is congenital or is acquired after trauma, if there is no local sign of infection, if the mass presents above the medial canthal tendon, or if it becomes firm when the infant is crying. If in doubt, x-rays of the skull and dacryocystograms should be obtained.

REFERENCES

1. Duke-Elder S: Textbook of Ophthalmology. St. Louis, Mosby, 1952, Vol 5, The Ocular Adnexae, p 5210
2. Lavin JR, Weil BA, Sorrana JE: Tratamiento de las obstrucciones congenitos de las vias lagrimales. Arch Oftal Buenos Aires 47:277, 1972
3. Korchmaros I. Saalay E, Fodor M, Jablonszky E: Spontaneous opening rate of the congenitally blocked nasolacrimal ducts. Recent Advances in the Lacrimal System. Tokyo, Asahi Press, 1980, pp 30-35
4. Werb A: Anatomia del sistema lagrimal y su importancia en cirugia. An address delivered at XI Congresso Argentino de Oftalmologia. November 1979

SUPPLEMENTAL BIBLIOGRAPHY

Duke-Elder S: Systems of Ophthalmology. London, Henry Kimpton, 1974, Vol 13, The Ocular Adnexa

Milder B: Functional block in the lacrimal drainage system. XVIII Concilium Ophthalmologica, Belgium, 1958

Weil BA et al.: Dacryocystitis. The lacrimal system. Proceedings of the First International Symposium. St. Louis, Mosby, 1971, pp 118-125

Weil BA: La Dacrio-cisto-rinostomia en el Nino. Arch Oftal Buenos Aires, 42:250, 1968

Weil BA et al.: La dacriocistografia. Arch Oftal Buenos Aires, 49:7, 1974

11

DISEASES OF THE LACRIMAL GLAND

BENJAMIN MILDER

Most pathologic processes are characterized by enlargement and/or displacement of the lacrimal gland. Signs and symptoms common to all lacrimal gland disease include fullness in the temporal half or one third of the upper eyelid, ptosis in the temporal half of the upper lid margin producing a characteristic S-shaped curve to the lid margin, and, frequently, elevation of the temporal half of the brow. The S curve of the upper lid margin is diagnostic for lacrimal gland disease and is not duplicated by any other upper lid abnormality. If symptoms of pain, lacrimation, and tenderness suggest an inflammatory process, the S curve will immediately identify the site of the inflammation or infection as being the lacrimal gland.

Acute inflammatory diseases of the lacrimal gland will be accompanied by pain, swelling, tenderness, and mucopurulent secretion in the conjunctival sac. In chronic inflammations, however, there may be no such inflammatory picture, and the only sign would be enlargement of the gland with characteristic appear-

ance of the lid margin. Chronic dacryoadenitis may be unilateral or bilateral. Apart from these clues, chronic inflammatory disease of the lacrimal gland can readily be confused with neoplasms.

Cystic lesions involving the lacrimal gland may be freely movable on palpation, as will be small neoplasms, but the cyst may be identified by transillumination. Larger neoplasms, benign or malignant, are usually firm, nontender masses, not readily displaced on palpation.

This brief description of the clinical manifestations of lacrimal gland disease points up the importance of further definitive diagnostic evaluation of enlargements of the gland.

CONGENITAL ABNORMALITIES

Anterior displacement or prolapse of the lacrimal gland may be seen in patients who have shallow bony orbits. The prolapse may be unilateral or bilateral and is usually accompanied by proptosis of the eye.

Spontaneous prolapse of the lacrimal gland may result from congenital weakness of the fascial support.[1] Prolapse of the gland may also result from trauma, usually a perforating injury in the vicinity of the lacrimal gland fossa.

The editors express their gratitude and appreciation to Professor Morton E. Smith, Department of Ophthalmology, Washington University School of Medicine, for his assistance in the preparation of this chapter and for the illustrations from the Department of Ocular Pathology.

CONGENITAL CYSTS OF THE LACRIMAL GLAND

Congenital cysts of the lacrimal gland are rare. Fullness of the temporal half of the upper lid area in an infant should suggest such a possibility. The suspected area may be revealed as cystic by transillumination or by everting the lid and visualizing the cystic palpebral lobe of the gland. Aspiration of the cyst will be therapeutic as well as provide confirmation of the diagnosis. If treatment is limited to aspiration of the cyst, recurrences are likely, and the cyst should be excised if it is cosmetically objectionable. If it is small, no treatment is necessary. Because of the early onset, congenital lacrimal gland cysts are likely to be confused with solid tumors.

Dermoid cysts may occur in the lacrimal gland, but they are quite rare. However, dermoid cysts occurring within the temporal orbit or under the superior orbital rim may produce a prolapse of a contiguous lacrimal gland. An apparent enlargement of the lacrimal gland occurring in the first two decades of life should suggest a possible contiguous dermoid cyst (Fig. 11-1).

LACRIMAL CYSTS

Lacrimal gland cysts (dacryops) (Figs. 11-2 and 11-3) can simulate solid tumors of the gland in their clinical picture and their slow development. Unlike the rare congenital cyst, the dac-

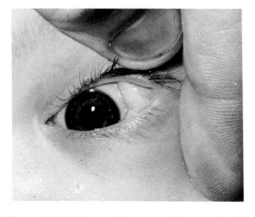

Figure 11-1. Dermoid tumor of temporal orbit. Portion of prolapsed lacrimal gland (palpebral lobe) can be seen on the surface of the tumor.

ryops is more likely to appear in the adult years. It is usually unilateral and may be of any size. The first indication of such a cyst is fullness in the temporal one third of the upper lid, with the characteristic S-shaped contour of the lid margin. The palpebral lobe is invariably the site of dacryops, and unless it is too large, the upper lid can be everted, revealing the leading edge of the dark-colored cyst. Such cysts may result from occlusion of the collecting ductules due to prior inflammation of the gland. However, more often than not, no history of dacryoadenitis can be elicited.

If the cyst is large, it should be excised for cosmetic reasons. It must be remembered that, in any excision of the palpebral lobe of the lacrimal gland, the ductules from the orbital lobe are transected, and there is the risk of lacrimal hyposecretion with keratitis sicca.

INFLAMMATIONS OF THE LACRIMAL GLAND

It is generally felt that half of all enlargements of the lacrimal gland are inflammatory, but Jakobiec and Jones[2] have suggested that, from their clinical impressions, inflammations probably account for as much as 75 percent of all enlargements of the gland.

Acute dacryoadenitis is usually unilateral (Fig. 11-4). At the onset, there is swelling of the temporal half of the upper lid with the characteristic S curve of the lid margin, some tenderness, and associated tearing. There is usually mucoid or mucopurulent secretion in the conjunctival sac. When the acute inflammation involves the orbital lobe alone or both lobes, pain is a prominent feature. As the inflammatory reaction progresses, the entire upper eyelid becomes edematous, tense, and tender, and the lid edema is accompanied by chemosis of the bulbar conjunctiva temporally. The ipsilateral preauricular lymph node may be enlarged and tender.

In *acute epidemic parotitis* (mumps), there may be an associated dacryoadenitis. In some few cases, the mumps virus may produce an acute dacryoadenitis without the usual parotid gland involvement. The chief pathologic finding is lymphocytic infiltration of the gland. This form of viral dacryoadenitis should be treated

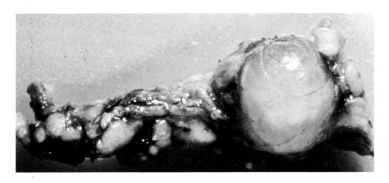

Figure 11-2. Dacryops. (*Washington University Reg. 82-663K4.*)

with supportive measures. It is self-limiting, lasting 2 to 4 weeks.

Epidemic dacryoadenitis in the absence of mumps has been considered to be influenzal in origin, since it is associated with the clinical picture of flu, but no specific organisms have been identified during these epidemics.[3]

Acute Bacterial Dacryoadenitis

This may occur as a result of exogenous invasion through the conjunctiva or may be metastatic from a remote site of infection via the bloodstream. Dacryoadenitis may be a sequela of trauma. It may also be present as one element in a generalized systemic infection. One of the authors (B.W.) found *Staphylococcus aureus* to be the most prevalent causative organism. Other infectious agents that have been identified are streptococci, the gonococcus, and the pneumococcus.

Treatment of Acute Dacryoadenitis. Acute dacryoadenitis is usually self-limiting, lasting from 4 to 8 weeks. The treatment of viral forms, such as mumps and infectious mononucleosis is symptomatic, requiring rest until the fever subsides. Application of ice packs to the swollen lacrimal gland may help reduce pain, which is often disabling. Codeine 30 mg and aspirin 600 mg every 4 hours may relieve discomfort. A barbiturate, such as phenobarbital 15 mg orally tid or qid, may be used to provide sedation.

If the causative agent is bacterial, smears and cultures of any discharge or tears from such infected glands are necessary to determine the etiologic organism and its drug sensitivity. A typical systemic antibiotic regimen that offers spectrum coverage for both gram-positive and gram-negative bacteria is a combination of gentamicin 4 mg/kg daily IM in three divided doses and a cephalosporin, such as cefazolin 1 g

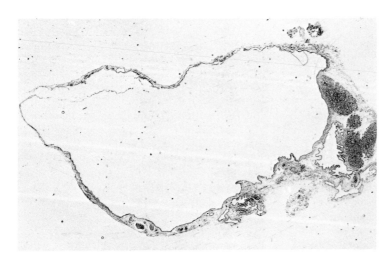

Figure 11-3. Dacryops. (*Washington University Reg. 82-615K5.*)

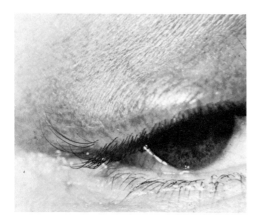

Figure 11-4. Acute dacryoadenitis.

every 4 hours IV, with probenecid 0.5 g PO four times daily. These drugs should be continued for 7 days. If the gland becomes abscessed, incision and drainage will hasten recovery.

If the dacryoadenitis is gonorrheal, specific antibiotics are prescribed. Penicillin is the drug of choice here, 4.8 million units of aqueous penicillin procaine B are given IM daily in divided doses and injected into at least two sites around the gland during the acute phase of the infection. To increase the antibiotic activity of penicillin, probenecid 1 g orally should be given at least 1 hour prior to injecting the penicillin in order to block renal excretion. When the gonococci are resistant or if the patient is allergic to penicillin, a total dose of 9.5 g of oral tetracycline is given as 1.5 g initially, followed by 0.5 g four times a day for 4 more days.

Fungal infection is an infrequent cause of dacryoadenitis, but such organisms as *Actinomyces, Histoplasma,* or *Nocardia* have been found in acutely inflamed lacrimal glands.

Chronic Dacryoadenitis
Chronic dacryoadenitis presents a much more serious diagnostic problem, because in any persisting enlargement of the lacrimal gland, there exists the possibility that the lesion is a tumor.

Chronic dacryocystitis presents no diagnostic problem when it follows upon an acute episode. In such cases, the condition may burn itself out over a period of months, with gradual regression of the enlarged gland. However, if the enlargement persists, biopsy may be necessary to confirm the diagnosis. The histology

may show a nonspecific pattern of lymphocytic infiltration (Fig. 11-5), or it may be granulomatous in nature (so-called pseudotumor).

SARCOID OF THE LACRIMAL GLAND

The lacrimal gland is the most common locus of sarcoidosis in and around the orbit. It may have a subacute onset, with moderate tenderness and tearing accompanying enlargement of the gland. More often, the condition develops as a silent enlargement. As a rule, the involvement of the lacrimal gland is one manifestation of generalized sarcoidosis with involvement of the lymph nodes and the nodes of the mediastinum as well as the lungs and other organs.

Sarcoid involvement of the lacrimal gland may be unilateral or bilateral, and a diagnosis will depend on biopsy. Histologically, there will be noncaseating granulomatous tubercles (Fig. 11-6), lymphocytic infiltration, giant cell nests, and replacement of the secretory acini by fibrosis.

In the treatment of the sarcoid, emphasis is placed on the use of corticosteroids. Results vary with the stage of the disease. Extirpation of the gland is indicated if the mass is deforming or symptomatic despite conservative treatment.

MIKULICZ SYNDROME

The term "Mikulicz syndrome" is archaic and could well join other eponyms nominated for oblivion. The term does not explain etiology and has been employed for a syndrome characterized by chronic simultaneous enlargement of the lacrimal and parotid glands, usually bilateral. However, the histologic features are those of a nonspecific granulomatous dacryoadenitis and may be due to sarcoidosis, syphilis, tuberculosis, mumps, or lymphoma.

PSEUDOTUMOR OF THE LACRIMAL GLAND

Pseudotumor, or chronic granuloma of the lacrimal gland, is a smoldering, slowly progressive inflammation of unknown etiology. It may be a

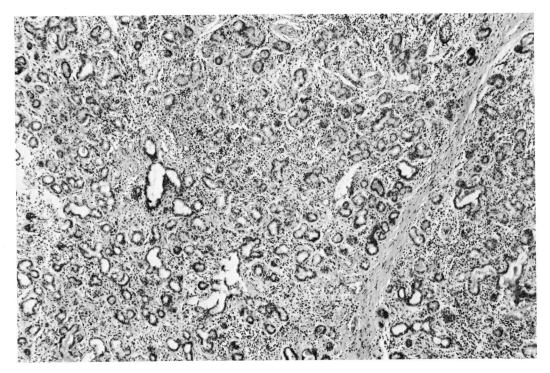

Figure 11-5. Chronic dacryoadenitis. An infiltration of lymphocytes has replaced most of the normal gland tissue. (*Washington University Reg. 82-671.*)

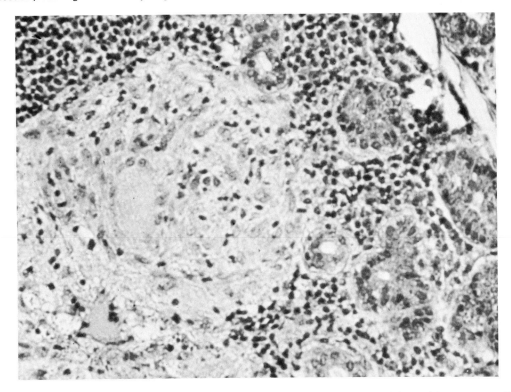

Figure 11-6. Noncaseating granulomatous tubercle of sarcoidosis. A few remaining acini are seen on the right side of the photo. (*Washington University Reg. 82-662P3.5.*)

sequela of a prior acute dacryoadenitis or part of the picture of systemic granulomatous disease.

Jakobiec and Jones[2] defined pseudotumor as an idiopathic granulomatous disease of the lacrimal gland. Idiopathic pseudotumor is usually unilateral. It comes on rapidly, with pain, moderate tenderness, proptosis, and lid edema, with the S curve of the upper lid margin characteristic of lacrimal gland disease. If the swelling of the gland progresses, the eyeball will be displaced downward. Histologically, the picture is one of chronic inflammation, with lymphocyte accumulations in follicles, reticulum cells, some plasma cells, and epithelioid giant cells, together with fibrovascular infiltration.

In the absence of acute signs and symptoms at the onset of the disease, pseudotumor presents a picture that must be differentiated from benign mixed tumor of the lacrimal gland, or possibly, Sjögren's syndrome. The sedimentation rate may be elevated. Pseudotumor shows no evidence of bone erosion on radiographic examination. B-scan ultrasound will reveal a mass with unencapsulated borders and an irregular shaggy outline.

The treatment of pseudotumor consists of large doses of steroids for up to 1 month, tapering gradually over a period of 3 to 6 months if necessary. Recurrences will necessitate further steroid therapy.

SJÖGREN'S SYNDROME

Although Sjögren's syndrome is now regarded as an autoimmune manifestation and is included in the family of so-called collagen diseases, the histopathology of Sjögren's syndrome is similar in many respects to that of pseudotumor. Chief features include dense lymphocytic accumulations, connective tissue proliferation, and eventually atrophy of the acinar elements. Although the histopathology of the two conditions may be similar, the two diseases are readily distinguishable, since Sjögren's syndrome has a characteristic clinical picture (See Chapter 21).

REFERENCES

1. Duke-Elder S: System of Ophthalmology. St. Louis, Mosby, 1952, Vol 5, p 4694
2. Jakobiec J, Jones I, In Duane TD: Clinical Ophthalmology. Hagerstown, Md, Harper & Row, 1980, Vol 2, Chap 35
3. Duke-Elder S: System of Ophthalmology. St. Louis, Mosby, 1952, Vol 5, p 5217

12

TUMORS OF THE LACRIMAL GLAND

BENJAMIN MILDER and MORTON E. SMITH

Tumors of the lacrimal gland are usually classified as either epithelial or lymphomatous.

I. Epithelial
  A. Benign
    1. Mixed tumor, benign
  B. Malignant
    1. Mixed tumor, malignant
    2. Adenoid cystic carcinoma
    3. Undifferentiated carcinoma
II. Lymphomatous
  A. Benign lymphoma (benign lymphoid hyperplasia)
  B. Malignant lymphoma
  C. Hodgkin's disease

All of these entities may have a similar appearance early in their clinical course, but since there are important differences in the appropriate treatment and ultimate prognosis, early diagnosis by biopsy is essential.

EPITHELIAL TUMORS

Benign Mixed Tumors

Benign mixed tumors, accounting for some 60 percent of all epithelial lacrimal gland tumors, are found in the young and midadult years (78 percent between the ages of 20 and 50).[1] These tumors are characterized by painless progressive enlargement of the lacrimal gland. The benign mixed tumor is a multiobulated, encapsulated growth which is usually adherent to the periosteum of the lacrimal gland fossa. Therefore, the tumors are fixed on palpation.

Forrest[2] emphasized the epithelial nature of the so-called mixed tumor and pointed out the importance of histologic differentiation in their treatment. Histologically, they contain tubular structures lined by a double layer of epithelium. These tubules are arranged in an irregularly anastomosing pattern in a myxoid stroma (Fig. 12-1). Pleomorphism is characteristic of both the epithelial and the connective tissue elements of these tumors, and there are wide variations between the relative proportions of the two elements.[3]

Benign mixed tumor is, by definition, nonmetastasizing. It is treated by removal of the tumor intact, within its capsule. If the tumor has broken through the capsule or if removal is incomplete, late recurrences can occur and have been reported as long as 22 years after the initial excision. In recurrences of these mixed tumors, there may be carcinomatous change with metastases.

The long-term prognosis for benign mixed

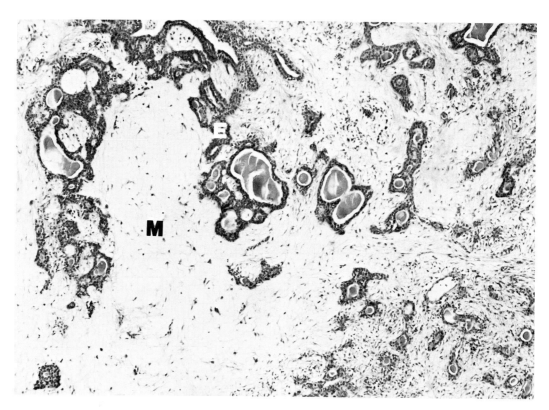

Figure 12-1. Benign mixed cell tumor. The epithelial tubules (E) lie within a myxoid stroma (M). (Washington University Reg. 82-670.)

tumor is excellent. In the report of Zimmerman et al.,[1] only 42 of the 116 lacrimal gland tumor patients were still living at the time of their review, and 39 of these 42 had a diagnosis of benign mixed tumor.

Malignant Mixed Tumor

Malignant mixed tumor may arise as a primary tumor of the lacrimal gland, or may manifest itself in a recurrence of a previously diagnosed benign mixed tumor. The malignant form has some clinical differentiating features. As a primary tumor, it tends to occur in older patients than the benign form (median age of 51 years, as compared to 34.5 years for the benign mixed tumor group). It develops more rapidly, and pain is frequently an early symptom.

Malignant mixed tumor occurs about one tenth as frequently as the benign form. Histologically, the malignant element of these tumors

is adenocarcinoma. Rarely are sarcomatous changes found (Fig. 12-2).

The prognosis for survival is poor. If there is no evidence of distant metastases, the treatment is by wide orbital exenteration supplemented by irradiation and chemotherapy.

Adenoid Cystic Carcinoma

Adenoid cystic carcinoma is the most frequent type of carcinoma of the lacrimal gland. It occurs at a younger age than other carcinomas (median age 37.5 years), and it is, therefore, likely to be confused, in its earlier stages, with benign mixed tumor.[1]

Epithelial tumors of the salivary glands are histologically similar to those in the lacrimal gland, and the two groups are classified in the same manner. However, in the salivary gland, the ratio of adenoid cystic carcinoma to mixed tumors is 1:31, while in the lacrimal gland the

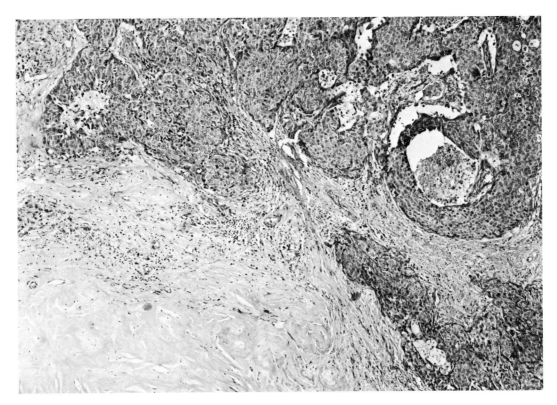

Figure 12-2. Malignant mixed tumor. The malignant element (upper right of photo) is adenocarcinoma. (Washington University Reg. 82-673.)

ratio is 1:2.7. Thus, adenoid cystic carcinoma is much more common, relatively, in the lacrimal gland than in the salivary gland.

Histologically, adenoid cystic carcinoma is unrelated to mixed tumor. The predominant cell type is a small, dense, basal cell, and these cell aggregates are separated by mucus-filled spaces producing a cribriform or Swiss cheese appearance (Figs. 12-3 and 12-4). Adenoid cystic carcinoma differs clinically from benign mixed tumor in several important respects. It grows more rapidly and is accompanied, early in the clinical course, by pain as a result of involvement of nerves and of surrounding tissues, including the adjacent bone. It is rapidly invasive and metastasizes rapidly. The prognosis for survival is poor. Treatment calls for wide exenteration along with irradiation and chemotherapy.

Because of the high degree of malignancy of these tumors, histologic studies should be undertaken as early as possible. Complete removal of the tumor is to be preferred. In such case, if the tumor proves to be a benign mixed tumor, the appropriate treatment will have been accomplished by excision of the mass in toto. If the tumor proves to be malignant, exenteration and further treatment measures can be undertaken. If the mass is too adherent to surrounding structures to remove en bloc or if there is evidence of bone invasion, a deep wedge biopsy should be made to establish the diagnosis.

Undifferentiated Carcinoma

Undifferentiated carcinoma of the lacrimal gland is found less frequently than is the adenoid cystic type. Their early clinical course is essentially the same, as is the poor prognosis and the urgent need for early biopsy confirmation of the diagnosis.

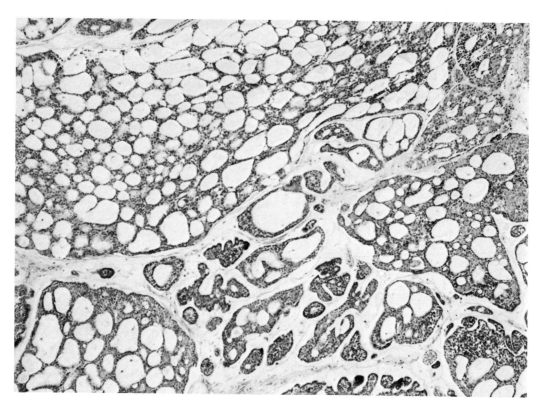

Figure 12-3. Adenoid cystic carcinoma. Note the Swiss cheese pattern. (Washington University Reg. 82-669.)

LYMPHOID TUMORS

Tumors that develop from cells of the reticuloendothelial system are regarded by Reese[4] as variants of a single neoplastic entity despite the widely differing histologic cell types. Lymphoid tumors may be benign or malignant, may be localized or diffuse. In all, such tumors make up only about 5 percent of all lacrimal gland neoplasms.[5]

Benign Lymphoid Hyperplasia

The benign lymphoid hyperplasias cause enlargement of the lacrimal gland and have a firm rubbery feel on palpation. Biopsy should be performed, and the pathologic diagnosis is established on the finding of germinal centers, mature rounded lymphocytes, and an admixture of other inflammatory cells, e.g., plasma cells and eosinophils. These lesions are localized to the gland and are not part of any systemic

disease. They respond dramatically to radiation therapy.

Malignant Lymphoma of the Lacrimal Gland

Lymphocytic Lymphoma. The lacrimal gland is the principal site of lymphoid tissue in the orbit. Hence, tumors arising in the gland are more likely to be lymphocytic lymphomas than reticulum cell tumors.

McGavic[6] reported a study of 21 lymphomatous tumors of the orbit with 15-year follow-up. Seven of his 21 patients had primary tumors of the lacrimal gland, and 3 additional tumors arose contiguous with the gland. Because these tumors are often very slow growing, 5-year survival rates do not necessarily indicate a cure. After 15 years, 25 percent of his patients were alive, and all of them had primary tumors that were not associated with other expressions of lymphomatous disease. Patients with lym-

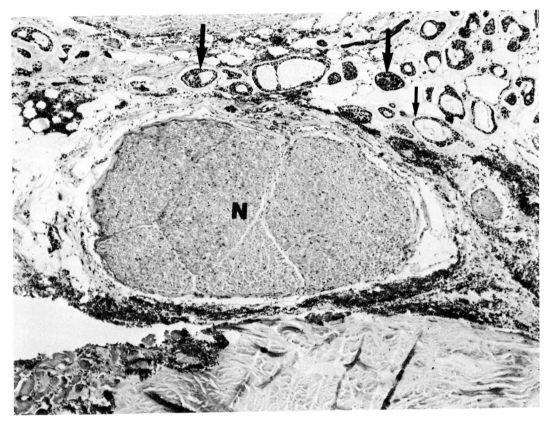

Figure 12-4. Adenoid cystic carcinoma. Tumor cells (arrows) surround an orbital nerve (N), causing pain. (Washington University Reg. 82-674.)

phocytic and giant follicle tumors had the longest survival rate (average 13 years), and those with Hodgkin's disease had the shortest survival (average 4 years).

Any of the malignant lymphomas may localize in the lacrimal gland. The lacrimal gland involvement is usually unilateral and manifests itself by swelling of the upper lid, enlargement of the gland, and usually proptosis of the eye. It is generally accepted that a lacrimal gland mass that is increasing in size must have early diagnostic biopsy. Since these lesions are part of a systemic process, the diagnostic study must include blood and bone marrow studies along with the search for other tumor foci.

For the lacrimal gland involvement, irradiation is the treatment of choice, since these tumors are highly radiosensitive. Surgery is indicated only to the extent of establishing the diagnosis. However, since these lesions are part of a systemic process, treatment must be directed to eradication of the multifocal aspects of the disease, and chemotherapy and radiation treatment are often used together. With local treatment (excision or irradiation of the lacrimal gland tumor), a possible complication is keratitis sicca.

Hodgkin's Disease

Hodgkin's disease is a multicentric form of malignant lymphoma in which the lymphocytic elements are the most prominent histologic feature. It involves cervical nodes, mediastinum, and, eventually, bones and viscera. Both lacrimal glands may be involved simultaneously. The disease is characterized by exacerbations and remissions.

The prognosis in Hodgkin's disease is, at

the present time, considerably less depressing than was the case only a few decades ago. If the lesions are localized to one side of the diaphragm, and if the patient does not have a febrile course and marked weight loss, radiotherapy is used. If the involvement is more extensive, radiotherapy is supplemented with chemotherapy. A combination of nitrogen mustard, vincristine, and procarbazine is used along with prednisone. Surgery has no place in the treatment of Hodgkin's disease except for diagnostic biopsy. Cure rates of up to 50 percent may be expected, even in advanced Hodgkin's disease. Prognosis is more favorable than for other malignant lymphomatous diseases.

REFERENCES

1. Zimmerman LE, Sanders TE, Ackerman LV: Epithelial tumor of the lacrimal gland. Int Ophthalmol Clin 2:353, 1962
2. Forrest AW: Epithelial lacrimal gland tumors: pathology as a guide to prognosis. Trans Am Acad Ophthalmol Otolaryngol 58:848, 1954
3. Hogan M, Zimmerman LE: Ophthalmic Pathology: Atlas and Textbook. Philadelphia, Saunders, 1962, p. 758
4. Reese AB: Tumors of the Eye, 2nd ed. New York, Hoeber (Harper & Row), 1963, pp. 465-67
5. Duke-Elder S: Systems of Ophthalmology. St. Louis, Mosby, 1952, Vol 5 p. 5265
8. McGavic JS: Lymphomatous tumors of the eye. Arch Ophthalmol 53:236, 1955.

SUPPLEMENTAL BIBLIOGRAPHY

Font R, Gamel J: Epithelial tumors of the lacrimal gland. In Jakobiec F (ed.): Ocular and Adnexal Tumors. Birmingham, Ala, Aesculapius Publishing Company, 1978

Stewart WB, Krokel GB, Wright JE: Lacrimal gland and fossa lesions: An approach to diagnosis and management. Ophthalmology 86:886, 1979.

13

THE DRY EYE

BERNARDO A. WEIL

HISTORY OF THE DRY EYE*

Severe xerophthalmia has been identified since remote antiquity. The disease of avitaminosis A was known since Hippocrates, but its cause was not suspected until the latter 19th century. Bitot (1859) described the clinical aspects and Garau Alemany (1881) established that fish and mammalian liver were curative. The pathology of degenerative change in the lacrimal gland in vitamin A deficiency was described by Mori (1921) and Yudkin (1922). Bloch (1924) and Goldblatt (1927) confirmed that vitamin A therapy cured hemeralopic xerophthalmia in man.

Leber described and named filamentary keratitis in 1882, and the following years, Fisher published the association between dry eye and arthritis deformans. The entire clinical picture of Sjögren's syndrome was described by Gougerot (1924) and Sjögren (1930).

Although the use of such things as saliva and egg white were known for a very long time, the first use of normal saline was reported by Berger in 1894. In 1908, Cantonnet introduced the term "artificial tears." More viscous solutions soon followed. These included mucin

Courtesy of Dr. Juan Murube del Castillo.

(Collins, 1931); gelatin (Gifford, 1943); methyl cellulose (1945) and polyvinyl alcohol (Kirshner, 1964).

THE DRY EYE

Why is it that a disease that was known 150 years ago[1] and that until not so long ago was considered to be an infrequent disorder should have become the most common ocular problem, apart from refractive errors? As many as 20 to 25 percent of patients who come to our eye clinic will have some symptom, sign, or evidence from clinical testing of the dry eye syndrome.

For many years, numerous causes of dry eye have been known. Among these causes are:

- Sjögren's syndrome
- Erythema multiforme
- Stevens-Johnson syndrome
- Ocular pemphigoid
- Lyell's syndrome
- Sarcoidosis
- Hypovitaminosis A
- Familial dysautonomia (Riley-Day)
- Congenital disorders of the lacrimal gland and its innervation

- Senile atrophy of the lacrimal gland
- Air pollution
- Hyposecretion secondary to contact lens wear
- Scarring secondary to inflammatory disorders
- Surgical removal of the lacrimal gland
- Cranial fractures with nerve damage
- Trigeminal nerve disorders
- Exaggerated palpebral lid openings with diminished blinking
- Rare systemic disorders associated with lacrimal hypofunction
- Drug-induced hyposecretion

Despite this impressive list of possible causes for the dry eye syndrome, this entity was not recognized as a common disorder until the advent of two modern-day insults—air pollution and contact lenses, especially soft lenses. Among the other mixed blessings of contemporary society, the widespread use of such therapeutic agents as anovulatory drugs and tranquilizers has added to the large number of patients with complaints of dry eye, especially in those who are already predisposed to lacrimal hyposecretion.

In addition to pollution of the environment (the residue of combustion of petroleum derivatives, chemical elements in suspension, and so on) we must also include the air from air conditioners, as well as the rate of air movement in such artificial environments. In winter and in summer alike, these devices maintain a very low level of humidity in the air.

There is no debating the great benefits brought about by contact lenses in terms of undistorted retinal images, improved field of vision, correction of irregular astigmatism and of keratoconus, as well as the overall aesthetic gratifications associated with contact lens wear. Unfortunately, it is no less true that there is a wide range of pathologic processes that can be induced by contact lenses, many of which will exacerbate a preexisting tendency for dry eyes. Problems in fitting and positioning of the contact lenses can result in metabolic changes in the corneal epithelium or in frank corneal erosions much more readily in the patient who has low or borderline tear secretion capability. Immunologic disturbances result from the antigenic effects of proteins adsorbed onto the contact lens and from the toxic sequelae in such

contact lens manufacture problems, as faulty polymerization.

It is possible that the active ingredients in various eye medications can increase in concentration in patients with hyposecretion. In such instances, dosages must be monitored so that adequate therapeutic levels are maintained without exacerbating the dry eye problem. Timolol[2] and the other beta blockers may induce dry eye problems. Some systemic medications, such as phenothiazines[3] and diazepam,[4] decrease tear secretion and produce dry eye symptoms.

Since all of these factors basically affect the stability of the precorneal tear film, they are likely to induce symptoms earlier and more intensely in patients who are actual or borderline hyposecretors.

Changes in hydration of the cornea with the use of high water content soft lenses can exacerbate the problems of the patient with borderline dry eye syndrome and can result in bacterial or fungal contamination.

THE PRECORNEAL TEAR FILM

The precorneal tear film consists of three layers. The anterior lipid layer is a product of the meibomian glands and the sebaceous and sweat glands of the lid margins. Mishima[5] has reported that if the lipid layer is absent or deficient, the rate of evaporation of tears can be multiplied some 10- to 20-fold.

The middle, aqueous layer is produced by the main lacrimal glands and the accessory lacrimal glands of Wolfring and Kraus. The corneal epithelium, normally hydrophobic, is rendered hydrophilic by the deepest layer of the precorneal tear film, the mucous layer. The middle aqueous layer, some 10μ thick, provides:

1. A flushing and buffering action of the corneal surface after contamination
2. The bulk of the lubricating material which facilitates movement of the lids over the conjunctiva and cornea
3. The maintenance of a high quality optical surface
4. The nutrition and immunologic defenses of the cornea

The mucous layer, in contact with the corneal epithelium, is an important factor in the cleansing of the conjunctiva and corneal irregularities. This hydrophilic layer is in contact with the aqueous layer, plays an important role in the stability of the entire tear film, and facilitates adequate wetting of the hydrophobic corneal epithelium.

The dry eye syndrome with associated corneal changes can be produced by excessive evaporation due to a deficient lipid layer, by aqueous layer deficiencies, by corneal irregularities, by discontinuity at the palpebral margins, and by alterations in the mucous layer. When there is absence or decrease of mucus in some dry eyes, the cornea is rendered hydrophobic. For this reason, the aqueous layer cannot spread itself evenly over the corneal surface, and dry areas develop, with possible later epithelial destruction. This assumption has been questioned by Dohlman et al.[6], who measured the mucous layer in patients with Stevens-Johnson syndrome and with benign pemphigoid of the mucous membrane. While mucus was decreased, it was questionable whether this reduction was sufficient to justify the instability of the tear film in these conditions. Electron microscopy of the corneal surface showed the existence of microvilli which maintained the tear film in a vertical orientation, thus favoring wettability.

Changes in pH from 7.5 will not produce symptoms or corneal changes over a range from 6.6 to 7.8. If the pH of tears is more acid or more alkaline than that range, the eye is susceptible to irritation.

Increased irritation may occur with changes in tonicity. When evaporation of tears is prevented, as occurs with the eyes closed, the tear film is isotonic with normal saline. The tonicity of tears is little influenced by increased tear flow, but when tear flow decreases, the tears become markedly hypertonic. Under normal conditions, an osmotic gradient across the cornea, from aqueous humor to epithelium, maintains deturgescence and optical clarity. However, when the tears become hypertonic as a result of decreased tear production, corneal drying occurs. This osmotic differential is the basis for the use of hypotonic solutions in the treatment of the dry eye syndrome.

BASIC AND REFLEX TEAR SECRETION

Lester Jones[9] has proposed that our total lacrimal secretory output is composed of basic and reflex tear secretion. In his view, the reflex secretors are the main lacrimal glands, under the control of the nervous system. The basic secretors are the accessory lacrimal glands, and these are not influenced by reflex innervational control but contribute to the formation of the tear film at a steady and constant rate. The basic secretors can provide the indispensable elements in the amounts required for the three layers. It is believed that the basic secretion is the only lacrimal supply in the newborn and during sleep.

CLINICAL PICTURE OF THE DRY EYE SYNDROME

The usual complaints associated with the dry eye syndrome are burning, aching, foreign body sensation, low threshold for conjunctival congestion, a feeling of dryness, and an accumulation of mucus in the conjunctival sac. Such a pattern of symptoms and signs, while not diagnostic, should cause the examiner to suspect lacrimal hyposecretion. The degree to which a patient experiences discomfort with tear deficiency varies greatly from patient to patient, and the dry eye syndrome must be thought of as a continuum from the mildest symptoms without obvious corneal change to the most severe corneal pathology, including ulceration and corneal perforation.

At all levels, the dry eye syndrome will be characterized not only by reduction in the amount of tear formation but also in conjunctival or corneal changes that can be demonstrated by clinical testing. It is possible for decreased quantities of lacrimal secretion to be associated with corneal-conjunctival normality and an absence of discomfort, as occurs in elderly patients. On the other hand, reduced tear film break-up time and corneal desiccation, or corneal and conjunctival keratinization, may occur in the presence of an adequate tear film, as occurs in some patients with vitamin A-protein deficiencies.

Thus, factors that can influence the dry eye syndrome include not only the amount of tears but also the character of each component of the tear film and the integrity of the cornea and the eyelid margins. The choice of treatment may depend on an appreciation of the specific causative defect.

DIAGNOSTIC TESTS

Rose Bengal Dye Test

This test provides a direct assessment of the degeneration of external tissue and an indirect measurement of tear volume deficiencies. Rose bengal stains dead or damaged cells, and the test response varies with the intensity of the injury. Dead cells will stain bright red, and the amount of staining of damaged cells will depend on the degree of damage.

The test is performed by placing a drop of 1 percent rose bengal dye in the conjunctival sac, followed immediately by irrigation with normal saline. Rose bengal may be irritating, and in some cases a 0.5 percent solution may be preferable. Certain topical anesthetics may alter the test findings. The corneal changes in the dry eye syndrome resulting from a diminished aqueous layer have a virtually pathognomonic rose bengal appearance (See Fig. 8-2). There is punctate staining of the cornea, usually in its lower two thirds. The bulbar conjunctiva stains brilliant red in the area corresponding to the palpebral aperture. It should be remembered that even in normal subjects the corneal epithelium is apt to take up some dye. Thus, a diagnosis of keratoconjunctivitis sicca should include both conjunctival and corneal staining.

Tests of Tear Quantity

Schirmer I Test. When the history and examination suggest dry eye, the Schirmer I test (Chapter 8) can be helpful in confirming the decrease in lacrimal secretion. There are several limitations to the test. It provides semiobjective information, the results of which may vary according to the investigator's technique and his interpretation. It provides semiquantitative data, indicating that tear flow is either probably normal or grossly subnormal. The diagnosis of dry eye cannot be confirmed or dismissed on the basis of the Schirmer I test alone, since quantity of tearing varies from day to day in a

given patient. The results of the test, furthermore, are not necessarily related to the severity of corneal damage.

Because the Schirmer I test measures both reflex and basic tear secretion, an eventual hyposecretion may be caused by defective secretion by the basic secreting glands, defective secretion by the reflex glands, or both. Instillation of an anesthetic into the conjunctival sac will annul the reflex secretion component. If the Schirmer I test is normal and the modification with anesthetic reveals diminished secretion, it would indicate that the reflex secretors are contributing the bulk of the fluid measured by the Schirmer I test. Proparacaine may be used for this purpose, although it does not completely anesthetize the conjunctiva. Cocaine does but is not used because it induces softening of the corneal epithelium. Therefore, either the reflex secretors have been overreacting in an attempt to compensate for the failure of basic secretion (pseudo-epiphora), or there may be an exaggerated reflex response to the paper test strips in the Schirmer I test.

Schirmer II Test. The Schirmer II test, designed to determine the amount of tears produced by the reflex secretors, is performed by aggressively stimulating the afferent arc of the lacrimal reflex. This may be accomplished by rubbing a cotton applicator lightly against the inferior turbinate of the nose. If this test reveals a substantial increase in tear outflow, as compared with the Schirmer I test, it would indicate that the tear replacement therapy can be augmented by, or changed to, some type of glandular stimulation. Several parasympathomimetic substances have been used. Nicotinic acid is said to increase tear secretion, presumably by its vasodilating action. Bromhexine has been employed in treatment of the dry eye syndrome.[10]

Lysozyme Activity Assay

Lysozyme is known to be reduced in the dry eye syndrome. In subjects sensitive to smog, a 60 percent reduction in the lysozyme activity has been reported. Lysozyme activity can be assayed by immunoelectrophoresis and by spectrophotometry. However, the method most suited to clinical practice is the agar diffusion method.[11] When lysozyme is significantly decreased, it indirectly suggests a reduced quantity of tears. Agarlysis assays will reveal this lysozyme deficiency in 99 percent of dry eye patients.

Tear Film Break-up Time

The average tear film break-up time (BUT)(Chapter 8) is 25 to 30 seconds. As the film breaks up, blinking serves to resurface the cornea before any desiccation can occur. Tear film BUT in the dry eye is defined as less than 10 seconds. In patients older than 70, the normal tear film BUT is shorter.

In performing the BUT test, the time from the last blink to the first dry spot is measured, examining the fluorescein-stained cornea at the slit lamp using a cobalt light. Several BUT measurements should be taken and averaged. Results longer than 25 seconds indicate that the patient does not have dry eye. Break-up in less than 15 seconds points to deficiencies in either the aqueous or mucous layer. The BUT is decreased when anesthetics are used. In some pathologic cases, an area of the cornea may never be covered by tear film. In such cases, the BUT would be nil.

Conjunctival Biopsy

When a mucin-deficient state is suspected, a conjunctival sample can be taken and stained with PAS stain (periodic acid-Schiff), and the goblet cells are identified and counted. In some cases they may be completely absent.

Osmotic Pressure of Tear Film

Recently, another method of diagnosing the dry eye syndrome has been reported.[12] Farris and Gilbard postulated that increased osmotic pressure of the tear film may play a part in the development of the dry eye syndrome. They have adapted the Mishima principle of determining tear film osmolarity with a microosmometer and found abnormal increases in concentration of salts in 85 to 95 percent of patients with dry eye syndrome.

TREATMENT OF DRY EYE SYNDROME

Treating individuals with dry eye syndrome can be one of the most frustrating problems that practicing ophthalmologists face. Not only is the diagnosis frequently missed, but treat-ment is not straightforward, and many of the current therapeutic modalities fail to help patients. The varying degrees of severity of dry eyes require different approaches. The so-called dry eye syndrome with senile dehydration of the cornea and conjunctival mucosa is more amenable to therapy than is the more severe end-state of keratoconjunctivitis sicca (Sjögren's syndrome) or neurogenic hyposecretion, such as that seen in the Riley-Day syndrome. Dry eye states following severe conjunctival scarring from ocular pemphigoid, Stevens-Johnson syndrome, trachoma, or chemical burns are also resistant to therapy.

With few exceptions, such as sarcoidosis and disseminated lupus erythematosus, tear flow is not improved by systemic therapy for the disorders associated with dry eye. For this reason, local treatment is today considered to be the cornerstone of therapy for the replacement or supplementation of natural moisture in the eye. Other measures employed include:

- Occlusion of the lacrimal outflow at the puncta
- Adjunctive lubricating, usually at bedtime
- Moisture-economizing measures (moist-chamber spectacles)
- Mucolytic agents
- Management of secondary infection
- Use of contact lenses
- Rarely, corticosteroid therapy

Tear Substitutes

Many different substitutes for natural tears have been used through the years. It has long been appreciated that any solution that differs greatly from natural tears in either tonicity or pH can cause irritation and pain. This observation led to the use of isotonic saline drops and Ringer-Locke solution. But such solutions provided relief for only very short periods of time. Subsequently, research was directed at solutions that approximated the natural tonicity and pH of the tears and that remained in the eye for longer periods of time. This was accomplished by introducing various polymers into artificial tear solutions. Even so, their presence in the eye is short-lived, and their instillation must be frequent. However, they are effective in improving the corneal changes and the patient's symptoms. Although compliance in therapy is an ever-present concern, the relief from discomfort afforded by tear substitutes tends to guarantee that they will be used as often as needed. Fortunately, there is little risk of toxicity or idiosyncrasy from these preparations.

The continuous infusion of tear solutions has been attempted to answer the problem of the short retention time of tear substitutes. The solution is infused into the conjunctival sac by way of intubation through a regular spectacle frame, using a miniature motor-driven pump delivery system.

Soluble artificial tear inserts, now available for general use, consist of an ocular wafer of succinylated collagen which dissolves over a period of hours after insertion, thereby providing time-released lubrication. These inserts have certain problems in terms of insertion and retention in the conjunctival sac. Patients who have mastered the insertion and retention problems obtain gratifying relief from these inserts.

Parasympathomimetic agents, such as neostigmine and diethylphenylphosphate, may provide some increase in tear flow. However, the user must deal with unwanted systemic effects from these agents, and their value is questionable over the long term.

Polack[13] has reported on the benefits of sodium hyaluronate (Healon) (0.1 percent) when tear replacement therapy has been ineffective. The drops must be instilled every hour initially, with gradual reduction of instillation as symptoms abate.

Methyl Cellulose. This synthetic colloid is reported to have a stable pH, a high degree of uniformity, and, in concentration under 1 percent, a refractive index similar to that of the tear film. It provides emollient action, reducing friction between the lids and cornea. An unfavorable feature of methyl cellulose is its viscosity, which has been responsible for blurring of vision and agglutination of the cilia as well as sticking together of the eyelids. It is also said to have a retardant effect on corneal wound healing. Diluting the methyl cellulose preparation reduces these unwanted side effects but shortens the duration of its effectiveness.

A rod-shaped, water-soluble, time-release hydroxypropylcellulose ophthalmic insert is available for insertion into the lower conjunctival cul de sac of dry eyes. This agent has been reported to prolong tear BUT, reduce rose bengal staining, and decrease foreign body sensation. The thickened tears produced by the hydroxypropylcellulose rod may reduce visual acuity and cause stickiness and irritation of the eyelids.

Some high-viscosity polymers may improve the dry eye syndrome by temporarily obstructing the lacrimal passages.

Polyvinyl Alcohol. Polyvinyl alcohol is a less viscous ingredient used to form tear substitutes. It is used in either 1.4 percent or 3 percent concentration for emollient properties. It has adhesive qualities to the cornea. No adverse effect on regeneration of the corneal epithelium has been noted. Polyvinyl alcohol is said to possess certain properties resembling those of mucin.

The surface tension of the natural tear film has been measured at 46 dynes/cm. The higher the surface activity, the lower the surface tension, and the more likely the substance is to spread. At present, it seems likely that improvements in eye drops will bring about solutions having ingredients with such potentiating properties. Commercial preparations used as tear supplements ordinarily include preservatives, such as benzalkonium chloride, EDTA (ethylenediaminetetraacetic acid), calcium chlorobutanol, and thimerosal. Some of these agents may be irritants. This is especially true of benzalkonium chloride and thimerosal.

Other Treatment

In severe cases of dry eye syndrome, ointments are used at night. When patients cannot compensate for increased drying when outdoors, protective sunglasses or moist chambers can be resorted to. Smoking should be discouraged.

Punctum plugs have been devised so that the potential benefits of permanent punctal occlusion can be evaluated. Cyanoacrylate glue has been used for the same purpose. It is applied to the punctum through a 30-gauge blunt needle. It is important to note that Sjögren's syndrome, as well as other causes of dry eye, may have remissions and exacerbations. Remissions may last for as much as 1 to 2 years. If the puncta have been sealed permanently, troublesome tearing could be present during such remissions. Occlusion of the lacrimal punctum is recommended only after all other treatments have failed, since it is irreversible.

When the vision is threatened by severe corneal damage, permanent closure of the puncta can be effected using cautery. Alternatively, the canaliculus may be dissected and ligated. Initial occlusion efforts should be directed at the lower puncta first. Then, if necessary, the upper puncta may be similarly occluded.

Surgical approaches include lateral tarsorrhaphy. Adhesions of the lateral one third of the lid margins may increase comfort in older individuals with severe keratoconjunctivitis sicca or in children with Riley-Day syndrome.

Contact Lenses

The use of contact lenses has saved the vision of many patients with dry eye. Molded hard scleral lenses and soft lenses have been used, depending upon individual requirements. The lenses have proved particularly valuable in patients with neuroparalytic keratitis. However, because of the increased potential for infection, the use of therapeutic contact lenses should be monitored carefully. Antibiotic drops, such as chloramphenicol, are used in conjunction with such contact lens therapy.

Mucolytic Agents

It has been reported that only 30 percent of dry eye patients require mucus-reducing therapy. Acetylcysteine, an agent originally used for treatment of excessive bronchial mucus, has been used for the dry eye patient. This agent is used in concentrations of 5 to 10 percent, and even as high as 20 percent. All such solutions are more or less unstable and have a relatively short life since the mucolytic agent rapidly inactivates. Oral mucolytic agents have no effect on the eye.

Systemic Therapeutic Devices

Corticosteroids have been administered either orally or parenterally in Sjögren's syndrome and other systemic disorders, such as sarcoidosis and erythema multiforme. Results have not been encouraging.

Salivary Glands

Attempts to substitute saliva for lacrimal secretions by transplanting Stensen's duct into the lower conjunctival fornix have met with little success. Excessive secretions during meals have been a troublesome complication. A stent is necessary to drain the secretions from the conjunctival sac into the antrum. The proteolytic enzyme components of the salivary secretion may add to the problems of the cornea.

IS THE LACRIMAL GLAND DISPENSABLE?

Based on the concept of the dual mechanism for the production of tears (basic secretion and reflex secretion), it has been proposed that adequate hydration of the cornea can be maintained by the basic secretors in the absence of the main lacrimal gland. Scherz and Dohlman[14] have reported keratoconjunctivitis sicca immediately after the removal of the lacrimal gland in a 43-year-old woman with normal eyes and satisfactory presurgery lacrimal function. On the nonoperated side, the eye continued normal for a period of 10 years. Eight similar cases are found in the literature. It was concluded that the basic secretors are not sufficient to avoid lacrimal insufficiency.

REFERENCES

1. Mackenzie W: Practical Treatment of Diseases of the Eye, 4th ed. London, Longman, 1854
2. Nielson NV, Eriksen JS: Timolol transitory manifestations of dry eyes in long-term treatment. Acta Ophthalmol 57:418, 1979
3. Siddal JR: Ocular toxic changes associated with chlorpromazine and thioridazine. Can J Ophthalmol 1:190, 1966
4. Saroux H, Martin P, Marax S, Offret N: Hyposecretion lacrymale et médicaments psychotropes. Ann Ocul (Paris) 209:193, 1976
5. Mishima S: Some physiologic aspects of the precorneal tear film. Arch Ophthalmol 73:233, 1965
6. Dohlman CH, Friend J, Kalevar V, et al.: The glycoprotein (mucus) content of tears from normals and dry eye patients. Exp Eye Res, 22:359, 1976
7. Singer JD, et al.: Hexosaminidase in tears and saliva for rapid identification of Tay-Sachs disease and its carriers. Lancet 2:116, 1973
8. Del Monte MA, et al.: Diagnosis of Fabry's disease by tear alpha-galactosidase A (letter). N Eng J Med 290:57, 1974

9. Jones LT: The lacrimal secretory system and its treatment. Am J Ophthalmol 62:47, 1966

10. Rossmann H: Treatment of decreased tear secretion with bromhexin eye drops. Dtsch Med Wochenschr 99:408, 1974

11. van Bijsterveld OP: The lysozyme agar diffusion test in the sicca syndrome. Ophthalmologica 167:429, 1973

12. Farris RL: Dry eye linked to many disorders. Ophthalmology Times, p. 66, May 1982

13. Polack FM: Treatment of Keratitis with Sodium Hyaluronidate (Healon). Scientific exhibit. American Academy of Ophthalmology, 1981, Atlanta, Ga

14. Scherz W, Dohlman CH: Is the lacrimal gland dispensable? Arch Ophthalmol 93:281, 1975

14

DISEASES OF THE UPPER EXCRETORY SYSTEM

BERNARDO A. WEIL

The lacrimal excretory system is a single entity, embryologically and histologically. The concept of dividing the excretory system into upper and lower components developed as a matter of convenience in diagnosis and treatment, and for no other reason. This chapter will consider diseases characteristic of the upper system—the puncta and canaliculi.

THE PUNCTUM

Malposition of the Punctum

Diseases that affect the eyelids and lid margins may result in malposition of the punctum, with resulting epiphora. Such diseases include marginal blepharitis, various forms of dermatitis, e.g., seborrheic, atopic, and neurodermatitis, and such collagen diseases as scleroderma. In all such dermatoses, although the punctum is not primarily involved, relief of the epiphora requires attention to the positioning and patency of the punctum (Fig. 14-1).

In the treatment of malposition of dermatologic origin, the treatment is first directed to the primary eyelid problem. Since any reduction in crusting of the lid margin, edema of the

lids, or eczematoid skin reaction can result in improvement in the position of the punctum, treatment of the primary skin problem may be adequate to relieve the epiphora. However, such skin problems may leave in their wake eversion and/or stenosis of the punctum.

If there is only moderate malposition of the punctum, inversion may be accomplished by *Ziegler cautery,* using a barrage of punctures applied to the nasal tarsus (Chapter 20). If there is a more severe ectropion of the punctum, a diamond-shaped or elliptical excision of conjunctiva and subconjunctival tissue is preferred (Chapter 20). In all of these methods, some later slippage is possible, and the procedure may have to be repeated. If there is ectropion of the lid margin as well as the punctum, the appropriate ectropion surgery may be combined with one of these punctum-repositioning procedures.

Beyond these measures, if the punctum is still not positioned for adequate access to the tear lake, apposition may be achieved by enlarging the punctal orifice on the posterior aspect of the lid. This is accomplished by the three-snip operation or by a punch punctumplasty (Figs. 14-2 and 14-3).

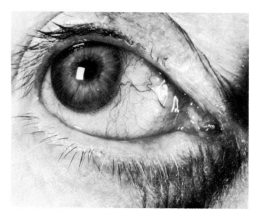

Figure 14-1. Eversion of lower lid punctum.

Stenosis of the Punctum

When the punctum is everted as a result of long-standing dermatoses of the lids, the orifice may be completely occluded, and, in some instances, the lacrimal papilla is so flattened that it may be difficult to identify. If the closure of the punctum is not complete, it can be dilated gently. In some few cases, repeated dilation may provide relief. All too often, however, the benefits of dilating are transient at best, and access to the outflow system requires a punctumplasty such as those mentioned above.

If the punctum cannot be identified and opened, the drainage of tears will require a conjunctivodacryocystorhinostomy. This procedure means that the surgeon abandons the upper excretory system in favor of a permanent stent,

such as the Jones Pyrex tube. Therefore, before proceeding to the Jones operation, an effort should be made to open the canaliculus for drainage of tears. In this procedure, the canaliculus is identified by transillumination, and it is entered by transecting the horizontal limb 3 to 4 mm nasal to the lacrimal papilla. The opening thus made is enlarged by the equivalent of a three-snip operation or similar procedure and is maintained open with the use of a Silastic tube or other form of stent over a 3- to 6-week period.

The punctal orifice may be the site of chronic inflammatory or neoplastic masses. Until the mass is removed for biopsy, it is often difficult to determine whether it arises from the lacrimal papilla or from the subjacent canaliculus. Granulomas may result from local irritation due to indwelling stents (Fig. 14-4). Solid tumors (Fig. 14-5) and papillomas (Fig. 14-6) may be encountered. It is appropriate to use Silastic intubation or other forms of stent to prevent cicatricial closure of the punctum after removal of such lesions.

THE CANALICULUS

Canalicular inflammation may be classified as mycotic or stenosing. Whatever the etiology of the inflammatory process—infection, chemical, or systemic—the end result may be partial or complete closure of the upper secretory system.

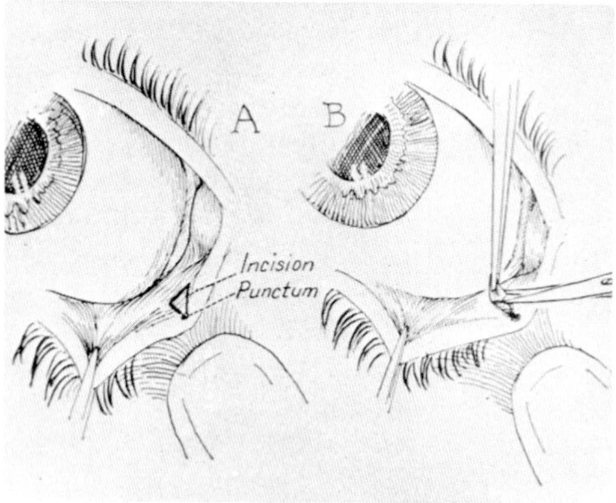

Figure 14-2. Three-snip punctumplasty.

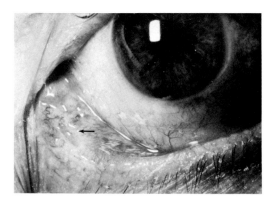

Figure 14-3. Holth punch punctumplasty. Note the cresent-shaped opening on the posterior lid margin.

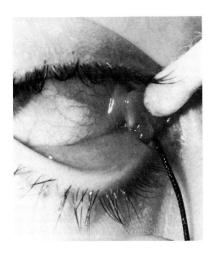

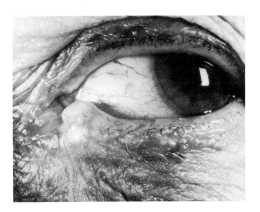

Figure 14-5. Tumor mass, lower punctum.

Figure 14-4. Granuloma, lower lid punctum, a complication of a silk indwelling stent.

Mycotic Canaliculitis[1]

The frequency of mycotic canaliculitis varies with climate and geography. In North America, such fungal infections are uncommon in the far west, in Canada, and in New England. They are much more common in farming areas in the middle west, especially in the Mississippi River valley. In the southern hemisphere, mycotic canaliculitis is not encountered frequently. We have seen about 30 cases in Argentina. The disease affects both sexes and is usually found in adult years. However, we have found this condition in a 10-year-old patient.

Acute inflammatory onset is rare. Usually the canaliculus harbors the infection for months or even years before it becomes clinically evident. Characteristically, it is unilateral, and the lower canaliculus is affected more than the upper. A smoldering unilateral conjunctivitis, particularly one confined to the nasal aspect of the eyes which does not respond to the usual topical antibiotics, should alert one to the possibility that the conjunctivitis is secondary to a fungal canaliculitis. In the characteristic picture of this disease, the punctum is patulous and pouting. Often thin white pus is seen at the punctum, and there is, of course, the associated conjunctivitis. There may be an appearance of fullness in the nasal third of the eyelid. Tenderness is absent or minimal, and light pressure over the canalicular region may produce addi-

tional pus or granules. Frequently, the diagnosis can be confirmed by instilling one drop of topical anesthetic into the conjunctival sac and then massaging the canaliculus lightly between two cotton applicators. In this manner, additional concretions may be expressed through the punctum (Figs. 14-7 to 14-10).

Radnot[2] had described an enormous dilatation of the canaliculus, particularly the ampulla as seen on the dacryocystogram, as a characteristic sign in mycotic canaliculitis. The lacrimal sac is not involved, as a rule, in mycotic canaliculitis, and the lacrimal passages are invariably permeable. The dacryocystogram will confirm normal outflow functions in the lower excretory system. In all of our cases, the

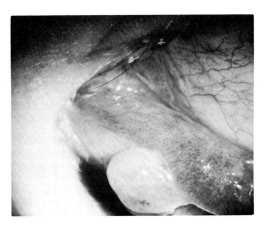

Figure 14-6. Tumor (papilloma with polypoid degeneration) distending the lower punctum.

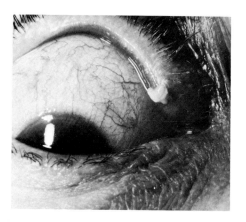

Figure 14-7. Fungal canaliculitis. Concretions expressed from upper punctum.

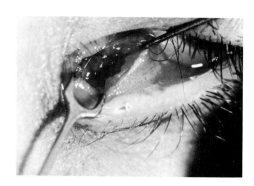

Figure 14-9. Fungal canaliculitis. Dilated canalicular ampulla from which stones have been removed (same patient as in Fig. 14-8).

causative agent was *Actinomyces israelii.* The diagnosis can be made with smears of the discharge. Gram stain will show many polymorphonuclear cells and fine, small, branching hyphae. The organism grows in an anaerobic medium, such as thioglycollate broth, after 7 to 10 days.

True fungi that infect the lacrimal system include such organisms as *Candida, Fusarium, Nocardia,* and *Aspergillus.* All of these can be diagnosed by inoculating the discharge into liquid thioglycollate broth or by performing a microscopic examination of the smear in a KOH hanging drop preparation. This is prepared by putting 1 drop of 10 to 20 percent KOH on a slide, adding the infected material to the drop, covering it with a coverslip, and looking

through the microscope for the glass rodlike hyphae of the fungi.

The treatment of fungal canaliculitis with medications instilled into the canaliculus has been disappointing. Possibly this is because adequate contact with the infected organism is not possible because of the numerous recesses and convolutions in the canalicular path. However, occasional success has been achieved using nystatin in a 1:20,000 suspension. This is instilled by drop into the conjunctival sac three times each day and irrigated into the canaliculus three times weekly.

The definitive treatment of fungal canaliculitis is surgery. In Argentina, surgical intervention resulted in a cure in every one of our cases, although it was necessary to repeat the procedure in a few patients once or twice. The

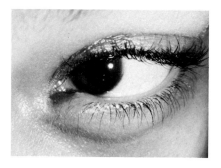

Figure 14-8. Fungal canaliculitis. Note the patulous punctum and the fullness of the nasal half of the lower lid.

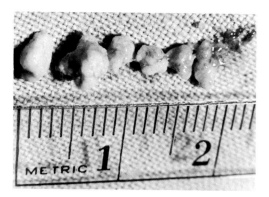

Figure 14-10. Stones removed from canaliculus (same patient as in Fig. 14-8).

therapeutic canaliculotomy is performed under local anesthesia.

We insert a 0 Bowman's probe through the punctum into the canaliculus. The roof of the canaliculus is slit beginning 2 mm medial to the punctum and continuing the incision for a distance of 5 to 8 mm. After opening the canaliculus, a 1 or 2 mm chalazion curette is used to clean the dilated canaliculus and its diverticuli as well as possible. Large quantities of white-yellow (sulfur) granules may be removed in this manner. After curetting the canaliculus, a Veirs rod is inserted, and the roof of the canaliculus is closed with interrupted 7-0 nonabsorbable sutures. The rod remains in place about 6 weeks to avoid secondary contraction and fibrosis.

In the United States, the method used for therapeutic canaliculotomies is somewhat different. Emphasis is placed on incising the horizontal limb of the canaliculus on the posterior surface. After removal of the concretions as completely as possible with the chalazion curette, the remaining mucosal lining is removed with tincture of iodine, and no attempt is made to close the incision. Invariably, this heals without compromising the lumen of the canaliculus. As is so often the case, common goals can be reached by different methods.

Stenosing Canaliculopathy[3]

The term "stenosing canaliculopathy" is used to identify those inflammatory diseases that basically consist in the cicatricial shrinking of the lumen of the canaliculus. The canalicular obstruction may be complete or incomplete. It may affect one or more of the lacrimal canaliculi. We have found the incidence of this disease to be 1 in 1,600 eye patients. That is, in approximately 200,000 listed eye diagnoses, there were 126 patients with stenosing canaliculopathy. In half of these, more than one canaliculus was affected.

When the etiologic factors could be identified, they were as follows:

1. Corneoconjunctival viral infection (herpes simplex), 13
2. Conjunctivitis due to bacterial infection, 11
3. Dacryocystitis, 11
4. Trachoma, 2
5. Sinusitis, 1

Although this series did not identify other causes, our colleagues have reported such cases following long-standing allergic conjunctivitis (pollenosis) and hypersensitivity to various topical medications. In more than half of our patients, there was no history or residual of prior pathologic process. Increasing epiphora was the only symptom. It appears that the largest number of cases of canalicular stenosis are the result of multiple low-grade or subclinical recurrences of herpes viral infection, as hypothesized by Sanford-Smith.[4] Werb cited two such cases following varicella and vaccinia infections.[5]

In the majority of our bacteriologic studies, we were unable to find pathogenic organisms. It is possible that in some patients,[4] iodo-deoxy-uridine (IDU) was responsible for the obstruction. However, in the same patients, it might be argued that the herpes itself was the responsible factor. In canalicular stenosis, slit lamp examination may reveal no sign of a punctum or a very phimotic one. The stenosis may proceed from the common canaliculus to the punctum or vice versa.

Histologic examination always shows the same picture: a canalicular lumen completely occluded by fibrosis with little or no cellular infiltration (Figs. 14-11 and 14-12).

The essential element in treatment of canalicular stenosis, where the obstruction is not complete, is the introduction of an obturator for an extended period of time. We use a Veirs rod and allow this to remain in the canaliculus for 40 to 60 days. A large proportion of the stenoses so treated will recur after the Veirs rod is removed. Although our results are poor, it is a simple treatment to employ, and the alternative is extended surgery (Jones conjunctivodacryocystorhinostomy). Therefore, we prefer to try the obturator method in incomplete closure cases. In North America, silicone intubation has, for the most part, supplanted the use of the Veirs rod for the treatment of partial stenoses. Using this method, the two free ends of the small caliber Silastic tube are fed through both the upper and lower canaliculus and then through the nasolacrimal duct and brought out of the nasal ostium in the inferior meatus of the nose. There, the two free ends are tied or sutured to the ala and permitted to remain in place for up to 3 months. The Quickert-Dryden Silastic tubes have swaged-on probes to facili-

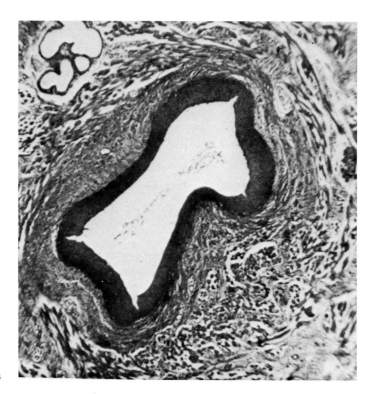

Figure 14-11. Normal canaliculus

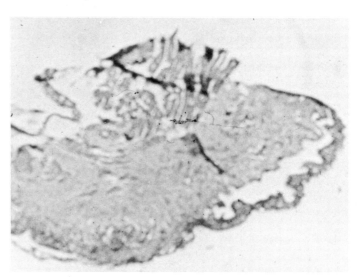

Figure 14-12. Stenosing canaliculopathy.

tate the passage of the tubing. Since it would
seem reasonable to employ the largest caliber
stent that can be used without distorting or
damaging the excretory passages, our preference is for the 1 mm (0.037 inches) outside diameter caliber. This size tubing provides optimum results in establishing and maintaining
patency of the canalicular lumen.

If, at the time of the examination, the canaliculus is completely stenosed, or if stenosis fol-

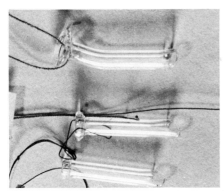

Figure 14-13. Jones Pyrex glass tubes used to maintain patency in conjunctivo-dacryocystorhinostomy.

lows conservative intubation treatment, an alternative tear pathway must be established. In such cases, our preference is for the conjunctivodacryocystorhinostomy of Jones with insertion of a Pyrex glass tube. When the problem is bilateral, the corrective procedures are performed during the same surgical session.

CONJUNCTIVO-DACRYOCYSTORHINOSTOMY

Conjunctivo-dacryocystorhinostomy employing the Jones Pyrex glass tubes has proven to be the most effective means of re-establishing tear outflow when the canalicular pathway cannot be restored. The Pyrex glass tube may be straight or angled and is available in any length. Tubes between 14 and 18 millimeters in length are most frequently employed. The tube has a collar at one end. This collar, preferably 4 millimeters in diameter, is placed at the inner canthus preventing the tube from slipping into the anastamotic passage (Fig. 14-13).

The technique for insertion of the Pyrex tube in not complicated. A dacryocystorhinostomy is performed in the usual fashion (see Chapter 17). After nasal mucosal and lacrimal sac flaps have been fashioned and the posterior flaps sutured, attention is directed to the nasal canthus. A portion of the caruncle, usually half to three-quarters, is resected as needed so that the Jones tube collar will lie snugly in the canthal angle. A Veirs trochar or long hypodermic needle is then passed from the canthal angle, two millimeters posterior to the muco-cutaneous junction, into the lacrimal sac cavity where it appears at the level of the internal punctum behind the anterior sac flap. The needle is carried beyond the sac, through the osteotomy into the middle meatus. Along this guide, a cataract knife is passed following the same track, manipulating the knife slightly up and down in order to enlarge the passage. A tube of proper length is threaded onto a probe, the probe passed along the same pathway and the Pyrex tube slid into place using the probe as a guide. The bevelled nasal end of the glass tube extends past the osteotomy into the nasal cavity for a distance of about one to two millimeters, staying well clear of the nasal septum. If the tube cannot be passed easily, the passage may be enlarged by inserting a small surgical ("mosquito") clamp and spreading gently.

Our preference is to use a tube which has a small hole in the collar, so that the tube can be fastened in place by suturing the collar to the nasal canthus for a period of two or three weeks. After insuring that the placement of the tube is correct (Fig. 14-14), the dacryocystorhinostomy

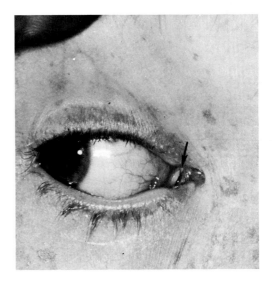

Figure 14-14. Correct placement of the collar of the Jones tube at the nasal angle.

is completed by closing the anterior mucosal flaps and completing the closure of the wound.

In cases where a dacryocystorhinostomy has been performed earlier, a Jones Pyrex glass tube can be inserted as a separate procedure. The caruncle is resected and the passageway is formed as described above, passing the guide needle and the knife through the previously formed osteotomy. It is essential, in any case, to visualize the tube in the nose for confirmation that it has been placed correctly.

REFERENCES

1. Francois J, et al.: Mycoses et pseudomycoses des voies lacrymales. Ann Ocul 199:1129, 1966
2. Radnot M, et al.: Die Roentgen Diagnostik der Tränenableitenden Wege. Budapest, Akademiai Kiado, p 124, 1966
3. Weil B, et al.: Canaliculopatia estenosante. Arch Oftal Buenos Aires 49:317, 1974
4. Sanford-Smith JH: Herpes simplex canalicular obstruction. Br J Ophthalmol 54:456, 1970
5. Werb A: In Rycroft P (ed.): Corneo-plastic Surgery: Proceeding II International Corneo-plastic Conference. London, Pergamon Press, p 87, 1969
6. Werb A: Reconstructive surgery of the lacrimal apparatus. Perspect Ophthalmol 151, 1968
7. Anderson RL, Edwards JJ: Indications, complications and results with silicone stents. Ophthalmology 86:1474, 1979
8. Davies P: Proximal obstruction of the inferior canaliculus. Proc Soc Med, 67:815, 1974
9. Metaireau JP, Legrignou A: Essais microchirurgicaux de repermeabilisation caniculaire par canaliculoplastie lacrymale. Bull Mem Soc Fr Ophthalmol 79:296, 1979

15

DISORDERS OF THE LOWER EXCRETORY SYSTEM

JOHN V. LINBERG

In this chapter we address clinical syndromes caused by pathology of the lacrimal sac and nasolacrimal duct. Congenital obstructions and abnormalities have been discussed as a separate unit (Chapter 10) and are not included here. The distal drainage system may be readily separated from the canaliculi in terms of anatomy and physiology, but these two systems frequently produce similar clinical signs and symptoms. This perspective is important, although canalicular problems have been treated separately (Chapter 14).

EPIPHORA

Tearing is probably the symptom most frequently associated with lacrimal obstruction, but the subject is considerably more complex. The term "epiphora" sometimes has been defined to specify only tearing related to lacrimal obstruction.[1] More commonly, "epiphora" is used to describe the phenomenon of tears spilling over the lid margin onto the face, from any cause. A large number of persons, perhaps one third, will offer this complaint during an ocular examination.[2] This should hardly be surprising, given that reflex lacrimal secretion is a normal response to physical and psychic stimuli. The healthiest lacrimal drainage apparatus is unable to cope with the maximal output of the lacrimal glands. Thus, a history of intermittent epiphora need not be pathologic and should stimulate an inquiry as to the frequency of such episodes and their environmental setting.

The clinical evaluation of simple epiphora should begin with inspection of the patient's face. While the exact mechanism of the lacrimal pump remains controversial, the normal functioning of the orbicularis muscle is a clear prerequisite. The observation of even slight brow ptosis, facial asymmetry, flattening of the nasolabial groove, or incomplete blink may be the only clue to a partial seventh nerve palsy. Mild facial palsy often produces nearly constant epiphora. More profound palsies will result in punctal eversion and lower lid ectropion.

Attention should be focused on the eyelids, as they must be normal in anatomy and function if the tears are to reach the drainage system.[3] Notching of the margin may allow tears to spill onto the face in the presence of a normal drainage system. Trichiasis is often a cause of reflex tearing. Laxity of the lower lids may cause a failure of the lacrimal pump, eversion of the puncta, or frank ectropion. Entropion may be intermittent and, therefore, a cause of intermittent epiphora.

A careful slit lamp examination is needed to rule out external disease that may account for reflex tearing. Special attention to signs of dry eyes can be worthwhile, as this is a remarkably frequent cause for epiphora. Ocular irritation is initiated by the poor quality or volume of the tear film, but this irritation then stimulates a copious flow of reflex lacrimation. The episode of epiphora ends either because these tears soothe the dry eye or perhaps because the lacrimal gland reaches a state of fatigue. The cycle may repeat itself many times during the course of a day.

The foregoing discussion may seem tangential to the subject of lacrimal sac problems, but it is necessary to establish a perspective on the problem of tearing. Most patients who complain of epiphora do not have a lacrimal obstruction, and indeed this is the clinician's real dilemma. An array of excellent clinical (Chapter 8) and radiologic (Chapter 9) tests will serve to document and localize an obstruction of the drainage system, but clinical judgment must be exercised in the selection of patients for these investigations. I have personally found the dye disappearance test to be a reliable and efficient method of identifying problems of lacrimal drainage. A drop of 2 percent fluorescein solution is instilled into each eye at a convenient point during the general ophthalmic examination. A few minutes later, the eyes are inspected for retention of dye. Prompt disappearance of the dye (seen in most cases) serves to document normal drainage and directs attention to other causes of tearing.

HALOS

Polychromatic halos are a rare but fascinating symptom of lacrimal obstruction. With stasis of tear flow, a collection of particulate matter and clumps of mucus will accumulate in the tear film. These particles produce fine irregularities of the tear film surface and result in diffraction of incoming light. The phenomenon is identical to that which produces the spectral halos of acute glaucoma or ultraviolet keratitis.[4, 5] An observant patient with lacrimal obstruction will occasionally note faint spectral rings around a bright point source of light. Colors are arranged with blue on the outside and red innermost.

The rings will disappear with blinking or irrigation of the eye.

CHRONIC DACRYOCYSTITIS

Canalicular obstruction usually causes epiphora as an isolated symptom, but obstruction of the distal drainage system is typically associated with some degree of lacrimal sac infection. Distal obstruction converts the sac into a stagnant pool, which is contaminated by debris from the environment, conjunctival flora, and secretions of the lacrimal mucosa. The resulting mixture is an ideal culture medium for bacteria, including anaerobes, and fungi. It is remarkable that many patients will tolerate such a condition for years without an episode of acute infection. Nonetheless, the presence of bacteria and fungi constitutes a threat to the eye. Minor corneal trauma may result in an infectious ulcer, and the chance of endophthalmitis is great if intraocular surgery becomes necessary. Lacrimal drainage should be reestablished before intraocular surgery is undertaken.

The obstructed lacrimal sac usually becomes dilated with time, producing a cystic mass at the medial canthus. Depending on the amount of ongoing infection and inflammation, the sac may or may not be tender. If the canaliculi are patent, the mucopurulent contents of the sac may be expressed from the puncta by digital pressure over the sac. The reflux of this thick yellow fluid from the puncta is essentially pathognomonic of an obstruction (Fig. 15-1).

With chronic inflammation, the opening of the common canaliculus into the sac may also close off. This event will often precipitate an acute dacryocystitis or produce a closed lacrimal sac mucocele. Lacrimal mucoceles gradually enlarge, as the secretions of the mucosa accumulate within the closed cyst. They may become quite large.

The most common organisms found in chronic dacryocystitis are *Staphylococcus*, pneumococcus, and beta-hemolytic *Streptococcus*, although a wide variety of pathogens may be responsible. *Haemophilus influenzae* is more frequent in children. Other gram-negative rods, such as *Pseudomonas aeruginosa, Klebsiella pneumoniae,* or enterobacteria will occasionally be cultured in adults.[6, 7]

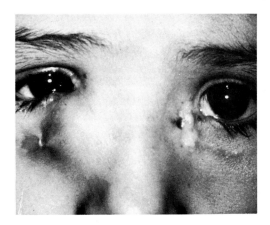

Figure 15-1. Chronic dacryocystitis. **Left.** Pyocele with fistulization at temporal edge. **Right.** Lacrimal fistula.

Anaerobic bacteria, especially *Actinomyces*, have been reported as a rare cause of dacryocystitis.[8, 9] Anaerobes prefer or require a low oxygen tension in order to multiply, and the lacrimal drainage system provides this environment. The lacrimal sac does not normally contain air, and the total volume of tear flow (containing oxygen) is quite small. Furthermore, the lacrimal system is continuous with the nasal passages and conjunctiva, both of which harbor anaerobes as normal flora.[10-13] Jones and Robinson[9] cultured a variety of anaerobes from washings of the normal lacrimal drainage system. Emergence of an anaerobic infection is encouraged by factors present in an obstructed lacrimal system, such as depletion of oxygen by growth of aerobic bacteria, foreign bodies (dacryoliths), and surgical manipulation (probing). Despite the presence of anaerobes in the flora of the sac and conditions that would encourage anaerobic growth, these organisms are a rare cause of dacryocystitis.

Fungi have been implicated in rare cases of chronic dacryocystitis, including *Candida* sp., *Aspergillus niger*, and chromoblastomycosis organisms.[14-16] Lacrimal washings from patients with lacrimal obstruction disclosed a population of numerous fungi.[17] Fungi seem to be important in the formation of some dacryoliths, as will be discussed later in this chapter.

Treatment of chronic dacryocystitis will not be successful for any length of time unless drainage of the sac is established or the sac is extirpated. In the present era of sophisticated lacrimal surgery, it should rarely be necessary to sacrifice the sac.[18] Topical antibiotics and frequent massage of the sac will serve to minimize the inflammation of chronic dacryocystitis until surgery can be undertaken.

ACUTE DACRYOCYSTITIS

Acute dacryocystitis is the most alarming and painful presentation of distal lacrimal obstruction and will bring the patient to the emergency room in extreme discomfort. An acute bacterial infection spreads from the lacrimal sac into surrounding tissue, producing edema, erythema, and tenderness in the medial canthus. Inflammation typically obstructs the opening of the common canaliculus into the sac, causing it to become distended with the infected contents. This distention of the sac within the confines of the lacrimal fossa and lacrimal fascia is the cause of severe pain (Fig. 15-2).

Unless the process is arrested by therapeutic intervention, the lacrimal sac will eventually decompress itself by forming a fistula (Fig. 15-3). Most often, this fistula will emerge from the skin just below the medial canthal tendon. Occasionally, the fistula will track into the orbit, resulting in cellulitis or abscess formation. The fistula can cross the floor of the orbit to emerge from the lateral aspect of the lower lid, confusing the diagnosis. Very rarely, the sac will

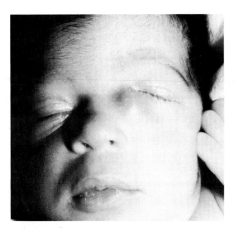

Figure 15-2. Acute dacryocystitis, left.

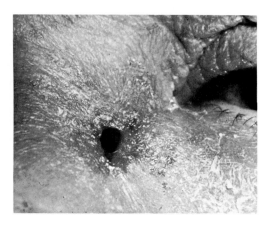

Figure 15-3. Fistula, left lacrimal sac, following an untreated dacryocystitis.

fistulize posteriorly into the anterior ethmoid air cells.[19]

The bacteria cultured from acute cases of dacryocystitis include *Staphylococcus,* beta-hemolytic *Streptococcus,* and the pneumococcus, although a variety of organisms may be found. Again, *Haemophilus influenzae* is frequent among children with acute dacryocystitis.

Therapy
The initial treatment of acute dacryocystitis is directed toward (1) control of the bacterial infection and (2) drainage and decompression of the lacrimal sac.

Broad-spectrum antibiotic coverage is necessitated by the variety of pathogens and the possibility of a mixed infection.[20] Occasionally, pus may be obtained from under the inferior turbinate or puncta, and a Gram's stain will be helpful. Cephalosporins offer good coverage with a single drug until culture reports are available. With children, it is important to treat for *Haemophilus,* and reports of ampicillin-resistant *Haemophilus* are now common. Third-generation cephalosporins, such as cefotaxime (Claforan), are effective against these resistant *Haemophilus* species. Local hot soaks are a worthwhile adjunct.

Some cases are relatively mild, and adults may be treated with oral antibiotics as outpatients. Most patients are quite uncomfortable, and hospitalization offers the advantage of intravenous antibiotic therapy and adequate nar-

cotic pain control. All infants and children should be hospitalized.

Drainage of the distended lacrimal sac is an important objective, as it provides relief of pain and aids in the control of infection. The opening of the common canaliculus into the sac is guarded by a mucosal fold, known as the valve of Rosenmüller. This flap or valve often prevents reflux from the sac, especially when it is inflamed. It is sometimes possible to open this valve by probing the common canaliculus, taking care not to force the probe. Anesthesia may be obtained by irrigating the canaliculi with cocaine solution and/or an infratrochlear nerve block. If this maneuver fails to drain the sac, an 18-gauge needle may be passed percutaneously into the sac. The point of entry should be low and, if possible, should be placed so as to lie in the path of a future DCR incision. Once the sac has been decompressed, the common canaliculus will usually open and provide continuous drainage.

Once the acute episode has resolved, a dacryocystorhinostomy is needed to prevent recurrences. Most patients will accept surgery after an unpleasant bout of dacryocystitis, and it is reasonable to proceed during the same hospitalization.

Differential Diagnosis
When the patient with a past history of tearing develops the florid symptoms of acute dacryocystitis, the diagnosis is obvious. In other cases, the past history is not helpful, with signs and symptoms sufficiently moderate to make the diagnosis difficult. The differential diagnosis is not lengthy (Table 15-1), but several possibilities should be considered.[21]

Frontal sinusitis usually presents with a long

TABLE 15-1. ACUTE MEDIAL CANTHAL INFLAMMATION

Differential Diagnosis
Ethmoidal sinusitis
Frontal sinusitis
Maxillary sinusitis
Facial cellulitis
Trauma
Acute dacryocystic retention
Acute dacryocystitis

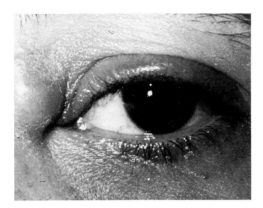

Figure 15-4. Abscess above medial canthal tendon, extrinsic to the sac. The lacrimal sac is not involved (note the absence of epiphora).

history of recurrent episodes. The inflammation tends to appear above the medial canthal tendon and spread across the upper lid, unlike dacryocystitis. The forehead may be tender to palpation, and the nasal examination may disclose pus emerging from the middle meatus. Reflex tearing is often present, secondary to trigeminal pain, but the drainage apparatus will be patent to irrigation. Radiographs will usually be diagnostic. Reinecke and Montgomery[22] described a fascinating case in which a frontal sinus mucocele fistulized into the superior canaliculus, causing chronic inflammation.

Ethmoid sinusitis is common in children[23] and presents with physical findings similar to those of frontal sinusitis. Again, the lacrimal drainage system will be patent, even in the presence of tearing, and radiographs will be diagnostic. It is important that this diagnosis be considered, as ethmoiditis has a tendency to fistulize into the orbit, causing an acute cellulitis or abscess. In the presence of orbital cellulitis, emergency drainage of ethmoiditis is indicated. In contrast, antibiotic therapy alone is usually adequate for acute dacryocystitis.

Maxillary sinusitis will rarely if ever present in the medial canthus, except for one situation. If the patient has previously undergone a blowout fracture repair, the implant may become infected, secondary to maxillary sinusitis, with signs in the lower lid.

Facial cellulitis of the medial canthus may result from an intranasal furuncle or minor

trauma. Although the pain and inflammation will mimic dacryocystitis and cause tearing, the lacrimal drainage system will be patent (Fig. 15-4).

Trauma should rarely cause diagnostic difficulty. Occasionally, a nasorbital fracture will acutely obstruct the nasolacrimal canal, causing an acute dacryocystitis.

Acute dacryocystic retention was recently described by Smith et al.[24] in a report of 11 cases. The patients had severe unilateral facial pain, which sometimes localized to the medial canthus. No evidence of swelling or erythema over the lacrimal sac was noted. The syndrome seemed to be caused by a sudden obstruction of the distal drainage apparatus, followed by distention of the sac and obstruction of the common canaliculus. The syndrome was treated by percutaneous aspiration of the sac, followed by probing of the canaliculus. Lacrimal casts could be identified in several cases. Why the lacrimal sac should be so painfully distended in the absence of infection is far from clear, but further reports should be forthcoming now that this syndrome has been characterized.

CAUSES OF OBSTRUCTION

While the preceding discussion has dealt with the clinical problems resulting from obstruction of the distal drainage system, the question of etiology has been avoided (Table 15-2). In fact, the cause of acquired obstructions in adults is unknown in a majority of patients. Women outnumber men with this condition by a ratio of at least 4:1,[25] but this only makes the question of etiology more obscure.

TABLE 15-2. CAUSES OF NASOLACRIMAL DUCT OBSTRUCTION

Congenital (Chapter 10)
Unknown
Foreign bodies (including melanin casts)
Trauma (including surgery)
Nasal disease
Infections
Lacrimal sac tumors (Chapter 16)
Sarcoidosis
Paget's disease
Midline granuloma

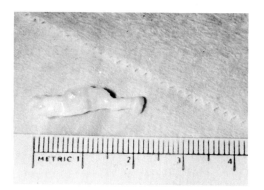

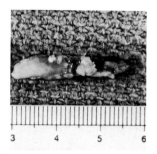

Figure 15-6. Partially calcified dacryolith of sac and duct.

Figure 15-5. Cast of lacrimal sac and duct expelled from nose (by sneezing).

Anatomists have pointed out that women generally have a narrower osseous nasolacrimal canal, but this may simply reflect the smaller stature of women.[26] Another study of patients with dacryocystitis revealed a preponderance of brachycephalic skulls, supposedly implying a longer and narrower nasolacrimal canal.[27] These theories really belong to another era and reflect our ignorance.

Among patients less than 50 years of age who undergo dacryocystorhinostomy for epiphora of unknown cause, about two thirds will have a dacryolith in the sac.[28] Whether these foreign bodies are always the cause of obstruction or are a result of stasis is not known.

Foreign Bodies of the Lacrimal Sac

A variety of exogenous and endogenous foreign bodies have been discovered within the lacrimal sac, usually at the time of surgery. Small exogenous objects, such as cilia, seeds, bristles, or vegetable debris, have been reported more frequently in the canaliculi, but this may reflect the greater accessibility of the canaliculi.[29] The contents of the sac are not seen except during surgery. Rarely, a cast of the sac will be discharged into the nose and retrieved by the patient. One such cast was found to contain cilia[30] (Fig. 15-5).

A variety of probes, stents, tubes, and broken instruments have found their way into the lacrimal sac through the efforts of our medical colleagues. Many of these have been tolerated for long periods or discharged through the nose.[29] Unfortunately, they can also cause a granulomatous reaction and obstruct the sac.[31] Larger foreign bodies may arise de novo in the lacrimal sac. Some of these are soft and amorphous, usually referred to as "casts" because their shape is formed by irregularities and folds of lacrimal mucosa. Other foreign bodies are stratified concretions termed "dacryoliths," showing some calcification (Fig. 15-6).

The clinical syndrome produced by these larger casts and concretions is often sufficiently distinct to allow a diagnosis prior to surgery. The hallmark of the syndrome is chronicity and extreme variability of signs, symptoms, and clinical tests.[28, 32] Epiphora is universal but intermittent in character. Scant purulent discharge from the puncta may be associated with mild tenderness and swelling at the medial canthus, suggesting a chronic low-grade dacryocystitis. This indolent inflammation is punctuated by episodes of acute dacryocystitis or at least exacerbations of the chronic cystitis.[28]

The incidence of lacrimal foreign bodies in patients requiring dacryocystorhinostomy is 15 to 20 percent.[28, 32, 33] Most patients are less than 50 years old, with a peak incidence between 40 and 50 years. Nearly two thirds of patients under 50 with lacrimal obstruction of unknown cause will be found to have lacrimal foreign bodies at surgery.[28, 32, 33] Several authorities have suggested an association between heavy smoking and lacrimal foreign bodies, but convincing statistical evidence has not been produced.

The foreign body appears to function as a variable ball valve, causing absolute obstruction at times but shifting to relieve the obstruction intermittently. For this reason, the clinical

Jones' dye tests will alternately document complete obstruction, functional block, or free drainage. Even calcified dacryoliths are usually radiolucent, but contrast dacryocystography should outline the foreign body (Fig. 15-2) (Chapter 16).

An external dacryocystorhinostomy is the usual approach to these patients, allowing removal of foreign bodies and establishing free drainage of the sac. Even if the nasolacrimal duct seems patent after extracting a dacryolith, it is wisest to complete the dacryocystorhinostomy. Patients who have expelled casts through the nose have been known to later develop new casts.[28] This has not been reported following a successful dacryocystorhinostomy.

Jones[28] has described a method of eliminating some foreign bodies from the sac without surgery. He first anesthetized the inferior turbinate with topical 5 percent cocaine solution and then applied a chalazion clamp to the lids, obstructing both canaliculi. With pressure over the lacrimal sac, some casts extruded under the inferior turbinate and were extracted with forceps.

The pathophysiology involved in the formation of lacrimal foreign bodies is not known. It is not even clear that they function primarily as a cause of obstruction or result secondary to stasis.

Some etiologic importance has been ascribed to the presence of yeast and fungi in foreign bodies, largely because canalicular concretions often consist almost entirely of fungi or *Actinomyces*. Subsequent reports have shown that many and perhaps most lacrimal foreign bodies do not contain fungi.[31, 32] It is known that assorted fungi may be cultured from obstructed lacrimal systems,[17] and it hardly seems surprising that a growing concretion should incorporate these organisms. One careful histologic examination of a dacryolith disclosed focal strata of the yeast forms, indicating that fungal contamination occurred during a short period in the growth of the concretion.[33]

This dacryolith was also found to contain a cilium at the center. The authors suggested that exogenous foreign bodies may form a nidus around which fibrin, cellular breakdown products, bacteria, fungi, and mucoprotein substance deposit to form the typical amorphous lacrimal foreign body.[33] Grönvall[34] reported a case of argyrosis in which a nidus of silver salt crystals was found at the center of a dacryolith, and Jones found a cilium in one cast he removed.[28] These are unusual reports, as most specimens do not contain a central nidus. A unique form of lacrimal cast has been observed in patients who use epinephrine chronically for glaucoma control. Spaeth[35] reported that 3 of 27 patients using epinephrine developed lacrimal obstruction secondary to melanin casts. In each case, the cast was passed after irrigation, and surgery was not required.

Trauma to Lacrimal Sac and Nasolacrimal Duct

Lacerations. Lacerations of the lids and canaliculi are relatively common, but it is exceedingly rare for such injuries to involve the distal drainage system. The sac lies deep in the medial canthus, protected by the nasal pyramid and anterior lacrimal crest. The medial canthal tendon protects the superior portion of the sac, which is also enclosed by dense lacrimal fascia. Even when a lid is avulsed from the medial canthus, the separation occurs external to the lacrimal fascia and leaves the sac intact.

Midfacial Fractures. The universal use of motorized vehicles has given rise to an increasing number of midfacial fractures, sometimes involving the lacrimal sac and nasolacrimal canal. In order to understand these fractures, it is necessary to consider the nature of the facial skeleton. While the brain is protected by a bony case of almost uniform strength, the facial skeleton consists of individual strong abutments or struts separated by relatively thin, fragile bone.

The distal lacrimal system lies on either side of the central nasal pyramid which consists of the nasal process of the frontal bone, nasal bones, and the alveolar process of the maxillae. Behind this pyramidal abutment lies the interorbital space, which offers little structural support. This space lies below the anterior cranial fossa, bounded on each side by the ethmoid plate of the medial orbital wall. The interorbital space contains the ethmoid air cells, middle and superior turbinates, and nasal septum. If a blow of sufficient force breaks the nasal pyramid free from the frontal bone above and malar processes below, it will be driven into the

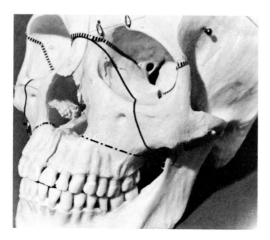

Figure 15-7. Naso-orbital fracture: The superior transverse fracture passes posteriorly along the medial orbital wall (dotted line) or just behind the posterior lacrimal crest (solid line). The inferior transverse fracture begins at the nasal aperture and passes laterally across the maxilla (interrupted line). These fractures allow mobilization of the central nasal pyramind of bone.

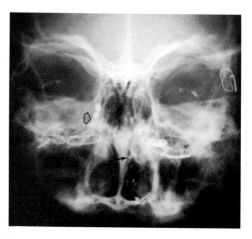

Figure 15-8. Midfacial and upper facial fractures (Le Fort III). **Right.** Complete block in region of sac-duct junction (open arrow). **Left.** Lateral diverticulum. Fistulization through fracture of nasolacrimal bony canal, into middle meatus (arrow).

interorbital space along the inclined plane of the base of the skull. This type of injury is termed a "naso-orbital fracture" and is frequently seen when the head strikes a dashboard or steering wheel.[36] As the nasal pyramid is driven into the interorbital space, the medial orbital walls are pushed apart, and overriding plates of bone may lacerate the lacrimal sac.[37] It is remarkable how rarely lacerations of the sac and canaliculi occur with this injury. Stranc[38] reported a series of 25 severe naso-orbital fractures without a single injury to the sac. Fragments of the interorbital space are quite fragile, while the dense lacrimal fascia protects the lacrimal mucosa.

The nasolacrimal duct is actually more vulnerable to injury from fracture lines that cross the canal. Still, the incidence is low; only 12 obstructions were seen in a series of 100 midfacial fractures.[39]

Fracture lines will follow predictable lines of weakness, and this pattern provides an explanation for the rarity of nasolacrimal injury in midfacial fractures. The high transverse fracture of the nasal pyramid begins with separation of the frontonasal suture. This fracture will then pass posteriorly along the upper edge of

the ethmoid plate or descend the medial wall of the orbit behind the posterior lacrimal crest to reach the inferior orbital margin. In either case, the lacrimal fossa is spared (Fig. 15-7).

The low transverse fracture of the naso-orbital complex begins at the nasal aperture near the floor of the nose. This line passes laterally across the maxilla and canine fossa. Medially, it extends posteriorly along the lateral wall of the nose just above the floor. Thus, the nasolacrimal canal escapes injury in most instances. If the lower fracture passes high enough along the lateral wall of the nose, it will cross the nasolacrimal canal, and a fistula may form into the maxillary sinus or ethmoid air cells.[40, 41] Such fistulas may provide adequate lacrimal drainage and be discovered only by bilateral dacryocystography (Fig. 15-8).

An unusual mechanism for lacrimal obstruction after an orbital blowout fracture was reported by Kohn et al.[42] They described migration of a large orbital floor implant resulting in compression and obstruction of the lacrimal sac as it entered the canal.

Surgical Trauma. Iatrogenic injury to the lacrimal drainage system has occurred after a variety of orbital, maxillary sinus, and rhinoplastic surgeries.

Transient epiphora is often seen immediately after rhinoplasty and is probably related to edema, which creates a functional block.[43] The sac can be damaged directly if the lateral osteotomies are performed at a low level. The other common mechanism of iatrogenic nasolacrimal injury is the incorrect placement of nasoantral windows.[44] A variety of procedures involving the maxillary sinus, including transantral orbital decompression,[45] require a nasoantral window in order to establish sinus drainage into the nose. The window should be placed under the middle of the inferior turbinate, safely distant from the ostia lacrimalis. The ostia lacrimalis shows considerable variation in its location under the inferior turbinate[46] and may be damaged by an anterior nasoantral window. Dacryocystography has demonstrated that the iatrogenic obstruction in these cases is at the distal nasolacrimal canal.[44, 45] Dacryocystorhinostomy is the treatment of choice once the obstruction is established. Silicone stents would probably serve to maintain a patent duct during healing if the error was observed promptly.

Radiation. The lacrimal sac and nasolacrimal duct appear to be immune to radiation, even at doses of 5,000 rads.[47]

Nasal Disease

Nasal disease is a straightforward cause of nasolacrimal obstruction. A deviated nasal septum may cause the inferior turbinate to press against the ostia lacrimalis. Nasal polyps, tumors, or hypertrophy of the inferior turbinate may produce a similar effect. Tumors of the sinuses or nasopharynx may involve the bony nasolacrimal canal and cause an obstruction. These conditions emphasize the need for a good nasal examination.

Following the division of ophthalmology and otolaryngology into separate subspecialties, the nasal examination of the patient with epiphora has been problematic.[48] Although the importance of a skilled intranasal examination is widely emphasized in texts and lectures, the actual teaching and experience provided to residents is limited. Consultation by an otolaryngologist may not resolve this problem as most otolaryngologists have limited knowledge of lacrimal physiology.

Rare Causes of Obstruction

Primary lacrimal sac tumors are discussed in Chapter 16. There are fewer than 200 reports of such tumors in the literature, which certainly qualifies them as a rare cause of obstruction.

Trachoma is rare in the United States but remains the leading cause of preventable blindness in the world. In countries of the Middle East, North Africa, and Southeast Asia, trachoma is an extremely common cause of distal lacrimal obstruction. In a recent report from Saudi Arabia, 19 percent of patients with signs of inactive severe trachoma had nasolacrimal obstruction.[49] Canalicular obstruction was even more common (38 percent).

Tuberculosis is another disease that rarely causes lacrimal obstruction in the United States, simply because the disease is now rare. Primary infection of the lacrimal sac has been reported,[50] although secondary involvement from lesions of the nose or skin is more common.[51, 52]

Leprosy causes extreme deformity of the facial tissues, and secondary involvement of the lacrimal system has been reported.[53]

Rhinosporidiosis is a fungal disease caused by *Rhinosporidium seeberi*. Friable growths may appear on the conjunctiva or in the lacrimal sac.[54] This infection is most common in India, but cases are seen in agricultural communities of the midwestern United States.

Parasites have been known to invade the lacrimal sac and have been reported in India and Africa.[55]

Sarcoidosis may involve any portion of the upper respiratory tract, and involvement of the lacrimal sac is seen in association with this presentation.[56, 57] Sarcoidosis of the sac is usually diagnosed only after a dacryocystorhinostomy has provided tissue for histopathology. It seems possible that sarcoid involvement of the sac would respond to systemic steroids. Chest x-rays, serum angiotensin-converting enzyme levels, and a careful nasal examination could establish the diagnosis prior to surgery.

Lethal midline lymphoma is a rare lethal disease causing progressive destruction of the nasopharynx and face. A case of lacrimal obstruction with recurrent dacryocystitis has been reported.[58]

Paget's disease causes abnormal growth and thickening of the facial skeleton, sometimes affecting only one bone (monostotic). Nasolacrimal obstruction has been reported, as has failure of a dacryocystorhinostomy because of pagetoid regrowth of bone.[59]

Pneumatocele of the lacrimal sac is a curiosity of the lacrimal sac. Normally, the opening of the nasolacrimal canal, ostia lacrimalis, is guarded by a flap of mucosa known as Hasner's valve. This flap acts as a valve and prevents the reflux of air during sneezing or forceful expiration. There is some anatomic variation to this valve,[60] which is sometimes incompetent. If the nose is blown, air may pass up the lacrimal drainage system and escape from the puncta. Duke-Elder and MacFaul[61] define this phenomenon as "ocular whistling" and state that 5 percent of normal persons are capable of this trick.

Occasionally, the air is unable to escape from the lacrimal sac, producing a tense pneumatocele and transient epiphora.[62] The air is rapidly absorbed into the bloodstream, and the patient learns to avoid the maneuver.

REFERENCES

1. Duke-Elder S, MacFaul PA: The ocular adnexa. Lacrimal, orbital and para-orbital diseases. In Duke-Elder S (ed): System of Ophthalmology. St. Louis, Mosby, 1974, Vol 8, p 675
2. Putterman AM: Evaluation of the lacrimal system. Eye Ear Nose Throat Mon 51:31, 1972
3. Jones LT: An anatomic approach to problems of the eyelids and lacrimal apparatus. Arch Ophthalmol 66:111, 1961
4. Duke-Elder WS: Halos. In Duke-Elder WS (ed): Foundations of Ophthalmology. St. Louis, Mosby, 1962, Vol 7, Chap 15, p 450
5. Duke-Elder WS: Pathological diffraction halos. Br J Ophthalmol 11:342, 1927
6. Pettit T: Lacrimal system inflammations. International Symposium on Ocular Inflammatory Diseases. Springfield, Il., Thomas, 1974
7. Sasaki T, Tanaka N, Odagiri Y, Itoh D, Takebayashi E: Microbial flora in dacryocystitis. Acta Soc Ophthalmol Jpn, 77:644, 1973 (Abstract)
8. Blanksma LJ, Slijper J: Actinomycotic dacryocystitis. Ophthalmolgica, 176:145, 1978
9. Jones DB, Robinson NM: Anaerobic ocular infections. Trans Am Acad Ophthalmol Otolaryngol 83:309, 1977
10. Watson ED, Hoffman NJ, Summers RW: Aerobic and anaerobic bacterial counts of nasal washings. J Bacteriol 83:144, 1962
11. Frederick J, Braude A: Anaerobic infection in the paranasal sinuses. N Engl J Med 290:135, 1974
12. Matuura H: Anaerobes in the bacterial flora of the conjunctival sac. Jpn J Ophthalmol 15:116, 1971
13. Perkins RE, Kundsin KB, Prat MV: Bacteriology of normal and infected conjunctiva. J Clin Microbiol 1:147, 1975
14. Halde C, Okumoto M: Ocular mycosis: A study of 82 cases. Proceedings XX International Congress of Ophthalmology, Munich, 1966, Amsterdam, Excerpta Medica, p 82
15. Fine M, Waring WS: Mycotic obstruction of the nasolacrimal duct (*Candida*). Arch Ophthalmol 38:39, 1974
16. Rosenvold LK: Dacryocystitis and blepharitis due to infection by *Aspergillus niger*. Am J Ophthalmol 25:588, 1942
17. Pine L, Shearin WA, Gonzales CA: Mycotic flora of lacrimal duct. Am J Ophthalmol 52:619, 1961
18. Jones BR: Syndromes of lacrimal obstruction and their management. Trans Ophthalmol Soc UK 93:581, 1973
19. Duke-Elder S, MacFaul PA: The ocular adnexa. Lacrimal, orbital and para-orbital diseases. In Duke-Elder S (ed): System of Ophthalmology. St. Louis, Mosby, 1974, Vol 8, p 706
20. Sood NN, Ratnaraj A, Balarman G, Madhavan HN: Chronic dacryocystitis. A clinicobacteriologic study. J All India Ophthalmol Soc 15(3):107, 1967
21. Healy GB, Strong MS: Acute periorbital swelling. Laryngoscope 82:1491, 1972
22. Reinecke RD, Montgomery WW: Frontal lacrimal fistula. Am J Ophthalmol 67(4):591, 1969
23. Haynes RE, Cramblett HG, Acute ethmoiditis. Am J Dis Child 114:261, 1967
24. Smith B, Tenzel RR, Buffam FV, Boynton JR: Acute dacryocystic retention. Arch Ophthalmol 94:1903, 1976
25. Veirs ER: Lacrimal Disorders. St. Louis, Mosby, 1976, p 73
26. Meller J: Diseases of the lacrimal apparatus. Trans. Ophthalmol Soc UK, 49:233, 1929
27. Avasthi P, Misra RM, Sood AK: Clinical and anatomic considerations of dacryocystitis. Int Surg 55:200, 1971
28. Jones LT: Tear sac foreign bodies. Am J Ophthalmol 60:111, 1965
29. Garfin SW: Etiology of dacryocystitis and epiphora. Arch Ophthalmol 27:167, 1942
30. Stallard HB: Case of chronic granuloma of the lacrimal sac. Br J Ophthalmol 24:457, 1940

31. Wilkins RB, Pressly JP: Diagnosis and incidence of lacrimal calculi. Ophthalmic Surg 11(11):787, 1980
32. Berlin AJ, Rath R, Rich L: Lacrimal system dacryoliths. Ophthalmic Surg 11(7):435, 1980
33. Jay JL, Lee WR: Dacryolith formation around an eyelash retained in the lacrimal sac. Br J Ophthalmol 60:722, 1976
34. Grönvall H: On argyrosis and concretion in the lacrimal sac. Acta Ophthalmol (Kbh) 21:247, 1944
35. Spaeth GL: Nasolacrimal duct obstruction caused by topical epinephrine. Arch Ophthalmol 77:355, 1967
36. Dingman RO, Grabb WC, and O'Neal RM: Management of injuries of the naso-orbital complex. Arch Surg 98:566, 1969
37. Converse JM, Smith B: Naso-orbital fractures. Trans Am Acad Ophthalmol Otolaryngol 67:622, 1963
38. Stranc MF: Pattern of lacrimal injuries in nasoethmoid fractures. Br J Plastic Surg 23:339, 1970
39. Campbell W: Radiology of the lacrimal system. Br J Radiol 37:1, 1964
40. Hendrickson DA, Cunningham RD, Veirs ER: Post-traumatic lacrimal-antral fistula: two cases. Ann Ophthalmol 9:475, 1977
41. Dayton GO Jr, Hanafee W: Lacrimal sac fistulas. Trans Am Ophthalmol Soc 78:301, 1980
42. Kohn R, Romano PE, Puklin JE: Lacrimal obstruction after migration of orbital floor implant. Am J Ophthalmol 82:934, 1976
43. Flowers RS, Anderson R: Injury to the lacrimal apparatus during rhinoplasty. Plast Reconstr Surg 42:577, 1968
44. Osguthorpe JD, Calcaterra TC: Nasolacrimal obstruction after maxillary sinus and rhinoplastic surgery. Arch Otolaryngol 105(5):264, 1979
45. Colvard DM, Waller RR, Neault RW, DeSanto LW: Lacrimal duct obstruction following transantral ethmoidal orbital decompression. Ophthalmic Surg 10(6):25, 1979
46. Schaeffer JP: Types of ostia nasolacrimalia. Am J Anat 13:183, 1912
47. Brizel HE, Sheils WC, Brown M: Effect of radiation on the nasolacrimal system as evaluated by dacryoscintigraphy. Radiology 116:373, 1975
48. Jones LT, Boyden G: The rhinologist's role in tear sac surgery. Trans Am Acad Ophthalmol Otolaryngol 34:654, 1951
49. Tabbara KF, Bobb AA: Lacrimal system complications in trachoma. Ophthalmology 87(4):298, 1980
50. Sigelman SC, Muller P: Primary tuberculosis of the lacrimal sac Arch Ophthalmol 65:450, 1961
51. Duke-Elder S, MacFaul PA: The ocular adnexa. Lacrimal, orbital and para-orbital diseases. In Duke-Elder S (ed): System of Ophthalmology. St. Louis, Mosby, 1974, Vol 8, p 725
52. Anderson SR: Tuberculosis dacryocystitis and lupus of the nose diagnosed as Boeck's disease. Acta Ophthalmol 25:455, 1947
53. Weerekoon L: Ocular leprosy in Ceylon. Br J Ophthalmol 53:457, 1969
54. Jain SC, Darbari BS, Bhatnagar BS: Ocular rhinosporidiosis. Eye Ear Nose Throat Mon 47:380, 1968
55. Kaplan CS, Freedman L, Elsdon-Dew R: A worm in the eye. S Afr Med J 30:791, 1956
56. Harris GJ, Williams GA, Clarke GP: Sarcoidosis of the lacrimal sac. Arch Ophthalmol 99:1198, 1981
57. Neault RW, Riley FC: Report of a case of dacryocystitis secondary to Boeck's sarcoid. Am J Ophthalmol 70:1011, 1970
58. Spalton DJ, O'Donnell PJ, Graham EM: Lethal midline lymphoma causing acute dacryocystitis. Br J Ophthalmol 65(7):503, 1981
59. Hurwitz JJ: Failed dacryocystorhinostomy in Paget's disease. Can J Ophthalmol 14(14): 291, 1979
60. Kuribayashi Y: Observation of the opening of the nasolacrimal duct. Jpn J Ophthalmol 1:96, 1957
61. Duke-Elder S, MacFaul PA: The ocular adnexa. Lacrimal, orbital and para-orbital diseases. In Duke-Elder S (ed): System of Ophthalmology St. Louis, Mosby, 1974, Vol 8, p 691
62. Levitt JM, Kravitz D: Lacrimal air anomalies. Arch Ophthalmol 61:9, 1959

16

TUMORS OF THE LACRIMAL EXCRETORY SYSTEM

BENJAMIN MILDER and MORTON E. SMITH

The lacrimal excretory system is so frequently obstructed as a result of infection and inflammation that it is easy to forget that interference with the outflow of tears may result from any type of pathologic process—congenital malformations, infection, trauma, and tumors.

Tumors involving the lacrimal sac and nasolacrimal duct are uncommon. The orbit, including lacrimal gland and lacrimal sac, is the site of only 1 of every 6,000 tumors.[1] In 1963, Radnot and Gall[2] were able to collect only 184 tumors of the excretory system in the world literature. In 1978, Flanagan and Stokes[3] reviewed three series of such tumors and reported a total of 212 cases. Of this number, 60 percent were malignant. Thus, although the incidence was low, the index of suspicion must be high, for early and accurate diagnosis is the key to successful management of these tumors.

Tumors of this system, benign and malignant, reflect the entire spectrum of histologic possibilities. Benign tumors that have been reported include papillomas and polyps within the lacrimal sac, granulomas and pseudotumors, hemangiomas, neurofibromas, and others. Benign epithelial lesions can undergo malignant degeneration. Malignancies include carcinomas, mesenchymal tumors, and malignant melanomas. The most disturbing fact about

tumors of the lacrimal sac is that all of them, initially, have the same clinical course and, at the outset, are frequently misdiagnosed as "chronic dacryocystitis." The classic diagnostic picture of a tumor of the lacrimal sac includes:

1. A history of recurring episodes of low-grade dacryocystitis
2. Unilateral epiphora
3. An irreducible mass, usually nontender
4. Functional block, that is, patency on irrigation in the presence of the epiphora
5. A characteristic dacryocystogram
6. Bleeding from the punctum, spontaneous or on probing

In most cases, when the patient first consults the ophthalmologist, the outflow system can be irrigated successfully. Therefore, there may be an unfortunate tendency to delay, to wait for the symptoms to abate with conservative therapy.

Tumors, benign or malignant, may arise within the lacrimal sac, but they may also arise from structures surrounding the lacrimal sac and duct. Such extrinsic tumors can produce the same clinical picture as a lacrimal sac neoplasm as a result of pressure on the sac. Dacryocystography provides the most effective diagnostic device for differentiating simple dacryocystitis from a tumor and for differentiating extrinsic from intrinsic involvement of the lacrimal sac. Therefore, in any patient with unilateral epiphora, a patent system, and a suspicious fullness in the region of the lacrimal sac, dacryocystography should not be delayed. While the precise histologic entity cannot be determined from the radiographic study, space-taking lesions will yield dacryocystograms that may be sufficiently characteristic and sufficiently different from the usual obstructive dacryocystitis as to be diagnostic. Further studies, including conventional tomography and computerized axial tomography, will provide guidelines for appropriate surgical intervention.

Histologically, almost any cell type may be found in lacrimal sac tumors. Epidermoid carcinoma is the most common malignant tumor, comprising 59 percent of all malignant tumors of the lacrimal sac.[4] They outnumber mesenchymal tumors by a ratio of 3:1. Reticuloses and melanoma make up only 12 percent of the lacrimal sac tumors.

Lacrimal sac malignancies have a 5-year survival rate of approximately 50 percent. Deaths are the result of metastases, most frequently to the lung, but also to other structures by way of the regional lymph glands.

From the standpoint of the clinician, it is convenient to classify lacrimal sac tumors as either intrinsic or extrinsic, benign or malignant. Table 16-1 lists the excretory system tumors that have been reported.

INTRINSIC TUMORS—BENIGN

Tumefaction in the region of the lacrimal sac, accompanied by epiphora and the inability to eliminate the fullness by digital compression, may suggest neoplasia but also may be nothing more than a mucocele or pyocele of the lacrimal sac. Such instances occur when there is complete closure at or below the sac-duct junction and the pressure of the fluid within the sac has produced a trapdoor closure of the valve of Rosenmüller at the internal punctum. It is often possible to insert a lacrimal probe through one canaliculus into the sac and, with the probe in place, evacuate the contents of the sac through the other canaliculus. When the sac is evac-

TABLE 16.1. EXCRETORY SYSTEM TUMORS

Intrinsic Tumors	Extrinsic Tumors
Benign	Benign
Polyps	Orbital cysts
Cysts	(dermoid, other)
Diverticula	Mucocele of sinuses
Granuloma—	Cavernous
pseudotumor	lymphangioma
Dacryolith	(nonmetastasizing
Mucocele of the	but invasive)
lacrimal sac	Fibrous
Benign epithelial	histiocytoma
tumors—	(nonmetastasizing
papillomata	but invasive)
Neurofibroma	Meningocele
Fibrous	
histiocytoma	
(nonmetastasizing)	
Malignant	Malignant
Epithelial	Carcinoma of
(epidermoid)	sinuses
carcinoma	(epidermoid-
Fibrous	transitional)
histiocytoma—	Fibrocarcinoma of
fibrosarcoma	orbit
Reticuloses	Metastatic lesions
Malignant	
melanoma	
Malignant	
lymphoma	

uated in this fashion, any attempt at irrigation will fill it and reproduce the swelling. The dacryocystogram will reveal a typical distended sac with smooth outline and a uniform distribution of the contrast agent and is unlikely to be confused with a neoplasm (Fig. 16-1).

Long-standing chronic dacryocystitis may be responsible for the formation of polyps, cysts, or granulomas within the sac and nasolacrimal duct. Such masses will not necessarily produce significant fullness in the lacrimal fossa if the system is patent. If not, the trapdoor mechanism may produce a distended, irreducible sac.

Dacryoliths result from stasis within the sac. It is significant that, in most instances, the system is patent and no tumefaction is visible, even with rather large stones. However, other characteristics that are invariably present include epiphora, mild deep tenderness, and functional block. The diagnosis of dacryolith is readily made from the dacryocystogram and

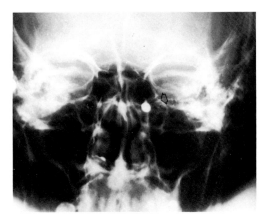

Figure 16-1. Obstructive dacryocystitis. Note the smooth, rounded outine of the left sac and the uniform density of the contrast agent filling the sac.

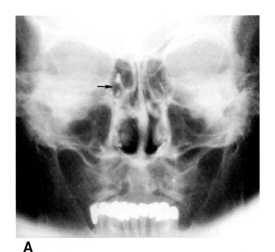

A

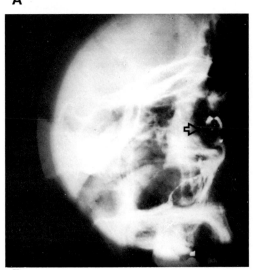

B

Figure 16-2. Dacryolith. **A.** Posteroanterior view, showing a patent system, and a reduplication of the sac outline, with central radiolucent area. **B.** Lateral view of sac, with rounded outline and central radiolucent area (dacryolith).

can be differentiated from other benign intrinsic space-taking lesions, such as polyps and granulomata. The dacryolith appears, on the dacryocystogram, as a radiolucent area in a distended sac (Fig. 16-2A). In lateral views (Fig. 16-2B), the contrast agent can be seen to line both sides of the radiolucent area and to appear in the duct and nasal cavity, while the polyp and granulomata are more likely to produce a deformity in the contrast shadow of the lacrimal sac. Figure 16-3 illustrates distortion of the lacrimal sac shadow by a granuloma arising from the anterior wall of the sac. This patient, a 45-year-old woman, had no symptoms other than unilateral intermittent tearing, and the only finding was slight, deep tenderness over the lacrimal sac. On the basis of the dacryocystogram, the sac was explored and a large benign granuloma was found, fastened to the anterior sac wall.

A *benign cyst* within the sac or duct can stimulate a malignancy. In one such patient who had a history of acute dacryocystitis, a nontender irreducible sac mass could be palpated. Dacryocystography (Fig. 16-4) revealed a filling defect in the lacrimal sac and an upper duct deformity characterized by marked narrowing of the nasolacrimal duct. At surgery, a follicular granulomatous mass was found in the sac, and below this, a large, clear cyst filled the entire nasolacrimal passage. The cyst was dissected from its attachment to the lateral wall of

the duct. This patient provided another demonstration of the importance of routine dacryocystography. Without the radiographic findings, the granuloma in the lacrimal sac would have been interpreted as the primary pathologic process. Actually, the cyst, developing slowly, was responsible for the stasis that spawned the lacrimal sac findings.

Neurofibroma is rarely encountered in the lacrimal drainage system[5] (Fig. 16-5). Such

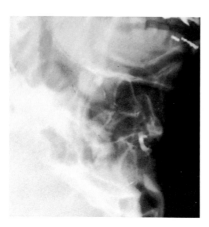

Figure 16-3. Dacryocystogram, lateral view, showing a radiolucent mass (granuloma) attached to anterior sac wall.

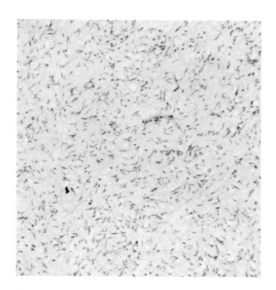

Figure 16-5. Neurofibroma of lacrimal sac.

growths are encapsulated and can be removed in toto, with an accompanying dacryocysto-rhinostomy.

Fibrous histiocytoma is a slowly growing, soft tissue tumor that does not metastasize but can be locally invasive.[6] Such a tumor, arising in the lacrimal sac, may extend into the orbit, and, conversely, lesions arising primarily in the orbit may impinge on the lacrimal sac. Such tumors present difficult problems for the pathologist because of variations in the cell types. There are differing proportions of fibrocytes and histiocytic cells, collagenous tissue, and spindle-shaped

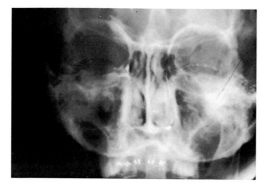

Figure 16-4. Cyst of right nasolacrimal duct. Flow of contrast agent interrupted by the rounded superior pole of the cyst.

cells. In one report,[7] a team of experts, viewing slides from the same patient, arrived at six different histologic diagnoses ranging from orbital pseudotumor to fibrosarcoma. Since fibrous histiocytomas are resistant to radiotherapy, local excision is the required treatment.

Although the treatment of each benign tumor must be predicated on the findings in the individual patient, the essential principles are surgical. These consist of removal of the mass and restoration of function. If there is obstruction and/or functional block, a dacryocysto-rhinostomy must accompany the removal of the lesion. Attempts by the author, in earlier years, to remove a stone or polyp without performing a dacryocystorhinostomy have met with failure. Although the presence of functional block can be inferred from the history of epiphora and the careful performance of fluorescein dye testing, the dacryocystogram will provide the definitive evidence by comparing the 0 time and 30-minute films (Chapter 9).

INTRINSIC TUMORS—MALIGNANT

Epithelial Carcinomas

The large majority of malignant tumors of the lacrimal sac are of epithelial origin. These tumors arise in the mucosal lining of the sac, and most of them are poorly differentiated, nonkeratinizing, epidermoid carcinomas. The classification of these epithelial tumors varies somewhat from investigator to investigator. Some prefer the term "transitional cell carcinoma" and grade the tumors in terms of malignancy, from transitional cell papilloma (benign) to transitional cell carcinoma, classified according to the anaplastic nature of the tumor.

Transitional cell tumors of the lacrimal sac are similar, histologically, to those found in the paranasal sinuses, and this similarity has, on occasion, led to confusion as to whether such an epithelial tumor of the sac was primary or arose secondarily from carcinoma of an adjacent sinus. Less frequent malignancies of the lacrimal sac include malignant melanoma, various types of sarcomas, hemangiopericytoma, and neurilemmoma.

Since the signs and symptoms tend to be the same for all lacrimal sac tumors, the initial steps and treatment will usually be the same for all. If a tumor is suspected on the basis of the examination findings and the dacryocystogram, histologic study by frozen section should be performed at surgery, using biopsy specimens taken from at least two different sites. It must be emphasized that the malignant nature of these tumors cannot be confirmed unless the histologic evidence is unmistakable from the frozen section. Failure to confirm the malignancy by frozen section does not rule out such a possibility. The surgeon must be guided, in part, by the gross appearance of the lesion at the operating table. If the tumor is well encapsulated and shells out easily in the capsule, an excisional biopsy will be the treatment of choice. Since lacrimal drainage function is usually compromised by the lesion, simple excision must be combined with the dacryocystorhinostomy in order to relieve the epiphora.

Epithelial (epidermoid) carcinoma requires wide local excision at the time of the initial surgery, and this should be preceded by irradiation. Schenck et al.[4] state that irradiation alone is not adequate therapy because of the proximity to bony structures and the potential for diffuse involvement of the mucosa. Recurrences of the tumor may be the result of extension down the nasolacrimal duct, undetected at the initial surgery. Minimal excision should include the upper and lower canaliculi, the lacrimal sac, the nasolacrimal duct, the bony lacrimal fossa, and the surrounding ethmoid air cells. Radical maxillectomy should be reserved for recurrences, and neck dissection should be employed if there are palpable cervical nodes. Figure 16-6 shows the histologic picture of an epidermoid carcinoma of the sac. This patient has had no recurrence years after treatment consisting of irradiation followed by excision of sac, nasal wall of orbit, antrum, and ethmoid sinuses[8] (Fig. 16-7).

A 71-year-old woman who exhibited all of the classic signs of a lacrimal sac tumor underwent surgical exploration. Frozen sections were reported as "chronic inflammation; no definite signs of neoplasia." The mass was removed, and the DCR was completed. The next day, histologic specimens were diagnosed as "epithelial carcinoma." Despite subsequent vigorous radiation therapy, the patient did not survive. This case points up the importance of interpreting negative frozen section findings cautiously. Although the early appearance of cervical nodes suggests that this patient had a poor prognosis in any event, it is possible that the dacryocystorhinostomy facilitated the spread of the tumor.

Spaeth[9] stated that there is a 50 percent mortality from lacrimal sac carcinomas. Metastases are most commonly cervical or pulmonary. Direct extension into the cranial cavity is possible.

Malignant Melanoma

Malignant melanoma of the lacrimal sac is rare. One such case in our practice had extension of the tumor into adjacent bony structures. The patient had undergone DCR some 5 years earlier, and at the time no biopsy was taken. The patient's subsequent course points up the importance of careful inspection of the lining of the lacrimal sac during every dacryocystorhinostomy and the desirability of taking a small portion of the sac for histologic study.

EXTRINSIC TUMORS—BENIGN

Any tumor in the region of the lacrimal sac can impinge on the sac and compromise its function. It can displace the sac, compress it, and

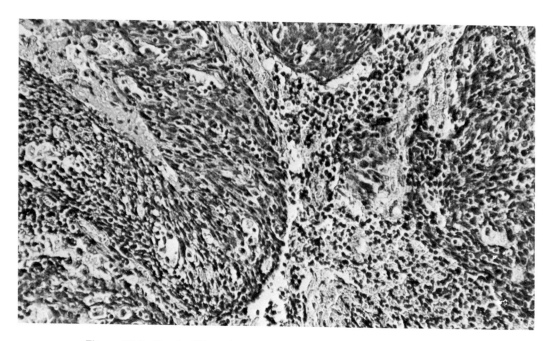

Figure 16-6. Poorly differentiated epidermoid carcinoma of the lacrimal sac.

invade it and can present a problem in differential diagnosis (Fig. 16-8).

As is true for any patient with unexplained epiphora, the successful resolution of the problem depends on a methodical and complete diagnostic evaluation. The clinical picture is almost always the same: epiphora, patency, and functional block. A mass may or may not be seen or felt. The dacryocystogram will reveal displacement, compression, or deformity of the lacrimal sac, while the concentration of the radiopaque material will be uniform within the sac. If there is a palpable or visible mass, the dacryocystogram can determine whether it is intrinsic or extrinsic to the sac. This information may be of aid in planning surgery. If the sac appears displaced or compressed but is not dilated or atonic, it may be possible to confront the primary mass without the necessity of performing a dacryocystorhinostomy.

If a mass is found or suspected at the initial examination, a careful examination of the nose and pharynx is indicated. Other useful diagnostic devices include conventional orbital tomography, CAT scanning, radiography of the paranasal sinuses, and a systemic review by an internist.

A 5-year-old patient who complained of tearing on the left side had a patent lacrimal system. The dacryocystogram revealed nasal displacement of the sac, without distention of the sac contrast shadow. The surgery was planned, on the basis of these findings, to spare the lacrimal system. An orbital cyst was dissected free, and the patient recovered normal outflow function (Fig. 16-9).

We have also found a mucocele of the ethmoid sinuses displacing the lacrimal sac.

The most dramatic illustration of the importance of dacryocystography in detecting extrinsic pressure on the lacrimal sac involved a 2-year-old boy who had epiphora and a tumefaction in the region of the right lacrimal sac. A diagnosis was made of dacryocystitis secondary to congenital dacryocystenosis. Dacryocystograms were not performed, but the surgeon proceeded directly to surgical intervention on the assumption that he was dealing with a distended lacrimal sac. When the surgical area was opened, there was an immediate flow of clear, cerebrospinal fluid from a meningocele. This could have been confirmed as being extrinsic to the lacrimal sac by dacryocystography. Fortunately, the child recovered.

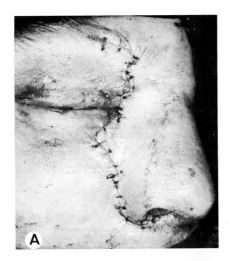

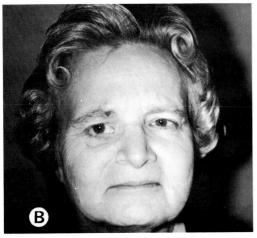

Figure 16-7. Epidermoid carcinoma of lacrimal sac. **A.** Closure after extensive resection of lacrimal sac, nasal bony orbit, antrum, and ethmoid sinuses. **B.** Same patient, 8 years later.

EXTRINSIC TUMORS—MALIGNANT

It is reasonable to conjecture that tumors of the orbit, especially metastatic lesions, would rarely manifest themselves as lacrimal problems. The proptosis and displacement of the globe, as well as disturbances in ocular rotations, would lead to the suspicion of an orbital mass long before it could impinge on the lacrimal excretory system. It has been suggested that it is rare for carcinomas of the paranasal sinuses to invade the lacrimal sac. However, such interactions are

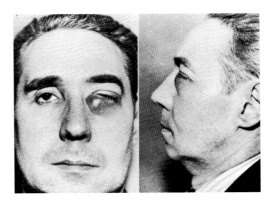

Figure 16-8. Myoblastoma of left orbit, resembling acute dacryocystitis. (*From Ingalls RG: Tumors of the Orbit and Allied Pseudo-Tumors, 1953 p 11. Courtesy of Charles C Thomas, Publisher, Springfield, Ill.*)

possible, and the site of origin can be confusing because of the similarity in the histopathology of carcinomas of the lacrimal sac and sinuses.

Probably because tumors in and about the lacrimal sac are so rare, there is a distressing tendency to procrastinate. One such missed or delayed diagnosis will serve to heighten our index of suspicion and hone our diagnostic methods. The presence of tumor should be sus-

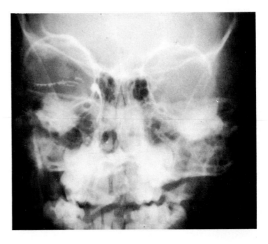

Figure 16-9. Dacryocystogram of a 5-year-old patient showing nasal displacement of the lacrimal sac due to an orbital cyst (posteroanterior view).

pected with unilateral epiphora, bouts of dacryocystitis, an irreducible mass, and bleeding from the punctum on manipulation. The dacryocystogram may well be definitive in determining if the lesion is extrinsic or intrinsic to the lacrimal sac. Careful inspection of the lacrimal sac at surgery and removal of tissue for biopsy are essential to the successful management of tumors of the excretory system.

REFERENCES

1. Ingalls RG: Tumors of the Orbit and Allied Pseudo-Tumors. Springfield, Ill, Charles C Thomas, 1953, p 11
2. Radnot M, Gall J: Tumoren des Tränensackes. II. Kongress der Europ. Ophthalm. Ges. Wien, June 1964. Ophthalmologica 151:1, 1966
3. Flanagan JC, Stokes DP: Lacrimal sac tumors. Ophthalmology, 85:1282, 1978
4. Schenck NL, Ogura JH, Pratt LL: Cancer of the lacrimal sac. Ann Otol 82:153, 1973
5. Milder B: Neurofibroma of the lacrimal sac. Am Ophthalmol, 53:703, 1962
6. Cole SH et al.: Fibrous histiocytoma of the lacrimal sac. Arch Ophthalmol 96:1647, 1978
7. Wachtel JG: Fibrous histiocytoma of the orbit. Presented at the Georgiana D Theobald Society XVII, 1976
8. Milder B, Smith ME: Carcinoma of the lacrimal sac. AmJ Ophthalmol 65:782, 1968
9. Spaeth EB: A surgical technique for lacrimal sac malignancy. Trans Ophthalmol Soc UK 89:351, 1969

17

SURGERY OF THE LACRIMAL SAC AND NASOLACRIMAL DUCT

ABRAHAM WERB

The fear of failure in the surgical treatment of epiphora can be effectively eliminated by familiarity with the anatomy of the region, an understanding of the physiology of lacrimal function and adequate examination of the system. Examination of the system, based on knowledge of it, will help the surgeon locate the site of obstruction so that he can achieve the obvious aim—restoration of function

ANESTHESIA

Surgery of the lacrimal sac is best performed under general anesthesia, but whenever possible, hypotensive anesthesia can be most helpful. This, however, should never be demanded and should always be left to the discretion of the anesthetist, thus eliminating any risk to the patient. There are other adjuncts that will help reduce troublesome bleeding. First is the avoidance of cutting major vessels or immediate ligation if they have to be cut. Second, the tilting of the head of the table 20 to 30° up from the horizontal helps reduce the venous pressure. Third, the nasal cavity can be packed for a short time with a solution of cocaine hydrochloride (4 to 10 percent) with epinephrine or lidocaine (4 percent) with 1:100,000 epineph-

rine. Finally, by working in the correct anatomic planes, much of the bleeding can be avoided. Under these conditions the injection of vasoconstricting solutions becomes unnecessary and thus eliminates the risk of distorting the anatomy of the surgical field.

In the United States, many surgeons prefer nerve block anesthesia using long-acting anesthetic agents. The infraorbital nerve and infratrochlear nerve are blocked, using bupivacaine hydrochloride (0.75 percent) combined with an equal volume of mepavicaine hydrochloride (2 percent), to which is added hyaluronidase (150 units for each 20 ml of the anesthetic mixture). With this nerve block anesthesia, distortion of the surgical site is avoided. Nerve block anesthesia is preceded by appropriate presurgical oral ataractics (Fig. 17-1).

THE INCISION

Some surgeons prefer to place a contact lens on the eye, in order to protect the cornea against the instrumentation and the surgical debris.

Exposure of the lacrimal sac requires a skin incision. The placement of the incision varies with different surgeons. The incision should provide adequate exposure of the surgical field,

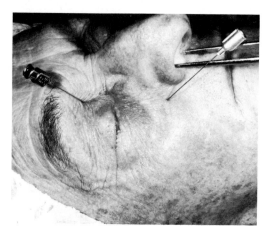

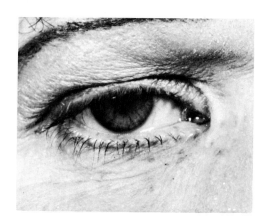

Figure 17-3. Bowstringing of DCR scar.

Figure 17-1. Local anesthesia for DCR. Cocaine (10 percent) cotton strip placed in middle meatus at anterior tip of middle turbinate; infratrochlear nerve block; infraorbital nerve block.

avoid excessive bleeding, and heal as invisibly as is cosmetically possible. Such an incision is best placed on the lateral wall of the nose just above the angular vein (Fig. 17-2). In that position there are only skin, peripheral rings of orbicularis, and periosteum. It is safe to take the incision down to bone in one sharp cut. This produces cleanly cut edges. The incision is straight and made at right angles to the skin surface. It must not extend above the medial canthal tendon or below the nasal bone. Curved incisions tend to heal with a bowstringing effect producing pseudoepicanthal folds (Fig. 17-3).

An alternative method of exposure is to

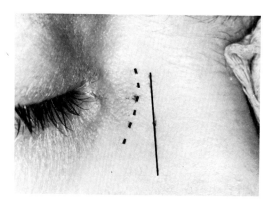

Figure 17-2. DCR incision (solid line). Dotted line indicates angular vein.

place the incision lateral to the angular vein so that the straight through-and-through incision impinges on the bone near the anterior lacrimal crest. Here, too, the incision must be held below the medial canthal tendon.

A straight incision which leads onto the nasal bone, permits the separation of the periosteum from the bone and thus keeps intact the layers between skin and periosteum. By separating the periosteum from the nasal bone, the insertion of the medial palpebral tendon is peeled off the bone simultaneously. This avoids the necessity of cutting it and subsequent replacement. When separating the periosteum from the bone, a small, sometimes troublesome, nutrient vessel at the sutura notha is encountered, which can be controlled by any form of hemostasis. A convenient method is to place the tapered end of the punctum dilator against the bleeding point and touch the punctum dilator with the cautery.

By reflecting the periosteum laterally with a Freer periosteal elevator, the first important landmark, the anterior lacrimal crest, is reached (Fig. 17-4), thus insuring correct orientation. The periosteum is firmly adherent to the crest, and at this point care is required. Failure to appreciate this anatomic relationship will result in inadvertent entry into the sac. This will produce unnecessary problems when the stage of fashioning the flaps is reached.

If the sac is distended and tense, it should be decompressed so as to improve the exposure. This can be performed by inserting a 19-gauge needle into the sac at or near the sac-duct junc-

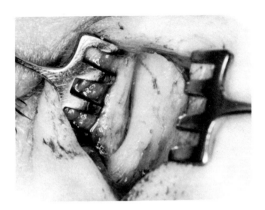

Figure 17-4. Anterior lacrimal crest exposed by reflecting the periosteum.

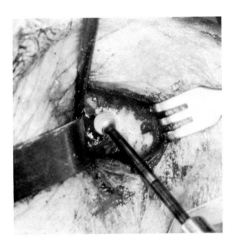

Figure 17-5. Removing the anterior lacrimal crest with a 4 mm high-speed burr. The osteotomy can be fashioned using the same tool.

tion and evacuating the contents of the sac by aspiration.

Another important anatomic variant is the shape of the crest. It can be very sharp or blunt. When sharp, the lacrimal fossa is deep, and the lacrimal sac housed in a deep fossa requires careful exposure. Only blunt dissection is recommended when a sharp crest is encountered. The sharp crest can be removed with a high-speed dental drill using a 3 or 4 mm diameter burr. Removing the crest in this fashion aids in exposure of the sac and the lacrimal fossa (Fig. 17-5).

A blunt crest presents no such problem, but it can cause some difficulty in identifying the sac as, in some cases, there may be no recognizable lacrimal fossa. If there is a question regarding the position of the sac, the sac may be gently irrigated through the upper or lower punctum and the increase in sac volume identified by light digital palpation. To ensure the correct topography, it is sometimes necessary to follow the anterior crest to the point where it becomes continuous as the inferior orbital margin. Once that point is reached, all doubts are dispelled.

The sac lying in the fossa has hardly any significant attachments and dislocates laterally quite easily with a periosteal elevator. Such dislocation need only be effected to the point of identifying the posterior lacrimal crest, which is the limit of the lacrimal fossa and, therefore, the lacrimal sac, and also the limit of the posterior margin of the eventual osteotomy.

THE OSTEOTOMY

There are strongly held views on how and where an osteotomy should be placed, as well as views on its size and shape. The object of the osteotomy is to enable the lacrimal sac to be anastomosed to the nasal mucosa. To achieve this, the intervening bone must be removed. The bone involved is that which constitutes the lacrimal fossa, i.e., a part of the frontal process of the maxilla and the lacrimal bone. No better view of it can be obtained than by its present exposure which seems to render unnecessary the use of other instruments placed in the invisible middle meatus of the nose. In questionable situations, a helpful guide is a focal transilluminator placed within the nose.

Having established the area of bone one has to remove, any discussion about the size of osteotomy seems irrelevant. Removing less than the anatomy indicates will cause surgical difficulties in flap preparation. The limits of the osteotomy are: posteriorly, the posterior lacrimal crest; inferiorly, the curve of the crest becoming the inferior orbital margin; superiorly, the fundus of the sac. There is, therefore, only one direction in which enlargement can take place and that is anteriorly. Dacryocystorhinostomy is unlikely to fail because the osteotomy is too large. Unhappily, however, failures do result from an osteotomy that is too small.

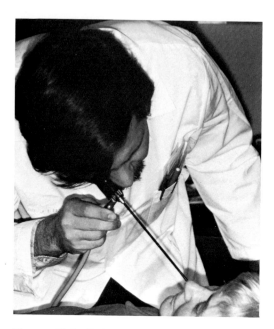

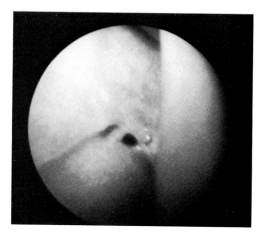

Figure 17-7. Dacryocystorhinostomy. Nasal osteum viewed with endoscope.

Figure 17-6. Endoscope tip is introduced just above the inferior turbinate. (*Courtesy of J.V. Linberg, MD, Department of Ophthalmology, Louisiana State University.*)

In a recent study,[1] measurements of the size of the intranasal DCR ostium were made at intervals up to 13 months following surgery. The ostium was visualized and photographed using a rigid endoscope with fiberoptic illumination, an instrument in common use by otolaryngologists. The ultimate mucosal aperture is quite small, averaging 1.75 mm. This small opening is adequate to the task of elimination of tears (Figs. 17-6 and 17-7). Its size seems to be independent of the size of the osteotomy. It follows, therefore, that the chief purpose of a large osteotomy is that it makes available adequate mucosal flaps for anastomosis.

It is the author's preference to create the osteotomy in the following manner. More often than not, the anterior lacrimal crest is angled enough to prevent the flat application of an Arruga trephine. For that reason, the trephine is placed just above the anterior lacrimal crest. Rotatory movements with this hand trephine will dislodge a disc of bone, carefully removed without damaging the underlying nasal mucosa (Fig. 17-8). This affords an entry point into the nasal cavity, and with a bone punch (Kerrison

or another type) the rest of the osteotomy is created to the limits already indicated. A variation may occur due to the presence of an anteriorly placed ethmoidal cell. In such cases, suspicion is aroused by the lacrimal bone's becoming thicker instead of thinner when removing bone posteriorly. If such a cell is encountered, it must be removed unless an adequate osteotomy can be fashioned without disturbing the ethmoidal cell. The mucosal lining of the sinus is, generally, darker, thinner, and more vascular than is the nasal mucosa.

The anatomy in this area is such that, with

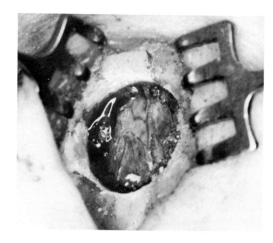

Figure 17-8. Osteotomy performed with 10 mm Arruga trephine. The nasal mucosa is intact.

a laterally shelving nasal mucosa and a medially shelving lacrimal sac, the two are close together at the posterior limit of the osteotomy. An intervening anterior ethmoidal air cell widens that gap and requires a wider posterior flap.

There is little to be said about the method of creating the bony opening. It has already been stated that a personal choice is a hand trephine and bone punch. There are surgeons who prefer dental burrs, mechanical saws, or, in removing the bone, even a hammer and chisel. Burrs measuring 2 to 5 mm in diameter, affixed to the slender handpiece of a high-speed (100,-000 to 250,000 rpm), air-driven drill, are ideal for controlling the size and shape of the osteotomy with little or no risk of damage to the nasal mucosa. However, the method used is of little consequence as long as the correct bone is removed and an adequate opening is created.

Views also exist on the shape of the osteotomy opening. Whether it is round or square is really unimportant. What might be mentioned in this context is that when an anterior flap does not hinge easily, a conversion of a round opening into a rectangular opening, by nibbling away the anterior corners, will definitely facilitate mobility of nasal mucosa. An adequate osteotomy is one in which the intervening bone between sac and nasal mucosa has been removed sufficiently to allow adequate formation and anastomosis of mucosal flaps.

THE ANASTOMOSIS

The formation of flaps is the next step in the operation. The sac should be dealt with first. There are various methods of entry into the sac, but it is, perhaps, more important to consider the aim and object of entry than the method. Ideally, the sac should provide an anterior and posterior flap. Sometimes its small size, other times inadvertent damage, may make this ideal difficult if not impossible. The nasal mucosa would, therefore, become the main source of flap formation, and it should be kept to the last.

Prior functional testing and dacryocystography will have resolved the question of the integrity of the canaliculi as well as the size of the lacrimal sac cavity. If, however, there is a question of preexisting obstruction in the canalicu-

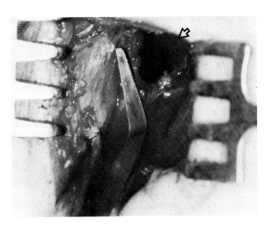

Figure 17-9. Opening the lacrimal sac. Initial entry is at the sac-duct junction. The osteotomy is at the right of the scissors blade (arrow).

lar system, a probe pushing blindly into the sac may be very misleading in locating the correct point of entry. In any case, it is the author's view that obstructions in the canalicular system should not be overcome blindly. Faced with an intact medial wall of sac, the safest point of entry is its junction with the nasolacrimal duct. This point is selected for incision, executed with the aid of specially designed scissors. The first cut is at right angles at the point where the duct descends into its canal (Fig. 17-9). Through this incision it is possible to insert one blade of the scissors into the lumen and then complete a vertical incision on the medial wall of the sac to reach the fundus of the sac. This will expose the interior of the sac.

If there is no indication of canalicular obstruction, a probe may be inserted gently through the canaliculus into the sac tenting the medial wall of the sac to facilitate entry into the sac. The initial incision is then enlarged with scissors. To confirm that one is inside the sac, a search is made to locate and identify the common opening. The common opening usually appears as a small slit. It may be hidden by surrounding valves, which in reality are folds of sac lining. If it is occluded by a membrane, it may, of course, be unidentifiable. In such circumstances it is necessary to pass canalicular probes into the canaliculi to indicate its site or its hidden position. Once it is identified, the interior of the sac is decidedly confirmed. If there is a question, one can instill a fluorescein stain or other colored solution into the sac through either canaliculus.

The question of identifying the common opening into the sac (the internal punctum) is highlighted because the outer coverings of the sac are loosely attached to its mucosal lining and if that plane is erroneously entered and not recognized, anastomosis between outer sac covering and nasal mucosa is doomed to failure. Another reason for devoting attention to the common opening is to ensure that there is nothing obstructing it, for it is obvious that even anastomosing sac to nose adequately will not ensure success unless the pathway is completely patent. It is most important that the interior of the sac be examined for polyps or other tissue masses, dacryoliths, mucous plugs, and cicatricial bands.

If in fashioning the sac flaps, one or the other is inadequate, a proportional flap must be tailored from the nasal mucosa, and it is to this structure that one's attention is directed at this stage. The nasal mucosa is highly vascular, and a certain amount of bleeding is possible. It can be minimized by the application of vasoconstricting plugs in the nose, or suction can be used to keep the field clear during the fashioning and suturing of flaps. Hemostasis can be achieved by infiltrating a local anesthetic mixture into the nasal mucosa using a small syringe and a 30-gauge needle. If the needle engages the mucosa and does not penetrate into the nasal cavity, the nasal mucosa is blanched and slightly thickened so that it is easier to suture. Small bleeders in the nasal mucosa can be controlled using cautery applied at the tip of a punctum dilator. The nasal flaps must match the sac flaps. A small posterior sac flap may require a larger nasal flap. The reverse holds true for the anterior flap.

The first incision into the nasal mucosa should be a small penetrating incision to establish position. A determination is made, with this initial incision, regarding the relative size of the anterior and posterior mucosal flaps, and this determination depends on the previously fashioned lacrimal sac flaps. In general, the practice is to make the anterior nasal mucosal flap twice as long as the posterior flap. The incision is then extended superiorly and inferiorly to the limits (and sometimes beyond) of the osteum (Fig. 17-

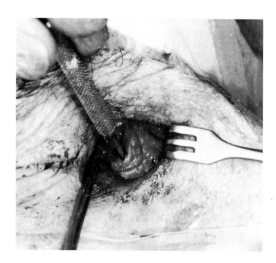

Figure 17-10. Incising the nasal mucosa. The anterior flap is wider than the posterior flap.

10). This incision into the mucosa tends to be limited by an elastic recoil at the ends of the incision, so that it is necessary to cut firmly against the edge of the osteotomy in order to achieve maximal length for the incision. Apposition to the posterior lacrimal sac flaps will usually be met with no tension, and suturing is easy. No hinging of flaps is necessary. Overly generous hinging may embarrass the blood supply. If, however, approximation of the anterior flaps is difficult, the osteum can be squared or enlarged anteriorly. This will make available more nasal mucosa. A further maneuver is to immobilize a small part of the lateral wall of the sac by slight hinging, taking care to not damage the entry of the canaliculi into the sac. Such a manipulation should seldom be necessary and follows earlier surgical error rather than a very contracted sac. A correctly placed nasal osteum will always be in the middle meatus, in front of the middle turbinate, which should never be in the way.

SUTURING THE MUCOSAL FLAPS

Controversy exists as to the necessity of the anterior and posterior flaps, the need to suture flaps, and, if so, how many sutures to use. Anterior and posterior flaps are desirable, and suturing of both is essential. This avoids the possibil-

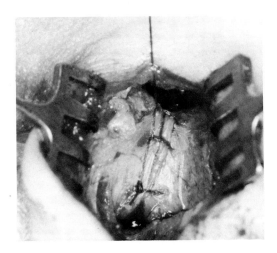

Figure 17-11. Anterior flaps closed with running locked suture technique.

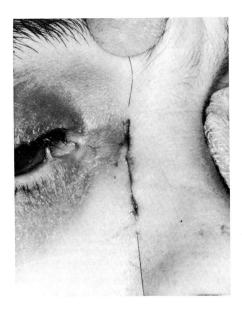

Figure 17-12. Subcuticular wound closure.

ity of granulation tissue occluding the opening. Current personal practice is the use of a continuous locked Dexon suture in both anterior and posterior flaps (Fig. 17-11). This replaces interrupted sutures, used for many years, and is found to be satisfactory. With adequate flap formation and suturing, the need for a foreign body of any kind to separate the anterior and posterior flap lines of union seems unnecessary, and the use of the rubber catheter or other stent for that purpose has been abandoned.

WOUND CLOSURE

Secure in the knowledge that adequate flaps have been apposed and fixed, all that remains is wound closure. A subcuticular nylon stitch, carefully placed, brings the skin wound together (Fig. 17-12). As a straight incision, it will heal invisibly as a hairline scar without the risk of bowstringing or suture marks of any kind. At this final stage of the operation, all bleeding will have ceased. Any blood clot in the nose is removed. The contact lens that was inserted at the beginning of the procedure to protect the cornea is removed. A light pad and bandage are applied and not removed for 48 hours unless the patient complains of pain or discomfort. We do not irrigate postoperatively under any circumstances, and topical medications or systemic an-

tibiotics are used only if indicated. Some surgeons prefer to irrigate the system gently on the third or fourth day, possibly as a form of reassurance therapy for both patient and surgeon.

COMPLICATIONS

Apart from the failure of the main object of DCR—elimination of symptoms of epiphora—there are certain undesirable occurrences that can be regarded as complications. Some are avoidable, others inevitable, and some unpredictable. The first group results from errors in technique.

1. The ideal hairline incision may turn out to be a bowstring or pseudoepicanthal fold. This can be avoided by placing it on the flat surface of the side of the nose and avoiding the curve of the inner canthal area. If the incision line has healed as a bowstring, Z-plasty will be necessary to correct it. By exercising care to the skin edges, it is possible to avoid further damage, such as burns and lacerations. In patients who have shown previous keloidal tendency, the possibility of this complication must be discussed with the patient. Keloid, however, is rare in the eyelids

and nasal canthal area. If the wound, post-operatively, appears unduly thickened, an injection of a repository corticosteroid into and alongside the scar may resolve the problem.

2. Damage to the sac during the process of dislocation from the lacrimal fossa can be avoided if the anatomic variations of the anterior lacrimal crest are borne in mind. If such damage has occurred that takes the form of perforation of the sac in an anterior position, resulting in a large posterior flap and a very tiny anterior flap, additional care must be taken in exposing the nasal mucosa. This is to ensure an intact surface so that corresponding tissue is available for matching nasal mucosal flaps.

3. If, during the process of creating the osteum, an anterior ethmoidal air cell is encountered, it must be removed in toto. Failure to recognize it may result in anastomosing sac to lining and eventual failure—or difficulty in bridging the posterior flap by virtue of the greater distance between sac and nasal cavity.

4. Damage to the nasal mucosa may occur during trephination. Small perforations of the mucosa will bleed excessively, and apart from the delay no major problems arise. However, larger tears in the mucosa require immediate repair. If access is difficult, the bony osteum must be enlarged anteriorly so that the defect can be adequately sutured. Failure to repair at this stage will jeopardize flap formation and endanger eventual success. Damage to the mucosa is uncommon when the ultra-high speed burr is used. With this device, careful attention should be given to maintaining contact between the burr and the bony edge of the osteotomy.

5. If the middle turbinate is exposed to the point where it interferes with the anastomosis, the osteum has been taken too far posteriorly. There is nothing to do but remove that part of it that is prominent. The anatomic position of the middle turbinate should never feature in a rhinostomy. When it does, it is not the turbinate that is in the wrong place!

6. Postoperative bleeding can be a serious problem. It can be immediate or delayed. During surgery, bleeding points should be dealt with, using either monopolar or bipo-

lar cautery. Small bleeders in the wall of the osteotomy may require the use of bone wax or, alternatively, simple pressure for several minutes to allow for clotting. Delayed hemorrhage can be quite serious. It always requires nasal packing and should always supersede the desire for noninterference with the anastomosis. In some cases, the help of a rhinologist may be necessary.

7. Infection is a very rare event, but its possibility must never be overlooked.

8. Failure of function, although listed last, is most important. When it occurs, the most important question to answer is "why?" This requires reinvestigation, and several possibilities exist:

    a. Some contributory cause to the epiphora other than nasolacrimal duct obstruction has been overlooked.

    b. Some technical error in the surgical performance may be the cause, e.g., inaccurate placement of the osteotomy, anastomosis to an anterior ethmoidal air cell. It is possible for the anterior and posterior anastomotic suture lines to adhere either from organization of an intervening blood clot or from collapse of anterior flaps due to excessive pressure during postoperative dressing. Whatever the cause, reoperation becomes essential.

REOPERATION

An interval should elapse before reentering the operative site. It is possible for function to return if the surgery was correctly performed and the failure was due to an unpredictable factor, such as hemorrhage into, or excessive trauma to, the orbicularis muscle. Spontaneous resolution can follow.

When reoperation is decided upon, general anesthesia is preferable. For those who use local nerve block anesthesia, the same technique as was employed primarily for a dacryocystorhinostomy can be used for reoperation. The exposure of the osteotomy site should be the first aim. This is best done by starting off on an intact bony surface on the lateral wall of the nose. The original skin incision may be used, but to reach the bone the incision must be gentle and stepwise until the bony surface is exposed. This will enable exposure of the whole circumference of the osteotomy. At all times, it is important to keep the nasal side of the tissue intact. To ensure identification of nasal mucosa, the bony osteum should be slightly enlarged beyond the original edge. Exposure of nasal mucosa will permit removal of excess scar tissue from its surface. Care must be taken not to perforate.

The connective tissue is incised to free the nasal mucosa. The lateral block of tissue will contain the lacrimal sac. With the aid of canalicular probes, the area can be identified and as much scar tissue as possible removed. The sac area is then opened, with the probes as guides, and the common opening is identified. As much of sac and mucosal flaps as possible should be fashioned. Essential to this operation is the introduction of canalicular tubes to act as scaffolding around which patent passages will heal and drain tears.

The choice of tube must be based on individual experience or the experience of others. A personal choice is for polyethylene because of its inertness and splint-ability. Others advocate silicone material, the rigidity of which will depend on the relationship between the outside diameter and the thickness of the wall of the silicone tube. Appropriate for canalicular intubation is silicone tubing with an inside diameter of 0.025 inches and outside diameter of 0.040 inches (1 mm). Silicone tubes of lesser caliber do not provide sufficient cross-sectional area for an adequate stent.

When such materials are to be introduced into the lacrimal system, patients should be warned that they are intended to remain for months and that the longer they remain in situ, the better the chance of success. The introduction of the polyethylene tube is a simple procedure. A guiding pliable metal bodkin carries a nylon thread over which the polyethylene is threaded. The bodkin is introduced through upper and lower canaliculi, with the two ends protruding through the nostril (Fig. 17-13). The two ends have a cuff of wider bore polyethelene over them and the cuff is pushed into the nostril, out of sight, and up to a point where the loop which links upper and lower canaliculi, does not jut out too far to irritate the eye.

When using silicone tubing, each end of the tube can be affixed to a stainless steel probe, using silicone glue, and this probe is introduced into the upper and lower canaliculi respec-

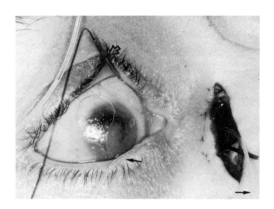

Figure 17-13. Polyethylene canalicular tubes act as a stent to maintain patency. The tube has been placed in the lower canaliculus (dark arrows), and the malleable metal bodkin is threaded through the upper canaliculus (light arrow).

tively. Additionally, such sets of Silastic tubing and stainless steel probes are available with the silicone swaged-on. However, most of these use silicone of smaller caliber than the size recommended above.*

If such a procedure is impossible surgically, due to inability to form flaps or locate the correct anatomical structures, then by-pass surgery is the only alternative to alleviate persistent epiphora.

SIMPLIFICATIONS AND SHORTCUTS IN DACRYOCYSTORHINOSTOMY

In the preceding pages, detailed descriptions of step by step stages of dacryocystorhinostomy are presented. The details, on the face of it, would appear to be simple enough, and no un-

---

* *For canalicular intubation, we use a Bowman probe which has a small fenestration at either end. This probe is introduced into the sac cavity through the canaliculus. A 00 nylon suture is threaded into the fenestration, and the probe is withdrawn. The nylon thus traverses the canaliculus from punctum to sac. The 1 mm silicone tube is then slid onto the nylon suture for a distance of 4 or 5 cm, clamped firmly to the suture, and drawn through the canaliculus by means of traction on the suture. The opposite end of the canalicular tube is brought into the sac through the other punctum and canaliculus, and then the two ends are brought through the osteotomy into the nose.*

necessary steps are advocated. However, the description does not depict the simplicity of the procedure when performed or observed.

Yet, "simplified" or "variations of" the standard dacryocystorhinostomy are described and advocated in the literature. One may well ask "what is simpler than simple?" A glance at the "simplified procedures" or the "variations" reveals not simplicity in performance but, rather, the omission of certain steps in the procedure. One such is to omit the suturing of posterior flaps. In some few cases, suturing may be a comparatively difficult maneuver to carry out, especially if one has encountered an anteriorly placed ethmoidal air cell or damaged either the sac or the nasal mucous membrane, or if there is excessive bleeding obscuring the field of operation. All this, however, is no reason for omitting this desirable step. Correct surgical apposition of mucosal flaps, as the guide for the reformation of an intact epithelium-lined passage, is a basic principle of good surgery—and the surgeon need settle for nothing less.

Another simplification is the omission of an indwelling catheter or tube for the purpose of separating the anterior and posterior flap suture lines. If the surgeon feels secure that the realignment of flaps at the end of the procedure is such that there is no contact of the suture lines and that there is no bleeding, there is justification for the omission of such an obturator. It will reduce operating time by several minutes and obviate the need for its subsequent removal and whatever discomfort it will cause the patient. But let no one underestimate the security it offers to those who use it. It not only separates suture lines but acts as a hemostat and thus contributes to the ultimate success. Our preference is for meticulous suturing of mucosal flaps and *no* internal stent.

There are "simplified" procedures that advocate "blind" intubation into the lacrimal system to avoid "cutting." To those who contemplate such procedures, a simple reminder is given of the right-angled turns that the lacrimal system makes from its commencement at the punctum to its termination under the inferior turbinate, not to mention the numerous folds within the lumen of the whole system. Feel and touch are no substitute for sight.

There is yet another variation which consists of transplanting the lower end of the sac after detaching it from its continuity with the nasolacrimal duct into the nose. It is claimed to be superior to the standard dacryocystorhinostomy by virtue of the absence of bleeding and easier suturing. It ignores the basic requirement of visual inspection of the interior of the sac and the possibility of taking appropriate action if an abnormality is encountered. The presence of a dacryolith or a mass of inspissated mucus (the precursor of the dacryolith) is sure to be missed. If the saving of time and lack of bleeding are the considered gains of such a procedure, it must be, in some cases, at the expense of success.

Varying techniques are to be respected as expressions of individual surgeons who feel that minor variations enhance their results. It matters little whether the incision is higher or lower, provided it gives good access and will heal in a cosmetically acceptable way. It matters little whether the bony osteum is circular or rectangular, provided it is correctly placed. Simplifying an operation not only implies that the original procedure is complicated but may discourage beginners from correctly performing an operation, introduced by Dupuys-Dutemps, which is satisfying and has stood the test of time.

SURGERY OF THE NASOLACRIMAL DUCT

Direct surgical approach to the nasolacrimal duct is difficult because of its anatomic inaccessibility. Therefore, when it is obstructed it is bypassed in favor of the easier sac-to-nose anastomosis. Obstructions can be either congenital or acquired.

In adults obstructions occur as the result of:

- Inflammatory occlusions
- Displacement following injuries
- Surgery in the vicinity of the inferior turbinate

These can be dealt with by conventional DCR. If dacryocystography has established that the obstruction is low in the nasolacrimal duct, the DCR will leave, inevitably, a cul de sac below. While there is a potential for failure of the DCR as the result of stasis in this dead space, it is interesting that such failures are infrequent. The risk of failure can be minimized to some extent by carrying the osteotomy inferiorly as far as possible in the middle meatus after removing the overhanging anterior lacrimal crest.

In adults, the nasolacrimal duct should not be probed. Such procedures are not successful and cause added trauma to the soft tissues. Obstructions following facial injuries (usually middle third fractures) can be irrigated and sometimes found to be emptying into the maxillary sinus. This shows that patency into the sinus is not an answer to tear drainage. Such malformations can be diagnosed by the usual lacrimal function testing and by dacryocystography. These problems are cured by DCR.

In the congenital form of nasolacrimal duct obstruction, probing is carried out not only to establish the site of obstruction but also to effect drainage (See chapter 10).

DCR carries such a high percentage of success that this type of lacrimal surgery is both highly desirable and strongly commended. The main surgical consideration is the patient's fitness, as age need be no barrier.

REFERENCE

Linberg JV: A study of the intranasal ostium created by external dacryocystorhinostomy. In press, 1983

18

INVOLUTIONAL CHANGES AND THE LACRIMAL SYSTEM

BERND SILVER

Abnormalities of eyelid position are frequent causes of tearing in the elderly. Such abnormalities may produce irritation resulting in reflex hypersecretion of tears. Tearing may result from eversion of the puncta, malposition of the lid margin, or failure of the lacrimal pump due to lid laxity.

The lacrimal pump is a delicate mechanism requiring that all factors must function correctly to provide adequate tear drainage. The punctum must be in proper position in the lacrimal lake to suck the tears into the ampulla. The punctum must be held in proper position by the tension of the lid against the globe. If the punctum or the lid falls away from the globe, the situation becomes similar to that which exists when the downspout of a house is pulled away from the gutter—water will spill over.

The support of the orbicularis muscle, tarsus, and tarsal tendons must be sufficient to hold the lid snugly against the globe. Failure of these factors has been described by Malcolm Bick[1] as "orbito-tarsal disparity." Additional senescent changes in the orbit may contribute to this disparity. Retrobulbar fat pads may sink posteriorly and inferiorly through attenuated fascia and thinned skin, producing baggy lids with fat prolapse. The lacrimal glands may

proptose into the lateral upper lid compartments, and the globe may fall back, producing a relative enophthalmos. The supratarsal sulcus may become exaggerated, and ptosis of the lids may result from loss of support by the globe.

If orbitotarsal disparity is sufficiently great, relaxation of the lower lid will be accompanied by an exaggerated tear lake, irritation, reflex hypersecretion of tears, and subjective complaint of a wet eye (Fig. 18-1). A similar effect can be demonstrated in the normal patient by gently pulling down on the lids and holding them away from the globe for several minutes. The discomfort will produce tearing in a short time.

The importance of orbicularis and lid relaxation in producing lacrimal insufficiency was documented by Mathur.[2] He attempted to treat the orbicularis insufficiency by galvanic stimulation. He achieved measurable increase in orbicularis tone, with modest subjective improvement. Our experience has shown that symptomatic relief is more frequently obtained by shortening the lid to correct the lid laxity. The lid-shortening procedure eliminates the separation between the lid margin and the globe and reduces or eliminates the excessive laking of tears. The subjective improvement

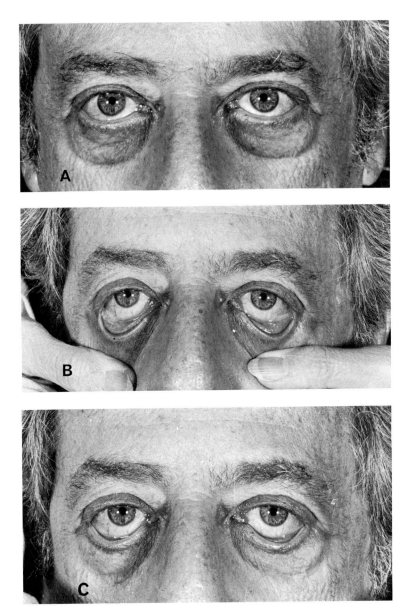

Figure 18-1. Patient demonstrating lower lid laxity. **A.** Looseness of lower lids permits formation of abnormal tear lake. **B.** Lower lids are pulled down. **C.** On release of lower lids, there is a sluggish, incomplete return of the lids toward the globe.

appears to be due to a reduction of the reflex hypersecretion and is independent of any improvement in the position of the puncta or the patency of the lacrimal passages. Tests of lacrimal outflow function are unchanged by this procedure.

PUNCTAL EVERSION

Eversion of the punctum is the mildest form of ectropion that develops in the aging lid. This may be present without significant ectropion of the rest of the lid. In the early stages, it is the

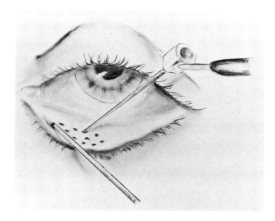

Figure 18-2. Ziegler cautery[3] consists of a series of fine, superficial tarsal burns from the area immediately below the punctum laterally to the center of the lid. Drawing illustrates application of electrocautery via a fine needle which just penetrated the surface of the tarsus. Note the lacrimal probe in place to warn surgeon of location of canaliculus and punctum.

result of relaxation of the tarsal tendons. It may be necessary to examine the patient under the slit lamp to appreciate a punctum that points vertically rather than posteriorly. Over a period of time there may be warping of the tarsus, which produces further eversion of the punctum. If the lid is pulled temporally to tighten it against the globe but the punctum fails to invert, warping of the tarsus has occurred. There are several methods for dealing with this problem. Some of these procedures are effective for only a few years, but they can easily be repeated. One must be careful to avoid vertical lid shortening with these techniques.

Ziegler Cautery

Cautery of the conjunctival surface of the tarsus is probably the simplest treatment for punctal eversion[3] (Fig. 18-2). A series of heat or electric cautery punctures is placed superficially along the surface of the tarsus just lateral to the punctum. If the cautery is restricted to the superficial layers of the tarsus, one can observe contraction of the surface of the tarsus, with reinversion of the punctum. Our preferred way of doing this is to insert the point of a fine hypodermic needle, such as a 25 or 27 gauge, just below the surface of the anesthetized tarsus. An electric cautery tip is touched against the hub of

the needle. The cautery reaction occurs at the point of the needle, with blanching of the tarsal surface and contraction of the tarsus back toward the eye. This cautery should be carried temporally as far as the center of the lid. A canalicular probe aids in everting the eyelid for this procedure and prevents placing the punctures in the ampulla or the canaliculus. Applying the cautery into the soft conjunctiva below the punctum produces very little effect. If the cautery penetrates too deeply, it can damage the marginal blood vessels and result in a slough of the lid margin. As the scar tissue heals, the tarsus may again evert. The procedure can be repeated.

Diamond Excision

A second method to resolve punctal eversion consists of excision of a horizontal spindle or diamond of tarsoconjunctiva below the punctum (Fig. 18-3). The widest vertical dimension of the spindle should be directly below the punctum. Vertical suturing of the wound pulls the punctum inferiorly and posteriorly against the globe. This is usually effective, but it is quite easy to develop full thickness vertical lid shortening without significant repositioning of the punctum.

PUNCTUM PLASTY

When the previously described simple procedures to reinvert the punctum fail, the use of punctum surgery may be considered. The punctum surgical procedures create a new, enlarged access to the tear lake. The simplest and probably the least effective is the one-snip operation, a simple vertical incision through the posterior aspect of the punctum. This incision usually heals very promptly. The three-snip operation creates a wider channel that remains open. This may be done more simply with a delicate Holth punch (Chapter 14).

ECTROPION

Ectropion of the lower lid is a further step in the progression of orbitotarsal disparity, with greater relaxation of the lower lid and its tendons. This may be made worse by frequent rubbing and pulling downward on the eyelid as

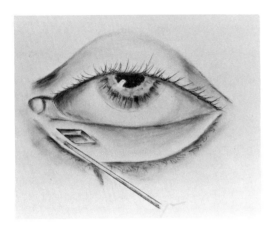

Figure 18-3. A horizontal diamond of tarsus is excised below the punctum. Closure tends to draw the punctum posteriorly into the lacrimal lake.

the patient wipes away tears. This entity may not produce significant symptoms until the condition has been present for a long time and gross ectropion exists. To correct the problem, the lid must be tightened against the eye by horizontal excision of the excessive lid tissue. The lid shortening may be done anywhere along the eyelids: nasally, centrally, or temporally.

Kuhnt-Szymanowski Operation

One of the oldest lid-shortening operations is the Kuhnt-Szymanowski[4, 5] operation, which was developed in the middle 1800s (Fig. 18-4). It worked adequately in the hands of a skilled surgeon who had at his disposal only the crude needles and sutures of 50 years ago. The Kuhnt-Szymanowski operation consists of splitting the lid into two layers along the gray line, then resecting the posterior tarsal lamella until

the lid is snug against the eye, followed by excision of the anterior lamella (skin and orbicularis) laterally at or beyond the lateral canthus. It was presumed that the intact anterior lamella would splint the resected tarsus and prevent traction or dehiscence of the tarsal wound. Unfortunately, a layer of scar tissue may form between the two layers during healing, causing the lashes to be misdirected posteriorly against the cornea, resulting in trichiasis.

Full-thickness Resection

Smith,[6] in the late 1950s, popularized full-thickness transmarginal lid resection for tumor removal, and this technique became popular for the correction of ectropion (Fig. 18-5). This operation was made possible by the development of modern fine needles and sutures. Smith was the first to recognize the possibility of accurately closing a lid margin wound without the development of vertical scarring and subsequent notching. The technique consists of an initial vertical lid incision, full thickness, performed by a razor blade knife to produce a sharply edged wound. The edges of the lid incision are overlapped until the lid margin is tight against the globe, and the excess lid is excised, again using a razor blade knife. By making the incisions perpendicular to the lid margin, accurate and precise reapposition of the lid margin can be achieved. Sutures, 6-0, with cataract quality needles are placed into the lid margin precisely 2.0 mm from the incision and 2.0 mm in depth on one side of the wound, passed across the defect, and redirected into the opposite side of the wound to emerge at the opposite lid margin in precisely the same position. A temporary knot is tied, the result is evaluated, and the suture is replaced until there is satisfactory apposition of the lid margin. Sutures can then be

Figure 18-4. Kuhnt-Szymanowski operation,[4, 5] demonstrating horizontal lid shortening after separation of the lid into two lamellae. The posterior lamella can be shortened anywhere along the length of the lid; the anterior lamella is shortened laterally.

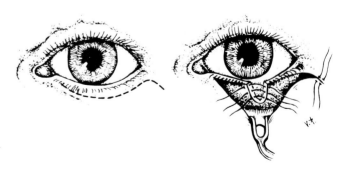

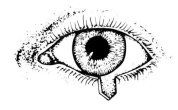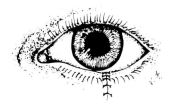

Figure 18-5. Horizontal lid shortening by full-thickness transmarginal resection, after Smith.[6] A horizontal section of the lid margin is resected, then reapproximated by meticulous anastomosis of lid margin landmarks.

placed through additional lid margin landmarks to reinforce accurate closure. Supporting sutures are placed deeply into the tarsus and the orbicularis to provide additional support. Marginal sutures are pulled forward and tied into a suture placed at the base of the skin defect to pull the marginal knots away from the globe so they will not irritate the cornea. The operation is best done with a loupe or surgical microscope to obtain a perfect anastomosis. Any separation of the wound will result in a widened scar, followed by contraction and notching of the lid margin. If this closure fails and the wound separates, further repair can be very difficult. For this reason and because of the difficulty in obtaining accurate lid margin repair, another operation, popularized by Bick,[1] became widely used.

Bick Operation

Possibly the best of the recent techniques was one revived by Malcolm Bick in 1966.[1] (Fig. 18-6). It was based on an operation described by Adam and later modified by von Ammon in the German literature of the middle 1800s. The entire lid resection is carried out at the lateral canthus. An inferior-temporal full-thickness lid incision is made with scissors. The severed end of the lid is pulled laterally until the lid is tight against the globe. The excess tissue is then resected in a V, and careful closure of the defect is performed. The cut end of the tarsus must be reanastomosed to the lateral canthal tendon or periosteum. Additional sutures are then used to close the rest of the wound, including orbicularis and skin. It is essential that the lid be carefully reattached to the tarsal tendon or periosteum of the lateral orbital rim, or the result will be a rounding of the lateral canthus. In the

event of a dehiscence, repeated repair can be performed easily, but often the lid will heal into proper position without additional surgery. There have been several modifications of this procedure. The scar can be placed into a more natural horizontal crease,[6] and a tongue of tarsus can be created and attached to the lateral canthal periosteum[7,8] to obtain additional tightening of the lid.

ENTROPION

The same orbitotarsal disparity that produces ectropion may also result in entropion. While the basic mechanism is similar, with relaxation of the lid and a relative enophthalmos, Jones et al. have suggested that the retractors of the lower lid have become stretched, permitting the lid to intort.[9] He has compared this with the dehiscence of the levator aponeurosis of the upper lid and has proposed that tucking the aponeurosis of the lower lid retractors will correct the entropion. Several factors are observed in the etiology of entropion. There may or may not be lid laxity, but there is almost always relaxation of the orbicularis with upward migration of this muscle over the tarsus toward the lid margin, producing intorsion of the lid. Once the lid turns in, irritation produces further spasm of the orbicularis muscle and additional entropion. Thus, a vicious cycle is set up. Because of the discomfort, these patients tend to seek help much sooner than the patient with ectropion.

Various operations have been proposed to correct entropion, which may be separated into two categories: (1) those that work by modifying the abnormal anatomy of the lid and (2) those that produce scar tissue barrier between orbicularis and the other layers of the eyelid. We will first consider operations that depend on the production of a scar tissue barrier. These operations depend on adhesions between skin and orbicularis muscle and between orbicularis muscle and underlying tarsus. Since scar tissue tends to soften and heal over a period of time,

the original abnormal anatomy may return, with recurrence of entropion.

Ziegler Cautery

Ziegler cautery[3] on the anterior lamella of the lid is a good example of a scar tissue barrier-type operation. This procedure consists of a se-

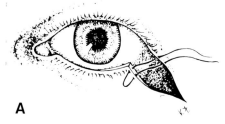

A

Figure 18-6. Horizontal lid resection after Bick.[1] **A.** Diagram demonstrates full-thickness lid resection at the lateral canthus, followed by careful reanastomosis of lower lid to lateral canthal tendon or periosteum of orbital margin. (*Cont.*)

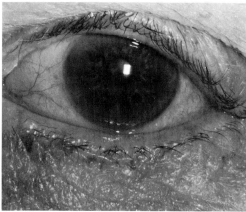

Figure 18-6. *Cont.* Photographs illustrating actual performance of Bick operation: **B.** Patient with lid laxity and punctal eversion.

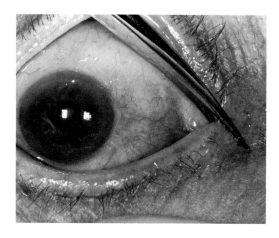

C. Incision of lid at lateral canthus performed with scissors.

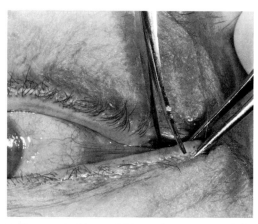

D. Free end of lower lid lapped over upper. Scissors poised to excise redundant lower lid at point of overlap.

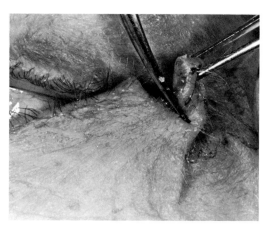

E. Scissors excising redundant lid tissue. (*Cont.*)

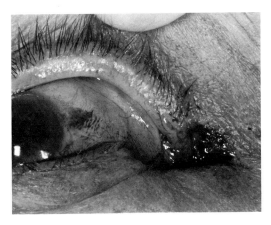

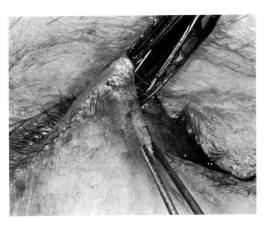

Figure 18-6. *Cont.* **F.** Resulting defect at lateral canthus.

G. Skin-orbicularis separated from underlying tarsus to permit easier insertion of suture into tarsus.

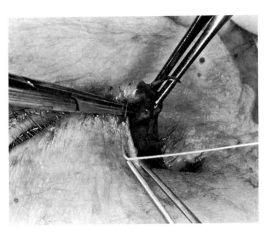

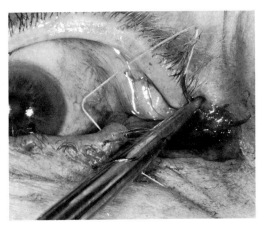

H. Suture being passed through anterior surface of tarsus, emerging at cut edge of lid.

I. Suture passed through stump of lateral canthal tendon.

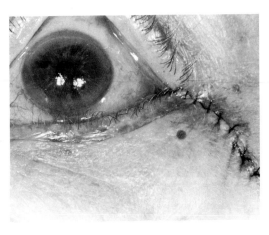

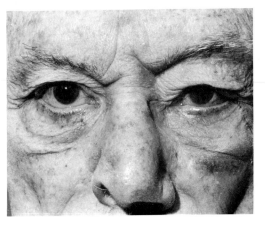

J. Tarsal sutures tied, and entire wound closed.

K. Early postoperative result with lower lid in good apposition against the globe.

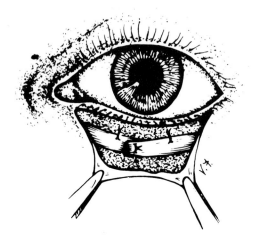

Figure 18-7. Wheeler orbicularis imbrication[11] operation consisting of elevation of horizontal strip of orbicularis, severing and shortening the muscle centrally, and then reattaching the orbicularis muscle to the base of the tarsus.

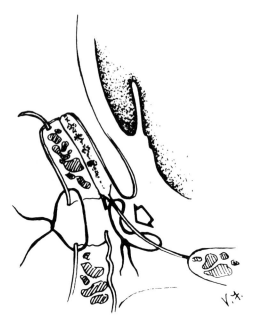

Figure 18-8. Aponeurosis tuck. Dissection is carried through an infraciliary incision inferiorly through the septum to the aponeurosis of the lower lid (see arrow), followed by a tucking of this structure.

ries of heat or electric cautery punctures through all layers of the lid—skin, orbicularis, and tarsus. The punctures may be applied in vertical or horizontal rows. A dense adhesion develops between these layers. It is intended that the horizontal scar barrier, placed near the lower border of the tarsus, will help evert the lid margin. If the punctures are performed timidly, postoperative edema occurs, and the entropion may return within a short time. If the punctures are applied too vigorously, there is the risk of vertical lid shortening, resulting in retraction of the lower lid and unsightly exposure of the inferior sclera (scleral show). The most significant problem following this procedure is the difficulty of performing a more definitive operation if there is a recurrence. This procedure is rarely performed by present-day oculoplastic surgeons.

Wheeler Imbrication

One of the two operations accredited to Wheeler is the orbicularis imbrication operation[10] (Fig. 18-7). An infraciliary incision is made through the skin, exposing the orbicularis muscle. A horizontal band of orbicularis muscle is then dissected free and elevated, severed in the center, and the cut ends are overlapped and shortened before being reattached to the lower border of the tarsus. Many modifications of this operation have been devised, including scrap-

ing all orbicularis free of the tarsus with a curette and placing additional sutures between skin, orbicularis, and tarsus in order to keep the orbicularis from reinverting the lid. This example of a scar tissue barrier operation has a 20 percent recurrence rate after the scar softens and the orbicularis is again free to roll up and force the lid back against the cornea. There is no permanent alteration in the lid anatomy resulting from this operation.

Aponeurosis Tuck

As a result of his hypothesis concerning the lower lid retractors, Jones[9] suggested an operation for tucking and shortening the aponeurosis of the lower lid (Fig. 18-8). This operation is performed through a horizontal infraciliary incision, followed by dissection along the border of the tarsus and orbital septum down to the retractors of the lower lid. The retractors are cautiously tucked to tighten them, avoiding vertical shortening of the lid. This is an operation with considerable dissection, and a scar tissue barrier develops. The recurrence rate equals that of the Wheeler imbrication operation. The author has achieved similar results by performing a sham operation for carrying out this operation without the aponeurosis tuck. The results of the aponeurosis tuck are improved considerably by performing the operation together with a horizontal lid shortening operation to tighten the lid against the globe. The hazard of this procedure is vertical lid shortening from overzealous aponeurosis tucking. When this occurs, restoration of the lid to normal level is very difficult and requires a lid recession procedure.

ENTROPION OPERATIONS THAT MODIFY ANATOMIC ABNORMALITIES

Bick Lid Resection

The Bick operation,[1] described for ectropion, produces a significant horizontal shortening of the lower lid by pulling it back against the globe, thus improving its stability. It is an excellent entropion operation. The few recurrences that have been observed appear to be in those patients who have had such long-standing entropion that the orbicularis muscle has become hypertrophied and continues to intort the lid despite increased lid stability.

Lateral Orbicularis Transplantation

The most definitive operation appears to be the Wheeler lateral orbicularis transplantation operation[10] (Fig. 18-9). In approximately 20 years of surgery, this author has observed only three recurrences, and these have been in patients who had had previous surgery with scarring of the posterior lamella.

This procedure commences with an infraciliary incision carried laterally and inferiorly. After the skin is dissected from the underlying muscle, the orbicularis muscle is freed from its attachment for the entire width of the lid except the nasal end, where the muscle is left attached. The lateral end is severed and transplanted downward, to be secured to the temporalis fascia over the malar bone. If it is noted that the lid is stretched and lax, a lid-shortening operation, such as the Bick, may be performed to avoid secondary ectropion. Removal of extra skin and fat before closure may be done for a cosmetically better result. This operation results in denervation of the orbicularis muscle and transforms it into a fibrous band wedged se-

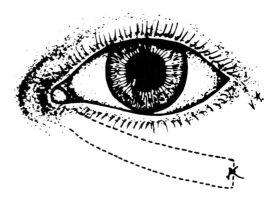

Figure 18-9. Wheeler lateral orbicularis[11] transplantation operation consisting of isolating the orbicularis muscle in a horizontal strip, severing it at the lateral end, then rotating and reattaching the severed end to the periosteum over the malar eminence.

curely against the lower border of the tarsus, keeping it from riding upward and turning the lid in again. It is interesting to observe such a patient when he squeezes his eye tightly. The orbital part of the orbicularis muscle attempts to ride upward but is prevented from doing so by the fibrotic orbicularis band. It is advisable to warn the patient that this is a very vascular area and that there may be extensive ecchymoses postoperatively.

Base-down Triangular Resection Procedure

Although the Ziegler cautery operation[3] is often used as an example of a simple operation with low morbidity, it has, as pointed out, a high incidence of recurrences. A simple operation that is more effective and with a lower morbidity is the base-down triangular tarsus resection (Fig. 18-10) described by Butler,[11] Fox,[12] and Kwitko.[13] This operation results in horizontal shortening of the base of the tarsus so that it is pulled snugly against the globe, everting the lid margin. This can be performed with the help of a chalazion clamp to stabilize the lid and reduce bleeding. It is even easier to perform with a chalazion forceps that has been modified by changing the plate to a ring. This results in a double ring clamp, and the closing suture can be passed through the full thickness of the tarsus and lid as a figure eight so that the closing knot can be tied on the skin surface where it will not irritate the cornea. The results are

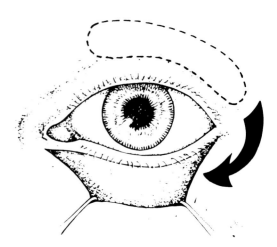

Figure 18-11. Diagrammatic illustration of skin transplant from upper lid into full-thickness defect created in lower lid to repair cicatricial ectropion.

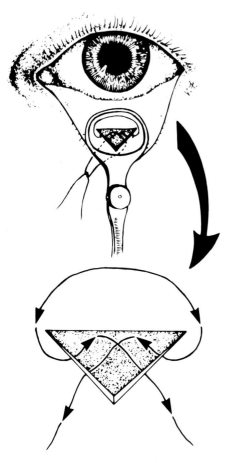

Figure 18-10. Triangular tarsal resection,[12-14] being performed with the aid of a modified chalazion clamp to avoid knots rubbing on the cornea, by passing the suture across the defect in a figure eight manner, then tying the suture on the external surface of the lid.

usually good for a period of some years postoperatively, following which, if the lid stretches again and instability recurs, the operation may be easily repeated.

CICATRICIAL EYELID DISEASES

Cicatricial Ectropion

There are a number of lid abnormalities produced by scarring processes, all of which may cause epiphora (Fig. 18-11). The damage may be in the anterior lamella of the lid (producing cicatricial ectropion), the posterior layer of the lid (producing cicatricial entropion), or from the entire thickness of the lid (producing vertical lid tissue shortage and scleral exposure).

Anterior lamellar defects may follow longstanding lid laxity in the elderly, removal of malignant tumors or benign lesions such as xanthelasmoas, extensive skin removal for blepharoplasty operations, burns or chemical injuries, or by cicatricial skin disease. With loss of tissue of the anterior lamella, a cicatricial ectropion develops that will produce considerable tearing. When possible, the original process should be treated and surgery avoided. Patients may respond to topical and sometimes even to injected steroids. However, when the scar has become permanent, surgery must be performed to replace the lost tissue. If the etiology of the ectropion is obscure, palpation of the skin of the lid and observation of the differences in lid level with the patient's mouth open and closed will help to establish the correct diagnosis of cicatricial ectropion.

Surgical treatment consists of replacing the lost tissue by skin grafts following incision or excision of scar tissue. The scar may be found to penetrate through the skin and orbicularis muscle down to the tarsus and orbital septum. The lid incision must be of sufficient depth so that the lid easily falls back into its normal position against the globe. A concomitant horizontal lid shortening operation may be necessary to counteract horizontal lid stretching. The ideal skin donor sites are from the opposite lid,

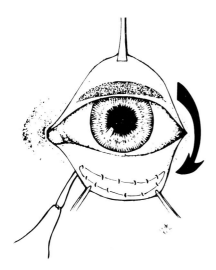

Figure 18-12. Tarsal transplant operation for cicatricial entropion transplants intact conjunctiva with supporting tarsus into a defect surgically created in the opposite scarred eyelid, forcing the lid margin away from the globe.

the retroauricular area, or the suproclavicular area. The recipient area should be kept immobile for a few days by a stent or other appropriate bandage. Permitting the graft to move risks the development of a hematoma under the graft, which will increase the risk of graft failure.

CICATRICIAL ENTROPION

Cicatricial entropion results from damage to the posterior lamella of the lid: tarsus and conjunctiva (Fig. 18-12). The causes include such chemicals as caustics and eye drops, trauma, autoimmune processes such as ocular pemphigoid, and Stevens-Johnson disease. The malrotation of the lid margin posteriorly makes it impossible for tears to enter the lacrimal system, produces corneal irritation by mechanical rubbing of skin and lids on the cornea, and causes discomfort due to exposure from vertical shortage of the lid. If the cause can be treated by medical means, such as antimetabolites or steroids, the results are often superior to surgical methods, since very often surgery produces its own complications. This is particularly true in Stevens-Johnson disease and ocular pemphi-

goid, where the surgical process seems to stimulate more scar formation. Surgical principles depend on the replacement of lost tissue. The ideal tissue is tarsus from the opposite lid. This is the only form of conjunctiva that has a firm base that resists contracture. Other sources include the nasal septum with attached mucous membrane and oral mucous membrane obtained from the inside of the cheek or lip. Nasal septum tends to be thick and may warp, while oral mucous membrane has no supporting stroma to resist shrinkage. The procedures consist of a horizontal incision through the contracture line of scarred lamella, everting the lid margin, and interposing the graft material into the bed created. If the grafted material is oral mucous membrane, it should be noted that we have replaced the sharp-edged windshield wiper effect of the normal lid margin with a soft, rubbery material which, while not irritating, fails to clean the cornea adequately.

REFERENCES

1. Bick MW: Surgical management of orbito-tarsal disparity. Arch Ophthalmol 75:386, 1966
2. Mathur SP: Lacrimal insufficiency in relation to the strength of orbicularis oculii muscle, and the effect after physiotherapy. Unpublished
3. Ziegler SL: Galvanocautery puncture in ectropion and entropion. JAMA 53:183, 1909
4. Kuhnt H: Beitrage zur operationen Augenhilkunder. Jean, G. Fischer, 1883, pp 45-55
5. Szymanowski J: Handbuch der Operationen chirugie. Berlin, Braunschweig, 1870, p 243
6. Smith B, Cherubini TD: Oculoplastic Surgery. St. Louis, Mosby, 1970, pp 93-94
7. Tenzel RR: Treatment of lagophthalmos of the lower lid. Arch Ophthalmol 81:366, 1969
8. Anderson RL, Gordy DD: The tarsal strip procedure. Arch Ophthalmol 97:2192, 1969
9. Jones LT, Reeh MV, Wobig JL: Senile entropion: a new concept for correction. Am J Ophthalmol 72:327, 1972
10. Wheeler JM: Spastic entropion correction by orbicularis transplantation. Am J Ophthalmol 22:477, 1939
11. Butler JBV: Simple operation for entropion. Arch Ophthalmol 40:665, 1948
12. Fox SA: Correction of senile entropion. Arch Ophthalmol 48:624, 1952
13. Kwitko M: A simplified treatment for entropion. Am J Ophthalmol 72:64, 1964

19

COMPLICATIONS OF LACRIMAL SURGERY

BENJAMIN MILDER

As in all surgery, the decision to perform a specific lacrimal operation on a specific patient involves balancing the risks against the potential benefits. One of the risk factors is lack of experience in dealing with the complications of such surgery. Fortunately, in lacrimal surgery, the incidence of complications is small, and the risk factor can be diminished by an awareness of such complications.

In this chapter, we discuss the complications encountered in the following surgical procedures:

1. Lacrimal probing in infants
2. Surgery of the canaliculi
3. Intubation techniques for occlusion of the internal punctum
4. Surgery for obstructions in the common canaliculus and internal punctum
5. Dacryocystorhinostomy

The surgeon must concern himself with the potential for complications in four areas:

1. Before surgery
2. At surgery, including anesthesia
3. Early postoperative period
4. Late postoperative period

LACRIMAL PROBING IN INFANTS

Preoperative Complications

In newborn infants, the incidence of nonpatent lacrimal drainage systems has been reported to be as high as 73 percent.[1] Korchmaros et al.[2] reported 54 percent obstructions at birth. After 12 weeks, 60 percent of these had opened spontaneously, and 10 percent of those remaining imperforate had an associated dacryocystitis. Thus, in their study, 4 percent of children with lacrimal obstruction at birth developed dacryocystitis. Since there is no general agreement about the percentage that open spontaneously, there are inevitable differences of opinion as to how early one should intervene with probing. Since not all infants exhibiting a wet eye have some form of congenital dacryostenosis, such infants should have the benefit of careful examination and a *short* period of observation. However, the practice of temporizing until the age of 6 to 12 months is not recommended, since the result may be a dacryocystitis which ultimately will require a major surgical procedure rather than a simple probing. If a period of observation and conservative treatment for 1 month does not result in relief of the tearing problem, irrigation/probing is recommended.

Operative Problems

Laceration of the lacrimal punctum is an avoidable complication. Before the age of 4 months, it may be possible to perform irrigation and probing without general anesthesia (Fig. 19-1). After that age, general anesthesia should be employed to avoid such a complication.

The current literature provides evidence that the upper punctum and canaliculus are functionally as important as the lower. However, clinically, it is our experience that damage to the lower punctum is more likely to result in persisting epiphora, and manipulations should be directed to the upper punctum.

In suspected dacryostenosis, irrigation should be attempted before using a lacrimal probe. If there is an obstruction at the sac-duct junction or below, reflux of irrigating solution through the lower punctum will provide adequate evidence of the integrity of the lower canaliculus. Furthermore, if distention of the lacrimal sac can be palpated during pulsed irrigation through the upper punctum, additional evidence is provided that the common canaliculus and internal punctum are intact. If preliminary irrigation can be accomplished successfully, probing can be avoided.

In addition to damage that may result from unexpected movements of the head, the punctum can be torn if it is dilated too rapidly or if the punctum dilator is tapered too bluntly. If the upper punctum is lacerated during lacrimal probing, no immediate repair effort is necessary. Epiphora is unlikely to result. If a lower punctum is involved and the tear extends more than 1 mm, the edges can be freshened and the laceration can be closed using 10-0 sutures over an indwelling obturator of small caliber. Such a repair is, of course, performed under the surgical microscope.

Bleeding from the punctum usually suggests iatrogenic damage to the canalicular or lacrimal mucosa. In the vast majority of successful probings, no such bleeding is encountered. No immediate manipulations to control this bleeding are necessary, since it invariably ceases within a few minutes. However, since the bleeding is an indication of mucosal trauma, there may be later cicatricial changes, and the infant should be kept under continuing observation for an extended period of time to be certain the system remains functional.

Subcutaneous infiltration of irrigating solution is

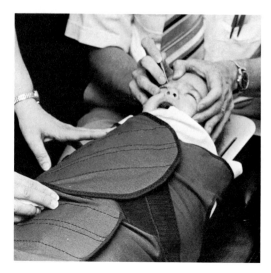

Figure 19-1. Papoose board provides head and body restraints for immobilization of infants.

also an indication of trauma to the lacrimal mucosa. This complication results from perforation of the canalicular mucosa or the common canaliculus. Although aqueous irrigating solutions are absorbed rather rapidly from the subcutaneous tissues, such manipulative trauma can result in canalicular stenosis. Therefore, an extended period of observation is indicated.

Pericystic cellulitis may occur as a complication of lacrimal probing if the manipulations are performed shortly after an exacerbation of dacryocystitis. If there are indications of recent, acute dacryocystitis, irrigation and probing should be delayed until the acute episode has subsided. Antibiotics should be used before undertaking the procedure.

Aspiration of the irrigating solution is a readily avoidable complication. This problem is uncommon if small amounts of irrigating solution are employed. The irrigant should be marked with fluorescein or another dye and recovered by inserting a small suction tube in the nose during irrigation.

Finally, the most annoying complication (for the surgeon) is to perform an uneventful probing and then be *unable to confirm the patency by irrigation*. At times, the probe may come to rest in the inferior meatus submucosally. If the probe cannot be visualized in the meatus using a nasal speculum, and if metal-on-metal contact cannot be demonstrated by passing a fine periosteal elevator into the vault of the meatus, the probe should be withdrawn and passed again after shrinking the nasal mucosa or out-fracturing the inferior turbinate.

Early Postoperative Complications

Following probing, the infant's parents may report the complications of bleeding or subcutaneous infiltration. A more disturbing postmanipulative complication is the presence of an acute exacerbation of dacryocystitis or of pericystic cellulitis. These problems are managed with appropriate antibiotic therapy.

Late Postoperative Complications

Persisting epiphora, after probing, is the most frequent problem encountered. Although lacrimal probing is a highly successful procedure, providing a cure in more than 90 percent of cases, there will be instances in which the surgeon feels that the probing was successful but the epiphora persists. A second probing will result in a cure in the majority of these patients. However, repeated probings increase the risks of mucosal damage and further stenosis. Therefore, since lacrimal probing is a blind procedure, the persistence of symptoms after two such efforts indicates the necessity for dacryocystography in order to visualize the site and character of the blockage. Based on this direct information, rather than the information of repeated failures, appropriate surgical intervention can be planned. If the dacryocystograms reveal an obstruction *without* associated dilation of the lacrimal sac, many surgeons will insert a silicone tube as a stent (Chapter 10) to maintain a patent outflow system. If this device is successful, a dacryocystorhinostomy can be avoided.

Stenosis of the punctum, resulting from earlier manipulations, may explain continuing epiphora after an apparently successful probing. This is an unlikely complication of the probing-irrigation procedure when performed through the upper punctum and canaliculus.

Chronic, persisting dacryocystitis is the ultimate fate of unsuccessful probing in congenital dacryostenosis. It is an unfortunate fact that a small percentage of lacrimal probings do not succeed. When epiphora is the only ongoing manifestation, the surgeon may delay definitive surgery. However, if chronic infection is present, the surgeon should provide relief by dac-

ryocystorhinostomy at the earliest practical time.

OCCLUSION OF CANALICULUS

Interruption of the outflow of tears resulting from disease or trauma to the canaliculus (particularly, the lower canaliculus) offers few diagnostic difficulties to the surgeon. Patency of the canaliculus may be restored if the problem is limited in its linear extent. A transection of the canaliculus is more readily repaired than is a 4 or 5 mm shelving laceration. When the stenosis is the result of infection or allergy, the only practical method of determining the extent of the involvement is to attempt to penetrate it. With this manipulation, a break in the mucosa is inevitable, and such complications as bleeding and subcutaneous infiltration of the irrigating solution are not uncommon.

If communication between the punctum and the lacrimal sac cannot be established with a sharp probe, silicone canalicular tubes or other obturators are unlikely to effect a permanently patent canalicular passage. Some substitution procedure, such as conjunctivodacryocystorhinostomy, will be necessary. However, if communication can be established by the use of obturators, that is the preferred method. Some form of obturator—silicone tubing or stainless steel canalicular rod—must be left in place for an extended period of time. In a clean, well-apposed laceration, the canaliculus may remain patent if the obturator is removed within a period of 2 months or less. If the stenosis is the result of more extensive trauma or of disease, a much longer time is necessary before the obturator is removed.

With prolonged use of stents such as silicone tubing, the chief problem is infection, although this is an infrequent complication. It is necessary to remove the tubing, treat the infection, and reinsert an alternative type of obturator.

INTERNAL PUNCTUM

The management of occlusion of the common canaliculus or internal punctum has become increasingly successful in the past two decades, largely as the result of the availability of silicone tubing for use as a stent to maintain patency. The soft, pliable, atraumatic quality of silicone enables the surgeon to leave this stent for extended periods of time. The insertion of such tubes has been simplified by commercially available probes with swaged-on silicone tubing. Unfortunately, as is the case with all new therapeutic devices, the indiscriminate use or use without rational diagnostic basis of the silicone tubes results in some failures and disappointments for the surgeon. However, when these intubation techniques are used for the internal punctum or common canaliculus, as originally described by Werb[3] and by Quickert and Dryden,[4] they are instrumental in restoring outflow function without the need for dacryorhinostomy surgical procedures.

The diagnosis of common canaliculus or internal punctum stenosis is made in three ways:

1. By irrigating through one punctum and observing reflux through the opposite, without irrigant entering the nose
2. By probing and finding that the probe does not enter the lacrimal sac but comes to a soft stop
3. By using dacryocystography to visualize the canaliculi and nothing further.

None of these techniques provides information regarding the state of the lacrimal sac or nasolacrimal duct beyond the closed internal punctum.

In the operative technique, the occlusion is penetrated by a sharp, stainless steel probe, Veirs trocar, or other sharp instrument introduced along the canaliculus. The penetrated closure is then dilated gently, and the silicone tube is introduced through both puncta and canaliculi, past the stenotic site, and into the inferior meatus of the nose by way of the nasolacrimal duct.

Operative Complications

Laceration of the Lacrimal Punctum. There is always a risk of lacerating the puncta when probes must be used of sufficient size to dilate the internal punctal stricture or when the more rigid stainless steel probes are employed. This problem can be minimized by slow, careful punctum dilation.

Misdirection of the Probes. If the occlusion of the common canaliculus or the internal punctum is quite dense, it is possible that the effort to penetrate the obstruction can create a false passage. Apart from the fact that the sac may be damaged in this manner, it may not be possible to pass the silicone tubing through the false passage.

A second complication is the creation of a false passage along the nasolacrimal duct. Because of the increased rigidity of the probes in some of the available intubation sets, problems may be encountered along the nasolacrimal duct, and the probe may emerge in the middle meatus or through the inferior turbinate. This problem can be avoided by careful inspection of the nasal structures and adequate shrinking of the nasal mucosa.

Intraoperative Bleeding. With the blind penetration of a stenotic area, there may be associated bleeding from the punctum or from the nose. This will present no great problem if it stops spontaneously, since the indwelling tube will maintain patency.

Postoperative Complications

Corneal Touch. Since the purpose of the indwelling tube is to maintain an opening, it follows that the larger the silicone tube, the larger the opening. However, the size of the tube is limited by the size of the dilated punctum. Even more important, when the tube is too large in diameter (or if the thickness of the walls of the tube is too great), the loop of tubing between the puncta will migrate out with movements of the eye. This larger loop will come in contact with the cornea when the eye is adducted, and it may produce erosion of the cornea and nasal bulbar conjuctiva. The loop can be repositioned by pushing it back in place and by pulling down on the nasal ends. If it tends to migrate upward again, it will be necessary to suture the nasal end of the tube to the ala nasi or to fasten a suture to the nasal end of the tube and tape this suture to the face at the nasolabial fold. In the absence of complications, it is neither necessary nor desirable to suture the nasal end of the tube to the nose.

Loss of the Nasal End of the Tube. The lower ends of the silicone tube are tied or sutured together and cut off flush with the external nares. In this fashion, it is an easy matter to locate the tube for removal. However, occasionally, the nasal end cannot be found. It may have fallen back posteriorly, in which case it can often be brought forward by having the patient blow his nose gently or by shrinking the nasal mucosa well and grasping the tube with a bayonet forceps. Less frequently, the tube will migrate up into the vault of the inferior meatus or even into the lower end of the nasolacrimal duct. The lower end of the tube can be replaced into the inferior meatus by introducing a slender probe into the tube at the canaliculus and moving the probe downward through the nasolacrimal duct.

Late Postoperative Complications

Infection. It is apparent that the indwelling obturator increases the possibility for a retrograde infection by way of the nasolacrimal duct. The surprising thing is that this is an infrequent occurrence. When the usual signs of infection are present, appropriate antibacterial drops and systemic antibiotics are indicated. Most often, the tube must be removed but can be reinserted later when the infection subsides.

Granulomas. Since canalicular tubes are usually removed after 3 weeks to 3 months, mucosal reaction to the silicone is uncommon. However, occasionally, a granuloma will be found at the punctum or even in the inferior meatus, and this is an indication for removal of the tube. Small granulomas can be excised, and topical corticosteroids will abort the mucosal reaction.

Late Closure of the Internal Punctum. The late closure of the stricture site, with recurrence of epiphora, suggests that the obturator tube was removed prematurely—no matter how long it had been left in place. It is not difficult to reinsert the tube, leaving it in place for a substantially longer period on the second attempt.

CONJUNCTIVO-DACRYOCYSTORHINOSTOMY

If lacrimal outflow cannot be restored using the punctum-canaliculus route, the alternate pathway for egress of tears is the conjunctivodacryo-cystorhinostomy. The essential requirement of this form of anastomosis is that the passage be maintained by some form of obturator, such as the Pyrex glass tube of Jones or the molded silicone tube of Reinecke.

As in all phases of lacrimal surgery, the best means of avoiding complications is adequate knowledge of the anatomy and physiology of the surgical field. The surgical niceties of this by-pass procedure are more easily seen than described, and even if the surgeon is well versed in the technique of dacryocystorhinostomy, he will benefit by observing this bypass procedure before trying his hand at it.

Operative Complications

Operative complications include those that are *usual for dacryocystorhinostomy.* In addition, however, there are two potential problems encountered in the conjunctivodacryocystorhinostomy procedure.

Incorrect Placement of the Osteotomy. In the usual dacryocystorhinostomy, the osteotomy is quite large and placed as far inferiorly as is compatible with careful surgical anastomosis. However, in conjunctivodacryocystorhinostomy, the emphasis on a large opening is less important than the location of the opening. It is not necessary to make this opening as low as possible. On the contrary, it should be centered not more than 4 mm lower than the lower border of the medial canthal tendon. Otherwise, the tube may be angled sharply downward rather than directly nasally. This could result in the funnel-shaped opening of the tube being tilted too far upward and not conducting tears freely.

Incorrect Placement of the Tube. Inadequate tear flow may also result from incorrect placement of the tube. In order that the mouth of the tube be positioned properly, an adequate portion of the caruncle should be resected. Sometimes, removal of the entire caruncle results in the tube slipping too deeply into the recess at the nasal canthus. The entry should be placed 2 mm posteriorly to the mucocutaneous junction at the nasal canthus. Removal of the anterior two thirds of the caruncle will usually permit the mouth of the tube to be seated properly. If insufficient caruncular tissue is removed, the mouth of the tube will sit too far away from the tear lake and will not function effectively for tear outflow. It is helpful to suture the mouth of the tube in its proper position for the first few weeks (Fig. 19-2).

When a scissors or small, curved hemostat is used to enlarge the passageway sufficiently to admit the obturator tube, there is a risk that the conjuctival orifice will be enlarged inferiorly and the tube will become seated so low that it rides on, or displaces, the lower lid margin. At times, it may even be covered entirely by the lower lid margin. This problem can be corrected by slitting the conjunctival opening upward with a cataract knife for the desired distance and then suturing the open lower end so that the tube is displaced upward and then anchored in its proper position. The reverse procedure can be performed when the mouth of the tube is seated too high. However, that is rarely a problem. The mouth of the tube may protrude

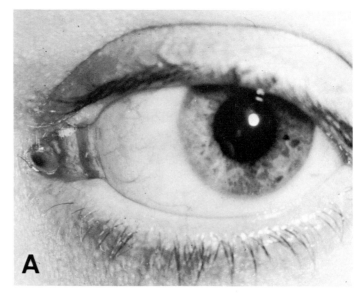

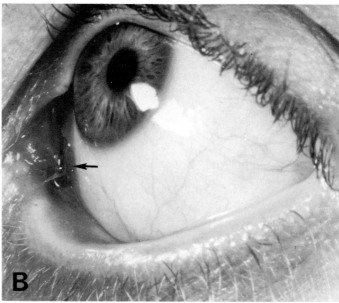

Figure 19-2. A. Incorrect position of Jones tube. The opening of the tube sits above the canthal tissues, out of the tear lake. **B.** Jones tube placed too far posteriorly.

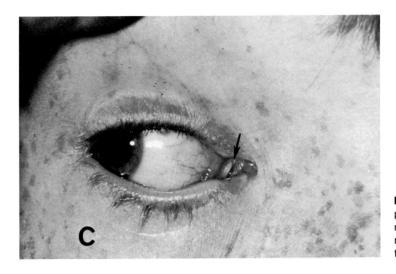

Figure 19-2. *Cont.* **C.** Correct position of Jones tube. The mouth of the tube sits in the nasal angle in contact with the tear lake.

from the nasal angle so that there is corneal touch with the eye in adduction. This complication will occur if the tube is too long, touching the nasal septum or middle turbinate, or if it is too short, slipping out of the nasal cavity through the osteotomy with eye movements. This problem is resolved by exchanging the tube for one of proper length.

If a silicone obturator tube (Reinecke) is employed, an improper placement of this tube may also negate an otherwise successful procedure. If the tube is placed too low at the nasal angle, the thin funnel mouth may be compressed by the lower lid. The lip of the silicone tube can be trimmed with scissors to enable it to conform adequately to its position in the nasal angle. However, unless this modification is performed carefully, sharp, cut edges of the silicone may impact on the conjunctiva and produce a local inflammatory reaction.

Early Postoperative Complications

Pyrex glass tubes may be lost early in the postoperative period by expulsion when sneezing or coughing. The patient must be instructed to immobilize the tube by applying light pressure over the closed lids at such times.

Late Postoperative Complications

Weil has reported on 178 Jones tube operations.[5] Among the late complications were 23 patients (13 percent) with granulomas, 20 (11 percent) with expulsion of the tube, and 17 (9.5 percent) in whom the tube was lost at the nasal

angle. There were also infrequent complications of chronic purulent discharge and breakage of the glass tube.

In the later postoperative period, the glass tube may be lost by sliding into the nasal cavity. When this occurs, the tube should be replaced promptly, using a tube with a larger collar, and it should be sutured into position for a period of several weeks. If the tube comes out repeatedly, after a year or more there may be sufficient relaxation of tissues in the surgical field so that the tube may be omitted entirely for a trial period.

Occasionally, the tube will migrate just enough to become covered partially or completely by conjunctiva. A slender punctum dilator is placed against the nasal end of the tube, gently forcing the tube upward into the nasal angle. When the mouth of the tube tents the conjunctiva, a small incision may be made to expose the tube. The collar should then be sutured so that it remains in fixed position until the tissues are stabilized around it. When the funnel of a silicone tube becomes buried, the same maneuver may be attempted, but it is less likely to be successful. The soft tube should then be grasped intranasally and removed from below. It may be replaced after incising the conjunctiva at the nasal canthus, or, alternatively, a glass tube may be substituted.

Clogging of the Tube. The most frequent complication of conjunctivodacryocystorhinostomy is clogging of the tube. Each patient is taught a daily routine of instilling an irrigating solution into the conjunctival sac and aspirating it into the nose, holding the nares closed. In addition, mucolytic drops may be employed. Despite these cleansing procedures, both types of tubes may become occluded with mucus in time. The mucus can be cleansed from the nasal end of the tube under direct visualization and then flushed out vigorously. However, it is best to remove the tube for thorough cleaning from time to time. The glass tubes develop scale on the surface, and this is removed by scrubbing the tube and sterilizing it before reinserting it. The interval of time varies from every 3 months to every year or longer.

Infection. Less commonly, infections occur within the anastomotic passage, and granulomas may develop (Fig. 19-3). Purulent drainage from the conjunctival orifice with either type of tube requires that the tube be removed and not reinserted until the infection has been eliminated. Bleeding at the orifice suggests a granulomatous reaction. The tube should be removed, the granuloma should be curetted or excised, and a steroid-antibiotic combination should be employed until the area is entirely quiet before resuming the tube. In general, a granuloma resulting from a silicone tube is an indication for changing to a Pyrex glass tube.

Corneal Ulcers. Corneal ulcers in association with these obturator tubes are uncommon. When they do occur and contact with the tube can be demonstrated in the inferior nasal quadrant of the cornea, the ulcer should be treated and the tube changed or repositioned or both.

Failure of the Operation
The most frustrating complication of conjunctivodacryocystorhinostomy is failure of the operation by closure of the anastomosis after removal of the tube. If the operation has succeeded and the patient obtains adequate tear flow through the glass or silicone tube for a few years, it is tempting to remove the tube and thereby eliminate the ongoing care required for all these operations. If the tear flow is compromised after removing the tube, the opening must be reestablished, using a sharp probe to identify the position of the osteotomy, then a cataract knife to reform the passage. The tube is then reinserted and remains permanently.

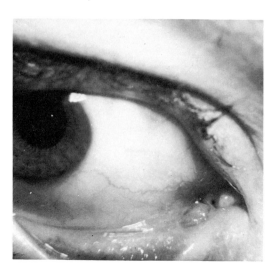

Figure 19-3. Granuloma at site of Jones tube (removed).

DACRYOCYSTORHINOSTOMY

The major complication of dacryocystorhinostomy is *failure.* Most disturbing is a poor functional result following a technically perfect operative procedure. The most frequent cause of this misfortune is failure to identify a problem in the upper portion of the excretory system. Problems involving the eyelid margins, stenosis of the lacrimal punctum or canaliculus, or diminished tonus of the orbicularis muscle—all may be responsible for persisting epiphora following dacryocystorhinostomy.

Such disturbing outcomes can be avoided if a careful external examination is performed and a careful search is made for possible causes of lacrimal hypersecretion. In addition, such intranasal problems as allergies, chronic inflammation, polyposis, and such structural abnormalities as deviated septum may spell the downfall of a routine dacryocystorhinostomy. Here again, failure may be avoided by careful preoperative examination.

Operative Complications
Local anesthesia avoids the risks and problems attendant on inhalation anesthesia and permits better hemostasis. Therefore, general anesthesia is reserved for children and the occasional overly apprehensive patient. The problem of having the operation last longer than the anes-

thesia may be resolved by employing one of the longer-acting anesthetic agents. At present, we employ bupivacaine hydrochloride (0.75 percent), combined with an equal volume of mepivacaine hydrochloride (2 percent), to which is added hyaluronidase (150 units for each 20 ml of the anesthetic mixture.) Infratrochlear and infraorbital nerve blocks provide adequate anesthesia for the surgery. During the administration of the infratrochlear block, retrobulbar hemorrhage is possible because of the proximity of the branches of the ophthalmic vessels. Such retrobulbar hemorrhages occur in 1 to 2 percent of anesthesias. If, after a short interval, there does not appear to be excessive intraorbital pressure, the operation may proceed. Here, the general surgical dictum applies: when in doubt, don't!

Intranasal anesthesia is effected using lidocaine hydrochloride (4 percent) with epinephrine hydrochloride (1:100,000). Alternatively, intranasal cocaine flakes or 10 percent cocaine solution may be employed. As with general anesthesia, those patients receiving local anesthesia should have an intravenous infusion started before the surgery so that emergency medications can be given without delay. Cardiac performance should be monitored.

Placement of the Skin Incision

It is said that successful dacryocystorhinostomy depends on three things—proper placement of the incision, control of bleeding, and a large osteotomy.

The position and length of the skin incision vary with different lacrimal surgeons. However, any incision for this operation should fulfill three basic requirements:

1. It should be so placed as to avoid troublesome bleeding
2. It should avoid damaging the lacrimal sac
3. It should result in a cosmetically satisfactory closure.

Adequate exposure of the lacrimal fossa may require that the anterior leaf of the medial canthal tendon be severed, and this may be done without compromising the final cosmetic or functional outcome of the operation. The skin incision need not be carried above the medial canthal tendon. If it is extended too far su-

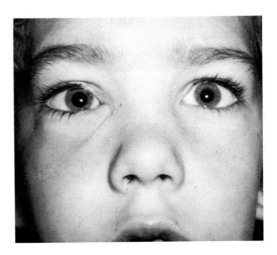

Figure 19-4. Incorrect placement of DCR incision: curvature is too great and extends too far laterally.

periorly, traction lines may result at the upper end of the scar.

Complications resulting from the incision can be avoided if the following principles are adhered to:

1. The incision should be straight rather than curved (Fig. 19-4)
2. The incision should be long enough for good visualization of the operative field
3. The incision should be made at right angles to the skin surface
4. The edges of the incision should not be handled with instruments
5. Caution should be exercised when using a drill or burr so that the skin edges are not burned

Bleeding during dacryocystorhinostomy interferes with good visualization and can lead to surgical errors. Hemorrhage can occur at three stages of the operation. At each stage, bleeding should be avoided if possible, and if it occurs, it should be controlled before proceeding to the next step. The first potential bleeding site is the skin incision and the underlying angular vein. Bleeding vessels should be located and, if they are small, cauterized with the bipolar cautery. Larger vessels should be clamped and either cauterized or suture-ligated.

The second troublesome site of bleeding is the osteotomy. Oozing from small vessels in the

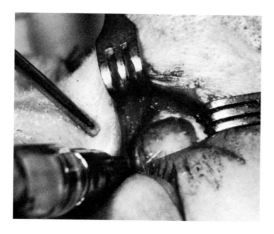

Figure 19-5. Infiltrating the nasal mucosa for hemostasis using a 30-gauge sharp needle.

cut edge of the bony window can be controlled by cautery. Occasionally, a small arterial bleeder will require the use of bone wax and pressure. Such bleeding from the osteotomy is less likely if the opening is kept as low as possible.

The third source of bleeding is the nasal mucosa. When the nasal mucosa is incised, even a modest amount of bleeding may make it difficult or impossible to complete a careful anastomosis. This complication can be minimized if, after completion of the osteotomy, the mucosa is infiltrated with a local anesthetic preparation containing a small amount of epinephrine (Fig. 19-5).

Placement of the osteotomy must be correct in order to achieve a successful dacryocystorhinostomy. It can be made with high-speed lacrimal burrs or drills, with rongeurs, or (rarely) with bone chisels. The bony window should straddle the anterior lacrimal crest, and it should be at least 12 by 15 mm. The proper osteotomy site can be identified by placing a transilluminator in the middle meatus. The light will diffuse through the area of the bone corresponding to the middle meatus, and the osteotomy can be started in that region. If the osteotomy site is properly chosen and the opening is large enough, nasal mucosal flaps may be fashioned without difficulty. Proper appositional requirements must be adhered to in forming the nasal and lacrimal sac flaps. That is, if the surgeon

finds that he has a large anterior flap of lacrimal sac mucosa available, he will match this with a small anterior nasal flap, and the reverse procedure will be followed with the posterior flaps. With careful anastomosis of flaps, it is unnecessary to insert packing or any other form of obturator in order to maintain patency of the anastomosis.

Finally, at the operating table, attention should be paid to careful *wound closure*. Small bleeders that persist after removal of the retractors should be controlled. The muscle and skin should be closed in separate layers.

Early Postoperative Complications

Nasal Bleeding. The most frequent complication encountered after the patient leaves the operating suite is nasal bleeding. Meticulous control of bleeders at surgery should avoid this problem. Unfortunately, such meticulous control is not always possible, especially in the elderly, the hypertensive, or the diabetic patient. Usually, such bleeding stops spontaneously within the first few hours. If it is mild, no treatment is required. If it is brisk or if it does not abate within 24 hours, the nose should be packed, introducing the pack well into the middle meatus. At times, a postnasal pack will be required. If, with this type of pressure, the bleeding is still not controlled, the anterior ethmoidal artery may be exposed in the nasal wall of the orbit and clipped. This seemingly dramatic method of controlling postoperative bleeding may be the only feasible method of managing intractable hemorrhage. If postoperative bleeding dissects between the anastomosis and the skin, the resulting hematoma will eventually tamponade the bleeding. The hematoma may then be evacuated through the skin incision. Such bleeding rarely compromises the surgical anastomosis. Some surgeons irrigate the surgical passage on the second or third postoperative day in order to remove any residual clots. This maneuver is usually unnecessary but is reassuring to patient and surgeon alike.

Wound Infection. This occurs infrequently but may be found in the early postoperative period. Since the surgical field, in this operation, is invariably contaminated, it is surprising that wound infections are rather uncommon. When they do occur, they usually involve the superficial layers of the wound closure. The absence of infection in the region of the mucosal anastomosis may be explained by the resumption of normal tear flow. If the patient has had a recent exacerbation of dacryocystitis, the preoperative use of antibiotics may help to avoid wound infections. The fewer the number of buried sutures employed in wound closure, the less likely will be this complication.

Late Postoperative Complications

Wound granulomas may form around buried sutures. If subcutaneous nodules persist after the early postoperative period (3 to 6 weeks), a repository corticosteroid may be injected at these sites to hasten their resolution. Generally, they will disappear in time.

A cosmetically unsatisfactory scar is any dacryocystorhinostomy scar that is visible. Of course, a visible scar may be unavoidable in some cases because of contamination of the site. However, incorrect placement of the incision will account for contraction of the scar, forming a tension band (bowstringing). Such bowstringing will result in a pseudoepicanthus (Fig. 17-3). There are several causes for bowstringing, including extending the incision above the medial canthal ligament, using a curvilinear rather than a straight incision, and placing the incision too close to the nasal angle. Those who prefer the one-step, through-and-through incision should allow a distance of no less than 3 to 4 mm from the angle.

If a tight scar with a thickened ridge and/or bowstringing should occur, massage and subcutaneous corticosteroid injections may be used. If the result is still unsatisfactory after 6 months or more, a Z-plasty revision, transposing skin flaps, will usually improve cosmesis. In some cases, it may be necessary to revise the scar by excision and skin grafting.

Trauma to the common canaliculus and internal punctum may occur during exploration of the sac, probing to verify the opening into the sac, or improper mucosal anastomosis. It is possible for traction on the sac, when suturing flaps, to cause closure of an otherwise normal internal punctum.

If there is a question as to the patency of the internal punctum during the operation, a silicone canalicular tube should be inserted to maintain patency. This tube should be no larger than 1 mm in outside diameter. After closure of the posterior mucosal flaps, each end of the tube is passed through one canaliculus, so that a short loop is formed between the two puncta. The two ends of the tube pass, together, through the internal punctum and are brought through the osteotomy into the nose, where they are fastened together. The anterior mucosal flaps are then closed, and the dacryocystorhinostomy is completed. After 3 to 6 weeks, the tube is cut between the puncta and drawn out through the nose.

Closure of the surgical anastomosis is the most common cause of failure of a dacryocystorhinostomy. When tearing recurs following the surgery, if the communication has closed on the osteotomy, the sac will distend on attempted irrigation, and probing will meet solid resistance at the osteotomy. These failures may be caused by several factors, including improper placement of the osteotomy—usually too far anterior, too small an osteotomy, a poor surgical anastomosis, residual bleeding, and pooling of mucopus in a residual dependent cul de sac.

There are three methods of managing a failed dacryocystorhinostomy resulting from closure of the anastomosis. Some failures can be converted into successes by introducing a sharp probe through the osteotomy site and dissecting away the barrier of scar tissue, intranasally, around the probe. A second method employs canalicular intubation after the method of Werb or Quickert. This may be combined with intranasal removal of scar tissue. The tube should remain in place for at least 3 months. Finally, in cases of closure at the osteotomy site, reoperation may be required. This somewhat tedious procedure requires that the new incision be dissected in layers, controlling bleeding carefully at each step, and that one edge of the existing osteotomy be identified and freed of periosteum. Using this as a starting point, the entire perimeter of the bony opening is dissected free, the scar tissue barrier is dissected away with a razor blade knife, and the osteotomy is enlarged slightly to provide fresh mucosal edges. A new anastomosis can then be made in the same fashion as the original dacryocystorhinostomy, and Silastic canalicular intubation can be used to maintain the new opening. These dissections are carried out with the surgical microscope.

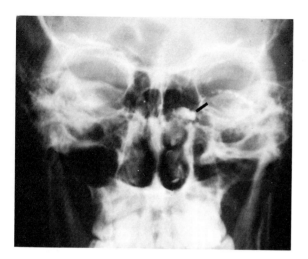

Figure 19-6. A. Failed DCR: the anastamosis is patent, but this 0 minute dacryocystogram shows a lateral diverticulum of the lacrimal sac.

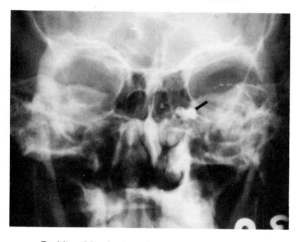

B. After 30 minutes, the diverticulum remains.

More disturbing than a complete scarring over of the original anastomosis is *functional block,* the persistence of epiphora in a patent system following a technically correct operation. If this complication occurs, a complete diagnostic survey should be undertaken, just as would be the case in a new lacrimal patient. The cause may be found, by means of Jones

testing, in some portion of the upper lacrimal system. If no obvious damage to the punctum or canaliculus is found, dacryocystography should be employed in every case. A residual cul de sac, a large flaccid remaining sac, or a previously unrecognized diverticulum (Fig. 19-6) may be at fault. The impaired functional state is identified by failure of the system to empty itself of the radiographic contrast agent. Visualizing the abnormality radiographically provides a basis for corrective surgery. If the remaining lacrimal sac is not unusual in size or shape, as seen in the dacryocystogram, it is wise to delay reoperation for 6 to 12 months, since some patients will regain adequate outflow function after that period of time.

Lacrimal surgery is not difficult from the standpoint of techniques. Complications may be avoided by careful preoperative diagnostic studies so that the therapeutic approach is based on a proper understanding of the site and nature of the pathology. Success rates are high, and complications are infrequent. When complications do occur, most failures can be converted into successes by intervention based on careful diagnostic evaluation.

REFERENCES

1. Cassady JV: Developmental anatomy of nasocrimal duct. Arch Ophthalmol 47:141, 1952
2. Korchmaros I, Szalay E, Fodor M Jablonszky E: Spontaneous opening rate of congenitally blocked nasolacrimal ducts. In Yamaguchi M, (ed): Recent Advances on the Lacrimal System, Tokyo, Asahi, 1978, pp 30–35
3. Werb A: Surgical technique. In Veirs ER: The Lacrimal System, Proceedings of the First International Symposium. St. Louis, Mosby, 1971, pp 145–149
4. Quickert M, Dryden R: Probes for intubation in lacrimal drainage. Trans Am Acad Ophthalmol Otolaryngol 74:431, 1970
5. Weil B: The Lester Jones operation: Conjunctivo-dacryocystorhinostomy with permanent prostheses. In Yamaguchi M, (ed): Recent Advances on the Lacrimal System. Tokyo, Asahi, 1978, pp 71–77

20

TRAUMA

BERNARDO WEIL

The ophthalmologist, by training as well as predilection, is inclined more toward surgical than medical solutions to the problems encountered in daily practice. This instant therapeutic device is not always feasible, and, in fact, the vast majority of the ophthalmologist's patients will be spared the terrors of the operating room. However, there is a significant group of lacrimal problems for which the only recourse is surgery, and prominent among these are the traumas involving the ocular adnexae.

THE LACRIMAL GLAND

Prolapse or avulsion of the lacrimal gland is a rare form of injury. It is usally the result of a penetrating wound in the superior temporal orbit. We have observed such injuries in children, where the orbit was entered by a sharp wood or metal object.

The treatment of such injuries requires three essentials. First, antibiotics are employed as prophylaxis against infection, or appropriate treatment is used if infection is already present.

Second, investigation for and removal of any foreign body in the orbit require the use of orbital x-rays, ultrasonography, and CT scanning to identify and localize the foreign body. Third, if the lacrimal gland is prolapsed, it must be repositioned surgically. If the prolapse of the lacrimal gland is not severe and if it does not pose a cosmetic problem, it need not be disturbed. However, if the palpebral lobe of the gland is visible in the lid aperture or if there is a visible tumefaction in the temporal third of the upper lid with or without associated ptosis, the gland should be repositioned. Such an operation is performed under either general or local anesthesia.

EYELIDS

When the eyelid margin has been disturbed by trauma, disease, or surgery, the accurate reapproximation of the lid margin is essential to avoid a tearing problem. A notch remaining in the lid margin will mean a small area of cornea that will be dry because of failure of complete apposition of the lids during blinking. The result ultimately will be reflex tearing. In addition, such notches may harbor misdirected cilia,

Figures 20-1, 20-2, 20-4, 20-5, 20-7, and 20-8 appear on Color Plate III at the end of this chapter.

which will be a further source of tearing. Whatever the cause, relief of the tearing will require that the lid margin be revised to eliminate the notch.

Scarring secondary to minor lower lid injury may cause ectropion of the punctum (Fig. 20-1, Color Plate III), and normal apposition of punctum to globe must be restored (Chapter 18). When injury to the eyelid involves loss of significant amounts of skin and subcutaneous tissue, deformity of the lid margins may result in epiphora (Fig. 20-2, Color Plate III). Skin grafting or other restorative procedures should be directed at reestablishing normal lid margin contour and normal contact with the globe, insofar as possible. If orbicularis muscle tone is lost in lid trauma, the lacrimal pump will be compromised, and anatomic restoration of the lid margin will not be sufficient to eliminate tearing. A Jones tube operation will be necessary, after the appropriate restorative surgery has been performed on the lids.

PUNCTUM

Although the punctum may suffer damage as part of extensive eyelid trauma, isolated injury to the punctum is rare. The usual cause is an iatrogenic injury and results from being overzealous in dilating the punctum. If the punctum is dilated too rapidly or too vigorously or if the dilator is tapered too bluntly, the result will be fine radial tears at the punctal orifice. A small amount of bleeding can occur, but, with or without the bleeding, varying degrees of stenosis may result. Attempts to treat punctal stenosis by repeated dilation can, therefore, lead to further stenosis. Ultimately, the problem of the stenosis will have to be resolved with a three-snip or punch punctum operation. Such operations represent a controlled form of punctal trauma in which tear elimination is preserved by placing the opening in contact with the tear lake.

When the nasal canthus has been subjected to irradiation, some degree of stenosis of the canaliculus can occur despite the best efforts of the radiologist. When dilation is used to identify or treat such canalicular stenosis, there is increased risk of damage to the punctum. Because of the loss of elasticity and the friable quality of tissues, the punctum and canaliculus

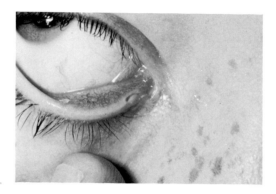

Figure 20-3. Laceration of canaliculus, lower lid (iatrogenic), with epiphora necessitating Jones tube conjunctivodacryocystorhinostomy.

are easily "cheese-wired," slit along the eyelid margin (Fig. 20-3).

Every ophthalmologist has encountered the infant or child with an elongated punctum—slit as much as 3 or 4 mm along the lid margin. The inclination to view this as a congenital oddity is rapidly dissipated when the parent reports that the child was treated for a tearing problem in infancy. If there is a significant amount of epiphora associated with such slitting of the punctum, the problem can be remedied by freshening the edges and approximating the canaliculus with 10-0 interrupted, nonabsorbable sutures. This procedure is performed under microscopic control, and a Silastic tube or other form of stent is allowed to remain in place for 3 to 6 weeks.

CANALICULUS

The more frequently encountered forms of trauma to the canaliculus will be considered separately.

1. Lacerations in the region of the nasal canthus, involving the canaliculus
2. Thermal, chemical, and radiation trauma
3. Iatrogenic trauma
4. Late sequelae of trauma[1]

Laceration of the Inner Canthus
Penetrating wounds or lacerations directly into the lacrimal sac are uncommon, but they usually result in cicatricial occlusion of the sac

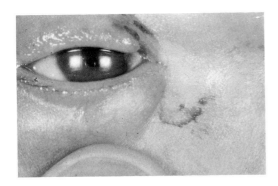

Figure 20-6. Laceration through lower lid margin and canaliculus.

and/or duct or external fistulization (Figs. 20-4 and 20-5, Color Plate III). Lacerations that involve the lower canaliculus are not uncommon. Although most of them occur within 1 to 4 mm from the lacrimal punctum, the traumatic force may not act directly over the site of the laceration. The most common mechanism is the hooking force exerted over the lower eyelid by a finger (as, for example, during a quarrel), by a branch of a tree, or by a dog bite. This locus resistentia minoris lies between the nasal end of the tarsus and the attachment of the medial canthal tendon. When sudden traction is exerted on the lid, it is more likely to give way at this point than at any other site (Fig. 20-6, Color Plate III).

When the canaliculus is transected more or less perpendicular to the axis, and particularly when it is near the punctum, repair of the laceration and restoration of function are not difficult. However, the seriousness of the wound increases if it is irregular, jagged, shelving, or near the common canaliculus (Fig. 20-7, Color Plate III).

The reparative procedure is not an emergency one. Surgical reconstruction should not be accomplished immediately unless both ends of the severed canaliculus are clearly visible. Fresh lacerations are often contaminated with blood or foreign material, and are edematous, and the ends are difficult if not impossible to visualize. A delay of 12 to 24 hours will not be harmful. As the edema subsides and tissues retract, the cut ends of the canaliculus will be exposed and simplify the repair. If there is any doubt, it is possible to wait as long as 3 or 4

days. Even if the severed surfaces are involved in adhesions, these are not difficult to separate during the surgical procedure. In some cases, the proximal and distal ends of the severed passage are clearly visible at the outset (Fig. 20-8, Color Plate III). In our experience, in severe lacerations, it is impossible to reconstruct a canaliculus by clean edge-to-edge suturing techniques if more than 8 days have elapsed since the injury.

In direct appositional repair of a severed canaliculus, there are three important surgical considerations to keep in mind.

1. Magnification—using the surgical microscope—is an absolute necessity.
2. Appropriate instrumentation is needed, and the instruments used here are those ordinarily employed in corneal surgery.
3. A stent is necessary in order to protect the integrity of the surgical repair until there is no further danger of stenosis as a result of scarring. After using various materials, we still prefer the Veirs rod. Its 10 mm length permits only the silk to emerge through the punctum and the vertical portion of the canaliculus. Veirs rods are manufactured by Davis and Geck and by Ethicon. The Davis and Geck rods undergo oxidation, and this phenomenon is usually noted by discoloration of the rod about 2 weeks after its insertion. This is not harmful to the healing process. The silk thread that emerges from the punctum is sometimes softened by tissue fluids and has been known to break in attempts to remove a Viers rod. In our view, up to the present time, the Viers rod is the best available element to protect the severed canaliculus. Once the reconstruction is accomplished, the rod must be kept in place for 4 to 6 weeks.

North of the equator, there seems to be a general preference for silicone intubation to provide the necessary stent during the healing. When silicone is used, it is threaded through both the injured and the intact canaliculus and brought through the nasolacrimal duct into the nose (Chapter 14). With silicone intubation the tube remains in place also for 4 to 6 weeks.

General anesthesia is preferred for canalicular repair as it permits comfortable, leisurely inspection of the wound as well as visualization and isolation of the severed ends of the canaliculus. If the nasal end of the severed canaliculus is difficult to identify, as is the case when there is jagged laceration or when the canaliculus has been severed close to the lacrimal sac, various techniques have been employed to identify the end. Techniques depending on such dyes as methylene blue should not be employed. These agents, instilled through the upper canaliculus, are intended to emerge through the cut end of the lower canaliculus, but the dye tends to escape into the nasolacrimal duct even when the sac is compressed and stain all of the surrounding tissues, rendering surgical exploration difficult or even impossible. Furthermore, we do not employ the pigtail probe because it may add to the trauma in the region. One agent that may aid visualization without staining the tissues is boiled milk instilled through the upper canaliculus.

It is important to remember that, in difficult cases, it is always possible to identify the severed end of the canaliculus with an open sky technique. That is, the sac may be opened and the canaliculus catheterized in retrograde fashion.

Once both ends have been visualized, a fixation suture is passed through the nasal cut end in order to retain identification, the Veirs rod is inserted, and the canaliculus is reapposed with three interrupted sutures using 10-0 nylon or other nonabsorbable material. One suture is placed anteriorly, and the others are placed posteriorly and superiorly. If all of the sutures cannot be placed properly, it is preferable that one firm suture be used for apposition rather than three tentative ones. The reconstruction of the eyelid is then completed with deep and superficial closure as needed, and the operation is concluded by fixation of the Veirs rod suture at a point 10 mm inferior and nasal to the lower punctum. In this way, the suture and metallic rod will form an angle of about 45°, and spontaneous extrusion of the rod is difficult. The Veirs rod suture must be left rather loose to avoid any possible eversion of the punctum or even slitting of the punctum and canaliculus from tension on the suture.

The Veirs rod procedure has few complications. Apart from possible extrusion of the rod prematurely, one minor complication is in-

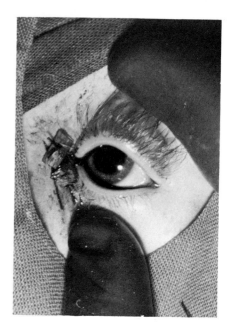

Figure 20-9. Following repair of a laceration through the left lower lid margin and canaliculus, a mattress suture is tied over rubber pads and anchored at nasocanthal tendon to eliminate traction on the wound.

fection in the skin at the site of the suture knot. This can be avoided by using a steroid-antibiotic ointment over the knot three or four times a day during the entire period. If there is spontaneous expulsion of the rod, it is reinserted, and a fixation suture is passed through the entire thickness of the eyelid 3 mm below the lid margin and tied over the nasal edge of the punctum in order to keep the rod from moving.

With the use of Silastic canalicular tube, as is preferred in North America, one end of the tube is threaded through the intact canaliculus and the other end through the severed canaliculus before suturing the cut ends of the severed canaliculus. In either case, a mattress suture should be employed, extending from the temporal aspect of the lid laceration to be anchored at the insertion of the medial canthal tendon. This relieves tension on the wound and on the canalicular closure during the healing period (Fig. 20-9).

Avulsion of the medial canthal tendon may occur as part of more extensive facial trauma (Fig.

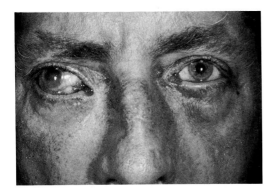

Figure 20-10. Traumatic avulsion of right medial canthal tendon. Note that the right medial palpebral angle is lower than the left, and the right nasocanthal distance is greater then the left.

20-10). In this form of trauma, the lacrimal excretory system is often damaged in the region of the internal punctum or the lacrimal sac itself. If these structures are damaged, a Silastic canalicular stent, fed through both puncta and canaliculi in the usual manner, should be employed. Even with such measures, the disruption of the lacrimal excretory system combined with the extensive damage at the nasal canthus may render the outflow system nonfunctional. With extensive damage in this area, the only recourse may be to permit healing and all of the necessary reconstructive procedures in the region of the nasal canthus and then, finally, to use a Jones tube procedure to effect drainage.

If there is no disturbance to the integrity of the canaliculus and sac in the presence of an avulsion, epiphora will still be present. The medial canthus will be displaced laterally (when compared with the intact side), and the punctum will not be positioned properly in the tear lake. The restoration of normal outflow will then depend upon reattachment of the avulsed medial canthal tendon, and this is accomplished either by direct suturing techniques or by transnasal wiring.

Thermal, Chemical, and Radiation Trauma

Burns at the inner canthus resulting from molten metals and other hot materials may injure or completely destroy the punctum and canaliculus. In such cases, prophylactic intubation is necessary in order to protect the integrity of the excretory system. The same precaution is necessary with chemical burns. If there is any question about possible late cicatricial retraction, the system should be intubated with silicone tubing, as described previously.

When radiotherapy is applied to the nasocanthal region (as for basal cell carcinoma), partial stenosis or complete obstruction of the upper passages is a possible complication. While it is true that proper techniques in radiation therapy should avoid this complication, it is a regrettable fact that the ophthalmologist must deal with the results of such complications, and routine prophylaxis would seem to be the most reasonable course. Silicone intubation should be performed before irradiation therapy as a routine in order to avoid possible late cicatricial stenoses.

Iatrogenic Trauma

Unfortunately, many obstructions of the upper lacrimal pathways have a history of previous instrumentation, either irrigation or probing or both. Without any doubt, these manipulations have been responsible for the lacrimal obstruction in many cases.

Because obstructions of the upper pathways are sometimes very difficult to treat, maximum care must be exerted to avoid such complications. For the lower canaliculus, probes must be blunt and atraumatic in order to avoid damage to the mucosal lining, with subsequent formation of adhesions. In adult patients, we use a very thin catheter in the lower canaliculus to check the permeability and not for the purpose of breaking adhesions, because this type of procedure is useless and generally harmful. Regrettably, it is still practiced all too frequently. In our view, therapeutic probing in adults should be abandoned since it leads to more problems than cures. We reserve therapeutic probing for congenital obstructions of the nasolacrimal duct, and such manipulations, in infants, are performed through the upper canaliculus.

There are other iatrogenic causes for stenosis in the upper passages. These include obstruction produced by surgery of small tumors situated at or near the lacrimal punctum and obstruction following removal of a chalazion near the lacrimal punctum or even following the application of chalazion forceps close to the nasal side of the lacrimal punctum.

Treatment of Late Sequelae of Canalicular Trauma

Many forms of trauma, treated or not, end with complete obstruction of the passages, just as occurs in such inflammatory diseases as herpes simplex. In such cases, the ophthalmologist must have a procedure for restoring lacrimal outflow. Since the upper system is involved, it is obvious that dacryocystorhinostomy does not provide a surgical solution.

For the past 12 years we have been performing the conjunctivodacryocystorhinostomy operation of Lester Jones. In the more than 300 such operations that we have performed, despite some complications, reoperations, reintubations, and despite occasional discomfort for both the patient and the doctor, it has proved to be the most successful surgical procedure available in complete stenosis. The prosthesis employed (the Pyrex tube) is generally considered to be a permanent-type prosthesis since only rarely can tear evacuation take place satisfactorily without the tube in place

To review briefly the indications for conjunctivodacryocystorhinostomy:

1. Trauma to the punctum or canaliculus for which lesser measures have been unsuccessful
2. Closure at the internal punctum or common canaliculus
3. A nonexistent tear sac
4. Repeated failure of a dacryocystorhinostomy, especially where the dacryocystogram shows a small residual lacrimal sac cavity
5. Tumors at the nasocanthal area that require wide extirpation
6. Severe middle facial trauma or surgery in which restoration of canalicular function is not possible
7. A symptomatic functional block following dacryocystorhinostomy
8. Complete orbicularis palsy
9. Extirpation of sac

Our indications for the Pyrex tube operation are quite in accord with those of Lester Jones. We feel that a dacryocystogram is essential in order to establish the precise location and extent of the pathology before undertaking such an operation. Our experience of more than 5,000 such diagnostic procedures has taught us that dacryocystography is the one indispensable diagnostic device. Even in cases of complete obstruction of the upper pathways, the roentgen examination will demonstrate, at the very least, the bony configurations that may assist in the planning of surgery and in avoiding technical difficulties. In some other cases, an apparently closed passageway is found to be open in some fashion that could not be discovered by syringing or probing. It is not uncommon that, in an apparent closure of a common canaliculus, the dacryocystogram reveals that the patient has actually a dilated tear sac with obstruction below the sac.

In conjunctivodacryocystorhinostomy, it is important that the patient be made aware that in about 50 percent of the cases the Pyrex tube must be changed one or more times and that in practically all cases the tube will be worn through the patient's entire life. To balance this, the patient can be assured that the final result will be functionally satisfactory. In 178 Jones operations performed between 1970 and 1978, with an average follow-up time of 28 months, our complete cure rate was 93.5 percent.[2, 3]

Although we do not routinely employ an ENT examination in every case, this is a common practice and strongly urged by colleagues in North America.

If the Pyrex glass tube must be replaced, this can be performed as an office procedure in many cases. However, pain and discomfort on the part of the patient may make this procedure sufficiently unpleasant that it is even necessary to resort to general anesthesia. This is certainly a routine necessity in children. The patient must be warned that all manipulations of the tube must be undertaken by the surgeon. The frequency with which tubes have to be removed for cleansing or to be changed can be reduced by daily sniffing of saline eyedrops through the tube. The normal saline drops are instilled into the conjunctival sac, the patient holds the nostrils closed and sniffs, thus drawing the saline through the tube and tending to keep it free of mucus.

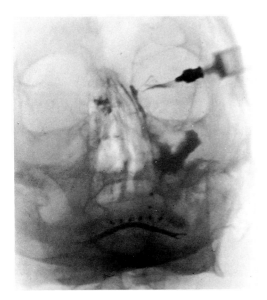

Figure 20-11. Traumatic fistulization of nasolacrimal duct into antrum (dacryocystogram).

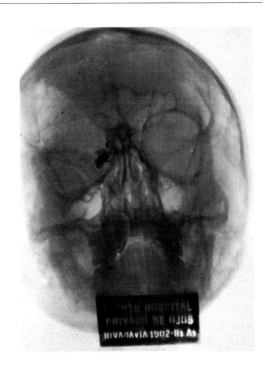

TRAUMA OF THE LOWER LACRIMAL PASSAGES

Interference with tear outflow and an associated dacryocystitis are increasingly common problems caused by automobile accidents. In midfacial trauma, craniofacial disjunction with retroposition of the face will often be accompanied by fractures through the bony nasolacrimal canal. Such displacement of facial bones can be for distances of several centimeters, but only a very small fracture in this area is required to damage the mucosal lining of the nasolacrimal duct and produce subsequent obstruction. Fistulization into the antrum or into the middle meatus of the nose is possible (Fig. 20-11).

Most often, in accidents of this type, there is multiple trauma, and care is generally devoted to more critical areas of injury. As the patient recovers, the epiphora becomes manifest. In some instances, a purulent dacryocystitis will make it impossible for the plastic surgeon to proceed with reconstructive or esthetic procedures because of the risk of infection. It sometimes occurs that because of the greater attention needed for other areas of injury, the lacrimal trauma is overlooked and multiple bone fractures come in contact with the suppurating sac. The end result is an osteomyelitis

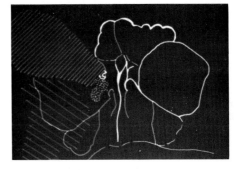

Figure 20-12. Trauma: Frontal defect with obstructive dacryocystitis (dacryocystogram).

(Fig. 20-12). In such extensive facial injuries there is usually bilateral involvement of the nasolacrimal ducts. Dacryocystograms are particularly important in such cases in order to identify the site of obstruction and any possible displacement of the infected lacrimal sac. Corrective surgery, dacryocystorhinostomy, should be performed as soon as possible.

Although the most common facial trauma in automobile accidents is the multiple midfacial fracture complex, it must be borne in mind that possible fronto-ethmoidal meningoceles can also occur as a result of trauma. This possibility can be ruled out readily by the use of the dacryocystogram. If there are lingering doubts, the neurosurgeon should be consulted prior to any proposed lacrimal surgery.

If multiple fractures result in telecanthus, the procedure of choice is some form of transnasal wiring. Since this problem is often combined with obstruction of the upper or lower lacrimal passages, it is our practice to perform the surgery on the lacrimal system at the same time as the transnasal wiring.

REFERENCES

1. Weil BA: Traumatisms of the Upper Lacrimal Ducts. Paper read at the Pan-American Association of Ophthalmology, 1972, Houston
2. Weil BA: Experiencia con la operacion de Lester Jones. Arch Oftal Buenos Aires 50:243, 1975
3. Weil BA: The Lester Jones operation conjunctivo-dacryocysto-rhinostomy with permanent prosthesis. Paper read, 1978, Buenos Aires

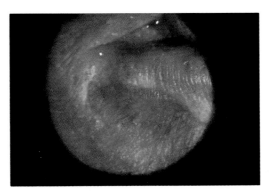

Figure 20-1. Everted punctum, secondary to trauma to lower lid.

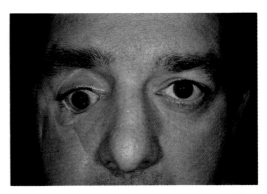

Figure 20-2. Right facial trauma, as a result of an automobile accident. Gross tissue loss involving lower eyelid, cicatricial ectropion with epiphora, and destruction of inferior bony orbital margin and floor of orbit.

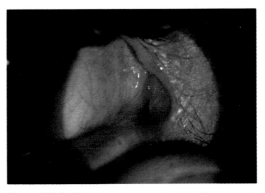

Figure 20-4. Fistulous communication from nasal angle to lacrimal sac, result of trauma.

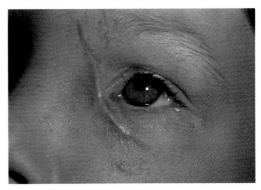

Figure 20-5. Healed laceration, left nasal, extending into lacrimal sac area, with occlusion of common canaliculus.

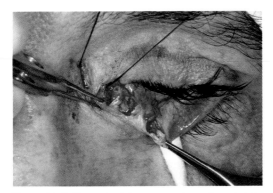

Figure 20-7. Extensive injury at nasal canthus. At left, the cut end of the common canaliculus. At right, the end of the severed lower canaliculus.

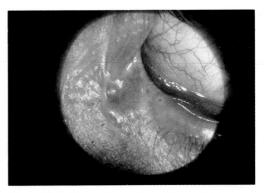

Figure 20-8. Healed laceration of lower lid showing exposed nasal end of the severed canaliculus.

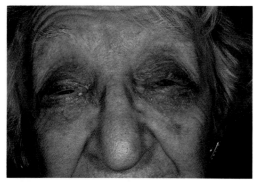

Figure 21-1. Dermatitis medicamentosa (neomycin sensitivity).

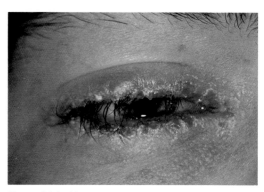

Figure 21-2. Marginal blepharitis, staphylococcal.

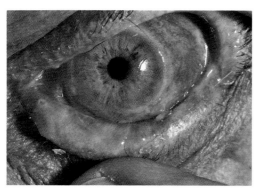

Figure 21-3. Pemphigoid.

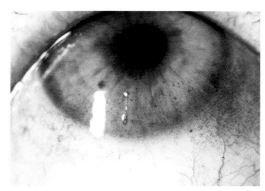

Figure 21-4. Keratitis sicca, in Sjögren's syndrome.

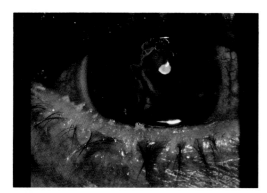

Figure 21-6. Herpes simplex, type I. Geographic corneal ulceration.

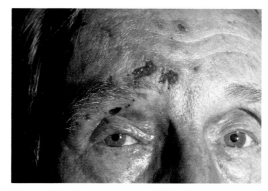

Figure 21-7. Herpes zoster ophthalmicus.

21

SYSTEMIC DISEASE AND THE LACRIMAL SYSTEM

BENJAMIN MILDER

This chapter, which considers the relationship between diseases of the lacrimal system and those of other organ systems, does not pretend to be an encyclopedic exercise in differential diagnosis. Rather, it is intended that lacrimal symptoms be looked at as possible manifestations of systemic disease. Indeed, the lacrimal signs and symptoms may be the earliest indication of a more generalized bodily disorder.

DERMATOLOGIC DISORDERS

Normal tear excretion requires accurate apposition of the eyelid margins and the puncta to the globe. It follows then that all skin diseases that can involve the eyelids may result in epiphora. Atopic dermatitis and all forms of eczematoid involvement of the skin, of whatever etiology—including such entities as psoriasis, seborrhea, and ichthyosis—may involve the eyelids and can induce sufficient retraction of the lid margin to interfere with normal tear outflow (Fig. 21-1, Color Plate IV). Furthermore, the spillage

Figures 21-1 through 21-4, 21-6, and 21-7 appear on Color Plate IV, between pages 196 and 197.

of tears over the lid margin usually aggravates the existing skin problem. The result is a vicious circle, broken up only by appropriate treatment of the underlying skin disease. Thus, all dermatoses that affect the eyelids may be the cause of impaired tear elimination.

Marginal Blepharitis

Marginal blepharitis (or blepharoconjunctivitis) is commonly seen in children and often persists into the adult years (Fig. 21-2, Color Plate IV). The etiologic agent is usually a staphylococcus, which bacterial invasion may be superimposed upon an existing seborrhea. As a result of the chronic inflammation of the lid margins and the frequently associated superficial punctate keratopathy, reflex lacrimation is inevitable. In the patient with blepharoconjunctivitis, the laking of tears along the lower lid margin tends to add to the inflammatory reaction.

Since the tearing is a secondary phenomenon, its elimination depends on treatment of the blepharitis with appropriate lid scrubs and topical antibiotics. Very often, treatment of a coexisting seborrhea of the scalp will ameliorate the blepharitis and result in a reduction of the tearing problem.

Pemphigoid

Pemphigoid is a disease characterized by sub-epidermal bullous formations and associated scarring or by a similar bullous formation in the submucosal layers of mucous membranes, again with subsequent scarring and shrinkage. Because of the devastating sequelae of the scarring process, the term "cicatricial pemphigoid" is used when the mucous membranes are the primary site of involvement. The form of pemphigoid limited to the skin is known as "bullous pemphigoid" and rarely involves the eyes.[1]

In cicatricial (submucosal) pemphigoid, although all of the body's mucosal structures may be affected, involvement of the conjunctiva may be the earliest manifestations, or the only one. Beginning as a conjunctivitis, often without visible bullae, the true nature of the disease may not be recognized until the scarring begins to manifest itself through fine traction lines in the palpebral conjunctivae and the fornices. A history of concomitant inflammation involving oral or genital mucosa will pinpoint the diagnosis. The disease is of unknown etiology, and although antibodies in the submucosal basement membrane suggest an immunologic mechanism, steroid therapy has not been effective. The conjunctival disease is chronic and progressive, with the scarring leading to tissue shrinkage and symblepharon formation. When it is confined to the eyes, the condition has been termed "essential shrinkage of the conjunctiva" (Fig. 21-3, Color Plate IV). The scarring seals the lacrimal gland ductules and inhibits accessory lacrimal gland secretion. Meibomian gland and goblet cell secretions are also lost, and the result is a dry eye with varying amounts of corneal destruction.

The treatment is that of a severe keratoconjunctivitis sicca and includes tear substitution products, therapeutic contact lenses, and appropriate eyelid surgery for the symblepharon. Unfortunately, since the disease is progressive, eyelid surgery does not usually provide definitive relief. Recently, sodium hyaluronate has been employed in 0.1 percent solution as a topical viscoelastic moistening agent in ocular cicatricial pemphigoid for relief of pain and improvement of vision.[2]

Pemphigus

Pemphigus is a bullous dermatitis occurring in middle-aged males. It is a severe, often lethal, disorder of unknown etiology. The eyes and lacrimal secretory apparatus are *not* usually involved in generalized pemphigus. However, the bullae and subsequent scarring on the face may produce cicatricial ectropion with secondary occlusion of the puncta and resulting epiphora.[3]

The term "ocular pemphigoid" is a confusing one since it is not a variant of pemphigus but a distinct and separate entity.

Erythema Multiforme (Stevens-Johnson Syndrome)

Erythema multiforme is an acute, inflammatory disease characterized by fever, malaise, and generalized rash involving the extremities and trunk. Characteristic lesions include intradermal bullae and dusky, ring-shaped, target patches. The eyes are involved in 50 percent of cases. It has been reported to be the result of various allergic reactions, infection by bacteria or viruses, and toxic reaction to various drugs.

The ocular involvement consists of acute conjunctivitis, often with pronounced edema and pseudomembranes, leaving behind a residue of symblepharon, shortening of the fornices, and submucosal scarring. The result is keratoconjunctivitis sicca, in varying degrees. The ocular sequelae of erythema multiforme are not unlike those of cicatricial pemphigoid. Eliciting the history of acute febrile onset with generalized rash will differentiate the two conditions.

Vigorous treatment of the acute conjunctivitis with antibiotics and steroids may limit the amount of later damage. The treatment of the dry eye residuals will depend on their severity.

COLLAGEN DISEASES

Failure of the lacrimal secretory mechanism may be the result of inflammation, atrophy, neurogenic deficit, or conjunctival scarring. Such a hyposecretion is a characteristic of a number of systemic diseases, and chief among these is the family of connective tissue disorders known as "the collagen diseases."

Sjögren's Syndrome

In Sjögren's syndrome, the keratoconjunctivitis sicca (KCS) is the predominant feature—at least, so it seems to the ophthalmologist, although not always to the patient. The KCS may vary in severity from burning and aching of the eyes or mild foreign body sensation with no more than minimal palpebral conjunctival hyperemia to the classic picture of the lusterless conjunctiva, ropy conjunctival discharge, filamentary and punctate keratitis, and even corneal ulceration (Fig. 21-4, Color Plate IV).

The diagnosis of KCS is established clinically by reduced Schirmer test values. However, since KCS is found in other diseases, e.g., leukemia, sarcoid, Riley-Day syndrome, the deficient Schirmer test values are not, in themselves, diagnostic of Sjögren's syndrome. In Sjögren's syndrome the patient's serum will exhibit a positive rheumatoid factor, positive antinuclear antibody (ANA) titer, and hyperglobulinemia. A salivary gland biopsy shows focal acinar degeneration with round cell infiltration and fibrosis.

Sjögren's syndrome characteristically appears in the fourth to sixth decade of life, and 80 percent of its victims are women. Confronted with the dramatic findings of KCS, the ophthalmologist runs the risk of not recognizing other manifestations of Sjögren's syndrome, i.e., dry mouth, difficulty in swallowing and chewing, inability to wear dentures, dysphonia, gastric achlorhydria, vaginitis, painful intercourse, and constipation. The gastric achlorhydria may be responsible for abdominal painful crises. Other manifestations may be generalized muscle weakness, hepatomegaly and adult celiac disease.

Sjögren's syndrome is associated with adult rheumatoid arthritis in 60 percent of patients. A positive rheumatoid factor and a positive ANA can be elicited in 90 percent of patients with Sjögren's syndrome. The entire Sjögren complex may accompany any of the collagen diseases. Sjögren's syndrome is, then, a generalized disorder in which the first encounter is most often with the ophthalmologist. Alert questioning can elicit the other manifestations.

Adult Rheumatoid Arthritis

Adult rheumatoid arthritis (ARA) is a progressive disease occurring chiefly in adult women, characterized by gradual onset and the development of enlarged painful joints. The disease results from an autoimmune mechanism in which circulating autoantibodies (rheumatoid factor) react with their own immunoglobulin to produce antigen-antibody complexes that generate an inflammatory response. Although Sjögren's syndrome is often a part of the picture of adult rheumatoid arthritis, there is evidence that Sjögren's syndrome with ARA is genetically different from Sjögren's syndrome without the accompanying arthritis. In the latter, the characteristics of Sjögren's syndrome are milder, and their onset is later. In Sjögren's syndrome without ARA, precipitating antibodies to a nuclear antigen are found in 68 percent of patients, but in Sjögren's syndrome associated with ARA, such precipitating antibodies are present in only 5 percent of patients. Furthermore, in Sjögren's syndrome with ARA, only a small percentage have positive human leukocyte antigen (HLA-B27). It appears that these are separate and distinct collagen diseases.[4]

In juvenile rheumatoid arthritis (Still's disease), KCS is uncommon.

Scleroderma

Scleroderma is a chronic progressive disease in which a fibrotic process results in hardening of the skin. When scleroderma involves the skin of the face, some loss of lid mobility may be responsible for epiphora. KCS has been reported, as with other collagen diseases.

Lupus Erythematosus

Lupus erythematosus (LE) is a generalized collagen disease affecting skin, pulmonary, cardiac, and renal tissues. The most characteristic skin manifestation is involvement of the nose and cheeks, often including the eyelids (butterfly lupus). When the eyelids are affected, there may be associated marginal blepharitis and resulting epiphora.

KCS or the complete Sjögren's complex

occurs in lupus patients, although not with the same frequency as in patients with ARA.

Perivasculitis

Perivasculitis takes several forms in the family of collagen disease. Periarteritis nodosa, giant cell arteritis, and Wegener's granulomatosis are different clinical expressions of necrotizing angiitis. K.C.S. may accompany any of these diseases. In Wegener's granulomatosis, dacryocystitis has been reported as a result of obstruction within the nasolacrimal duct.

MYOPATHIES

Any of the muscular dystrophies that produce ptosis and orbicularis weakness may have epiphora as a consequence. The infrequent mention of this symptom in the literature may simply be an indication that it is not of major concern to the nonophthalmologic observer.

Myasthenia Gravis

Myasthenia gravis (MG) is a chronic disease, usually beginning in the young adult years. Its chief clinical feature is excessive fatigability of striated muscle. Its earliest manifestations, in approximately half of patients, are ocular, and these findings usually consist of ptosis and diplopia.[5] Other characteristic findings in MG, such as weakness in the extremities and difficulties in swallowing, may not appear for many years after the involvement of the ocular muscles.

Since weakness of the orbicularis oculi muscles is an early sign of MG, it might be expected that epiphora would be a constant finding. Although little mention is made of this symptom in the neuro-ophthalmologic literature, this author has observed laking of tears and subjective complaint of epiphora in patients with MG.

It is interesting to speculate on the role of therapy for MG and its relation to lacrimal secretion. For some decades, anticholinesterase drugs have been the basic therapeutic tools in MG. Although moderate dosages seem to be effective in improving the blepharoptosis, considerably higher therapeutic levels are necessary to influence ocular motility, and in some cases, increased tear production has been observed with

the administration of Mestinon (pyridostigmine bromide) in dosages of 360 mg per day.[6] Since corticosteroids have been added to the therapeutic regimen, lower dosages of Mestinon are required, and lacrimation is not a significant problem.

Myotonic Dystrophy

Myotonic dystrophy is a hereditary degenerative muscular disorder characterized by periods of myotonia, and these episodes may be the earliest sign of the disease. The classic ocular finding is the polychromatic granular cataract. Increased tear secretion has been reported[7] and has been explained as being due to sympathicotonia. However, some investigators have found reduced Schirmer test values in 50 percent of cases.[8]

OSSEOUS DISORDERS

Paget's Disease

Paget's disease is a bony disorder characterized by progressive bony hypertrophy accompanied by absorption of cancellous bone. One of the chief sites of involvement is the skull. Increased bone formation in and around the orbits results in proptosis with the associated reflex tearing. Progressive obliteration of the bony nasolacrimal canal may interfere with tear excretion and result in dacryocystitis.

INTRACRANIAL VASCULAR DISORDERS

The internal carotid artery may be the site of vascular insufficiency, due to arteriosclerosis, embolism, or thrombosis. When one of the sequelae of carotid insufficiency is facial weakness, epiphora will be an associated symptom. The same type of facial weakness may result from interruption of the transverse arterial branches of the basilar artery. These vessels supply the nucleus of the seventh cranial nerve.

Histamine Headache (Cluster Headache)

Histamine headache is a severe unilateral headache of short duration. It usually is nocturnal, characterized by severe pain, profuse tearing, and redness of the eye.[9] The headaches may be repetitive, with long intervals between the clusters. The lacrimation is characteristic and serves to assist in differentiating the histamine headache from true migraine, since tearing is not often a symptom in the latter.

Parkinsonism (Paralysis Agitans)

The parkinson syndrome has been attributed to a variety of central nervous system insults—encephalitis due to infectious organisms, exogenous toxins, and, most frequently, as a manifestation of cerebral arteriosclerosis in older adults. In addition to the palsy of the extremities, the most noteworthy feature is immobile facies, with an associated decrease in the frequency of blinking. The reduced blink rate will be responsible for mechanical impairment of tear outflow, and the frequent superficial punctate keratopathy will produce increased reflex lacrimation. In some cases, antiparkinsonism drugs may be responsible for decreased tear formation.

ENDOCRINE DISORDERS

Thyroid Dysfunction

It could well be argued that Grave's disease, thyrotoxicosis, has been the subject of wider study in the past 40 years than any other medical entity. During that period of time, we have moved from a clear understanding of the hormonal basis for this disease, with emphasis on the thyroid-stimulating hormone of the anterior pituitary and the antithyrotropic substance of the thyroid gland, to a more sophisticated concept that Grave's disease is an autoimmune disorder. This immunologic concept was built on the premise that long-acting thyroid stimulator (LATS), a circulating immunoglobulin produced by lymphocytes, was the principal factor in the genesis of hyperthyroidism. This notion, in turn, fell by the wayside as subsequent investigations demonstrated that there was no direct relationship between LATS and the onset or severity of the disease. Finally, the disease is now considered by many investigators to be an expression of delayed hypersensitivity, resulting from thymic-dependent lymphocytes stimulating the thyroid cells directly.

The explanations for the eye changes in hyperthyroid disease have undergone a corresponding metamorphosis—from the concept of two separate entities, thyrotoxic and thyrotropic (or pituitary) exophthalmic findings, through the notion that all of the eye changes represent stages in a continuum of a single disease process, and, finally, to the more recently held concept that thyroid ophthalmopathy is an autoimmune disorder, with possible links to rheumatoid arthritis and lupus erythematosus.

It is with this concept that the lacrimal glands enter the picture. All of the orbital tissues, including the lacrimal gland, exhibit infiltration with inflammatory cells—lymphocytes, plasma cells—and with interstitial edema and increase in collagen fibers. From the events of the past 40 years, it is evident that the matter of the pathogenesis of thyroid ophthalmopathy is not yet settled.

There is some tendency to think of the eye changes as a disease entity apart from the hyperthyroidism itself, since the classic eye changes can precede, coincide with, or follow the onset of the other manifestations of thyroid disease. From a clinical standpoint, epiphora is not often associated with the earliest signs—lid retraction, lid lag, and mild proptosis. However, tearing due to reflex stimulation or to impaired outflow is an almost constant complaint, coinciding with the appearance of the characteristic signs of ophthalmopathy—greater proptosis, bulbar injection, chemosis, tenseness of the orbital tissues, and limitations of muscle excursions. The reduced blink rate and accompanying reduced amplitude of lid excursions result in exposure keratitis and in impaired tear outflow. This is quickly demonstrated by the fluorescein dye disappearance test. Superimposed on the impaired outflow, the keratitis and conjunctival chemosis may generate increased reflex tearing. Uncommonly, secretory activity may diminish, but this occurs only if the lacrimal gland tissue has become extensively involved in the infiltrative pathogenic process (Fig. 21-5).

Advanced thyroid ophthalmopathy is treated primarily with massive doses of corticosteroids in order to keep the inflammatory phase of the orbital pathology under control until the disease process runs its course, usually within a year or less. Relief from the epiphora may be gained by the use of the usual corneal protective measures—tear supplements, protective topical ointments, and, when necessary, angle tarsorrhaphy to reduce the corneal exposure problem. Vision may be threatened by corneal exposure or by optic nerve involvement resulting from the inflammatory pathologic process or possibly from optic nerve traction associated with maximal proptosis. In such instances, surgical decompression of the orbit is the indicated procedure. With control of the exophthalmos and the inflammatory reaction, relief from the epiphora may be expected.

Hypoparathyroidism

Hypoparathyroidism may result from removal of the parathyroid glands or may be idiopathic. Cataract is the principal finding in hypoparathyroidism, but blepharospasm, either intermittent or sustained, is also reported. A reflex response to the blepharospasm is increased lacrimation.

METABOLIC DISORDERS

Familial Dysautonomia (Riley-Day Syndrome)

Familial dysautonomia is a transmitted disease in which there is deficiency of dopamine-β-hydroxylase. It has been associated with ectodermal anhydrotic dysplasia. Alacrima is a constant feature of this condition. With this there is an associated corneal hypesthesia and severe keratitis sicca as a consequence.

Diabetes Mellitus

Despite the widespread clinical ramifications of diabetes mellitus, few if any abnormalities of the lacrimal system are associated with this disease. Epiphora is noted as a consequence of diabetic facial nerve neuropathy. Marginal blepharitis, with accompanying reflex tearing, is not uncommon in older diabetic patients.

ALLERGIC DISORDERS

Vasomotor Rhinitis

Although allergic disorders are antigenically specific, the physiologic basis is the same for all hypersensitivity diseases. The antigen-antibody

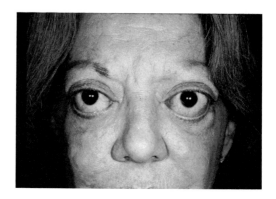

Figure 21-5. Thyroid ophthalmopathy.

reaction involves the liberation of toxic substances, chiefly histamine and other vasoactive amines. Depending on the concentration, these toxic amines may initiate reversible swelling through the transport of sodium and potassium across the cell membranes, or irreversible destruction through vasodilation and the liberation of proteolytic enzymes. The key element in the tissue response is extracellular edema.

In the large segment of the population plagued by pollinosis, the most frequent symptoms are watery eyes and stuffy nose. Vasomotor rhinitis can, of course, be an expression of sensitization to allergens other than pollen, but the clinical picture is the same. The common clinical characteristic of allergic disorders is the intermittent nature of the symptoms—diurnal, from day to day, or seasonal. The picture is a reversible one. Allergy is a systemic disease, and most patients will have some malaise, fatigue, or drowsiness as part of the picture of pollinosis.

The tearing may be secondary to conjunctival folliculosis or to an allergic conjunctivitis. In drug hypersensitivities, the tearing may be associated with edema of the excretory passages, especially the canaliculi. It would seem logical that the same response would occur with folliculosis, although little mention is made in the literature of this possibility.

Treatment of lacrimation in pollen allergy may require no local eye care. The symptoms will abate with antihistamine treatment or with antihistamine-vasoconstrictor combinations. These may be used on the nasal mucous membranes or taken systemically. In seasonal cases, a short course of systemic corticosteroids can be employed when there is no medical contraindication. Recently, corticosteroids with no appreciable systemic absorption have become available for topical nasal application as a spray mist. Of course, avoidance of the allergenic environment is the first therapeutic measure. However, if the chief manifestations are limited to lacrimation, itching of the eyes, and conjunctivitis, topical medications are the treatments of choice. Vasoconstrictor eyedrops with or without an antihistamine may be employed. Topical corticosteroids are helpful if used on a short-term basis. In some instances, all that is necessary is to use cold compresses to control the itching.

INFECTIOUS DISEASES

In general, the lacrimal system is not usually associated with primary infections of the other systems. Lungs, gastrointestinal tract, and bladder are the repositories of varied infections, unrelated to lacrimal disease. There are, however, some notable exceptions. Among these are lues, gonorrhea, and tuberculosis.

Gonorrhea
The gonococcus has been identified as the infectious organism in acute dacryoadenitis, usually as the result of metastatic spread of the organism. Clinically the symptoms are swelling of the upper lid, especially the temporal third, tenderness over the temporal third of the lid, tearing, and purulent secretion. Other bacteria have been implicated in acute dacryoadenitis.

Management of acute infectious dacryoadenitis consists of identifying the primary cause and specific antibiotic therapy directed at the cause. If there is localized abscess formation in the lacrimal gland, incision and drainage may be necessary.

Tuberculosis
Tuberculosis is reported to be one of the most frequent causes of chronic dacryoadenitis. The lacrimal gland infection has its origin in remote primary sites via the circulation. Dacryoadenitis is an uncommon clinical entity. Acute dacryoadenitis is usually unilateral, while chronic dacryoadenitis more frequently is bilateral.

In every case of chronic dacryoadenitis, a general medical etiologic survey is indicated. However, in the presence of known pulmonary tuberculosis, the persistence of a chronic smoldering dacryoadenitis is an indication for diagnostic biopsy. Such a biopsy may be the only means of differentiating among tuberculosis, sarcoid, lues, and even more remote etiologic entities, such as mycotic infections.

Tuberculous infiltration of the lacrimal sac is uncommon but can occur by retrograde invasion from the nose. Treatment of tuberculous dacryocystitis usually involves extirpation of the lacrimal sac and reconstruction of the tear drainage avenue by conjunctivorhinostomy, maintaining patency with the Jones tube or other conduit. Unfortunately, since tuberculous dacryocystitis is a rare entity, the disease usually escapes diagnosis until a dacryocystorhinostomy has been performed. It is desirable to remove a small portion of the lacrimal sac for laboratory study in all cases of dacryocystorhinostomy. The diagnosis of tuberculous dacryocystitis is made by histologic study.

Viral Diseases
In *herpes simplex, type I,* the classic eye manifestations are corneal (Fig. 21-6, Color Plate IV). The lacrimal gland has been identified as one possible factor in recurrent ocular herpes. Recurrences may be the result of latent herpes virus in the lacrimal gland.

One of the sequelae of herpes simplex infection is canalicular stenosis. Since the canalicular stenosis does not occur concomitantly with the active corneal disease as a rule, the relationship to the herpes simplex is not readily apparent. It is interesting that in many patients with otherwise unexplained canalicular stenosis, a history can be obtained of earlier herpetic infection.

Herpes Zoster. Herpes zoster may be responsible for ulcerative lesions on the eyelid margins resulting in reflex tearing. When keratoiritis is present, tearing will be associated (Fig. 21-7, Color Plate IV).

Mumps. Mumps is recognized as one of the more frequent causes of acute dacryoadenitis. It usually occurs at the same time as the parotitis.

It is bilateral, and it regresses as the mumps symptoms disappear.

Measles. Measles is another exanthematous disease that can be associated with pronounced lid edema and with dacryocystitis. Here, too, the disease tends to resolve spontaneously.

Upper Respiratory Disease

In epidemic keratoconjunctivitis, tearing is a consequence of the corneal pathology. The disease is associated with the adenoviruses, most frequently type 8. The various influenza viruses are less likely to cause keratopathy, but tearing is usual during these upper respiratory infections, epidemic or nonepidemic. Analysis of tears in these patients revealed low antibody titers. It has been demonstrated that upper respiratory infection can produce antibody in tears, but these tear antibody titers are generally low.[10, 11]

TUMORS OF THE LACRIMAL SYSTEM

This subject is discussed in Chapter 16. However, it is important to remember that the most common cause of lacrimal gland swelling is tumor, not inflammation. Metastatic carcinoma of the lacrimal sac is rare in comparison to carcinomas of the sac which are primary or which are the result of direct invasion from contiguous structures.

HEMATOLOGIC DISORDERS

Leukemia

Leukemia is a form of malignancy in which the circulating white blood cells undergo neoplastic change. The degree of malignancy can vary widely. Lymphocytic leukemia, occurring in older age groups, is generally characterized by a less aggressive symptomatic picture than the myelogenous form of leukemia. The leukemic patient exhibits a picture of generalized weakness and malaise, often with elevated temperature. Characteristic systemic findings are enlarged lymph nodes, spleen, and liver, and hemorrhages involving the skin and mucous membranes.

It is estimated that 50 to 70 percent of leukemic patients have ocular involvement.[12] Leukemic infiltration occurs in the bones of the skull and the orbital bones and may infiltrate the lacrimal gland and other orbital tissues. With involvement of the orbit, proptosis is a frequent finding. When there is involvement of the lacrimal gland, it is usually a late finding, and a diagnosis will have been established by hematologic study.

SUMMARY

It is evident that lacrimation and epiphora tend to rank very low on the attention-getting scale of the internist and, to some extent, of the ophthalmologist. The presence of tearing, so very troublesome to the patient who is suffering from it, should alert the ophthalmologist to the need for a methodical diagnostic evaluation of the lacrimal problem, but along with this should go an awareness that such symptoms may be related to a systemic disorder.

REFERENCES

1. Whitmore PV: Skin and mucous membrane disorders. In Duane TD: Clinical Ophthalmology. Hagerstown, Harper & Row, 1980, Vol. 5, Chap. 27, pp 2-3
2. Polak FM: Treatment of Keratitis Sicca with Sodium Hyaluronate (Healon). Atlanta, Ga., American Academy of Ophthalmology, 1981
3. Duane TD: Clinical Ophthalmology. Hagerstown, Md, Harper & Row, 1980, Vol 5, Chap 27, p 1
4. Gold DH: Ocular manifestations of connective tissue (collagen) diseases. In Duane TD: Clinical Ophthalmology. Hagerstown, Md, Harper & Row, 1980, Vol 5, Chap 26, p 3
5. Walsh FB, Hoyt WF: Clinical Neuro-ophthalmology. Baltimore, Williams & Wilkins, 1969, p 1283
6. Burde R: Personal communication, 1981
7. Walsh FB, Hoyd WF: Clinical Neuro-ophthalmology. Baltimore, Williams & Wilkins, 1969, p 1269
8. Duane TD: Clinical Ophthalmology. vol V, Chap 29, p 2, Hagerstown, Md, Harper & Row, 1980, Vol 5, Chap 29 p 2

9. Walsh FB, Hoyt WF: Clinical Neuro-ophthal-mology. Baltimore, Williams & Wilkins, 1969, p 408

10. Knopf HLS, Bertrow DM, Kapikian AZ: Demonstration and characterization of antibody in tears following intranasal vaccination Inv Ophth 9:727, 1970

11. Knopf HLS, Hierholzer JC: Clinical and immunological response in patients with viral keratoconjunctivitis. Am J Ophthalmol 80:670, 1975

12. Walsh FB, Hoyt WF: Clinical Neuro-ophthal-mology. Baltimore, Williams & Wilkins, 1969, p 2316

22

A CLASSIFICATION OF LACRIMAL DISORDERS

BERNARDO A. WEIL

It was the intent of the authors and contributors to this book that the subject of dacryology be dealt with in considerable detail. This classification of lacrimal disorders will serve two purposes: it will provide a summary of the wide spectrum of information contained in these chapters, and it will serve as a guide in the differential diagnosis of disorders of the lacrimal system. Reference is made to the chapters in which each subject is discussed.

I. Disorders of the secretory system (lacrimation)
   A. Hypersecretion. Disorders due to excessive production of tears in the presence of a normal excretory system (Chapters 5 and 11)
      1. Primary hypersecretion. Congenital disorders, with excessive production of tears from a histologically normal lacrimal gland (Chapter 10)
      2. Secondary hypersecretion
         a. Dacryoadenitis. Inflammation of the lacrimal gland (Chapter 11)
         b. Reflex hypersecretion due to inflammation of the lids, orbit, conjunctiva, cornea, or uveal tract (Chapters 5 and 11)

   c. Tumors of the lacrimal gland and of the orbit (Chapter 13)
   d. Central nervous system stimulation of the lacrimal gland (Chapter 5)
      i. Psychic
      ii. Voluntary
      iii. Corticomeningeal lesions
   e. Neurogenic or peripheral nervous system causes of hypersecretion (Chapter 11)
      i. Trigeminal irritation may be the mechanism for 2a and 2b, but the cause may be located higher up in the central nervous system
      ii. Retinal stimulation by light
      iii. Irritation of the facial nerve or the sphenopalatine ganglion
      iv. Paradoxical reflexes, gustatory or masticatory lacrimal reflexes, crocodile tears
      v. Sympathetic stimulation
      vi. Reflex lacrimation accompanying physiologic acts, such as laughter or emesis
   f. Symptomatic lacrimation associated with systemic disease:

thyrotoxicosis, encephalitis, hypophyseal tumors, tabes (Chapter 21)

   g. Medication: reactive hypersecretion after prolonged use of miotics, vasodilators, etc. (Chapter 7)

   h. Physical or chemical stimulation: cold temperatures, wind, excessive light, x-rays, ultraviolet light, chemical pollution, etc. (Chapter 11)

B. Hyposecretion (the dry eye)
  1. Congenital absence of the lacrimal gland (as in cryptophthalmos) (Chapter 10)
  2. Alacrima
    a. Congenital (Chapter 10)
    b. Familial dysautonomia (Riley-Day syndrome) (Chapter 10)
    c. Anhydrotic ectodermal dysplasia (Chapter 10)
    d. Acquired secondary alacrima (Sjögren's syndrome), Stevens-Johnson syndrome, pemphigus, and pemphigoid disorders (Chapter 21)

II. Disorders of the excretory system (epiphora)
Normal secretion of tears in the presence of impaired excretory function
A. Patent excretory passages
  1. Abnormality of the upper excretory system (Chapters 10 and 14)
    a. Congenital absence of puncta or canaliculi (Chapter 10)

    b. Malposition of eyelid margins (ectropion or entropion)
    c. Stenosis or malposition of puncta
  2. Functional block (Chapters 9, 13, and 15)
    a. Lacrimal pump failure
    b. Partial stenosis of lacrimal excretory passages
    c. Dacryolith
B. Obstructed excretory passages
  1. Upper lacrimal passages (lid margins, puncta, canaliculi, common canaliculus, and internal punctum (Rosenmüller's valve) (Chapter 14)
    a. Etiology of complete obstruction in the upper excretory system: congenital, inflammatory, traumatic, or neoplastic
  2. Lower lacrimal passages (lacrimal sac, nasolacrimal duct, and plica semilunaris [Hasner's valve]) (Chapters 15, 16, 17, and 20)
    a. Etiology of complete closure of the lower passages: congenital, inflammatory, traumatic, or neoplastic

REFERENCES

1. Duke-Elder S: System of Ophthalmology. The Ocular Adnexa. London, Henry Kimpton, 1974, Vol 13
2. Weil BA: Las Epiforas. Orientacion Diagnostica. Arch Oftal Buenos Aires 41:84, 1966
3. Weil BA: Las Epiforas. Orientacion Terapeutica. Arch Oftal Buenos Aires 41:195, 1966

POSTSCRIPT

A WORD FOR THE RESEARCHER IN DACRYOLOGY

When it comes to shedding tears,
The crocodile outshines his peers!
Although his talents are no greater
Than his lookalike, the alligator,
The crocodile gets the attention
And the alligator, little mention.

And despite their lacrimal proclivity,
They're looked upon with negativity
In every research institution
Where they could make a contribution,
For scientists are most discerning
In those higher seats of learning.

Consider the investigator
Of the crocodile or alligator—
While he may think to gain some status
By work on their tear apparatus,
Man's long been known for his insistence
That alligators keep their distance.

If one should venture near those creatures
To study, at close range, their features,
The odds would be, on who's the braver,
In the alligator's favor . . .
And were one rash enough to try it,
He could be on that reptile's diet.

In dacryology researches,
There seems to be no way to purchase
The one appropriate appliance
On which we can place full reliance
To guarantee us our survival
On a crocodile's arrival.

So . . . unless you have the sheer audacity
To test a crocodile's voracity
In your research work on tearing,
If a crocodile's appearing,
Do as this author recommends . . .
Use a telescopic lens!

—Benjamin Milder

INDEX